PHARMACOLOGY FOR THE
EMS PROVIDER

4TH EDITION

PHARMACOLOGY FOR THE
EMS PROVIDER

4TH EDITION

RICHARD K. BECK, MS, NREMT-P
Associate Dean of Academic Affairs, EMS
Broward College Ft. Lauderdale, Florida

JILL SHELTON, PHARM D, BCNSP
Consulting Editor
Clinical Specialist
Huntsville Hospital
Huntsville, Alabama

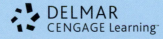
DELMAR
CENGAGE Learning™

Australia • Brazil • Japan • Korea • Mexico • Singapore • Spain • United Kingdom • United States

DELMAR
CENGAGE Learning™

**Pharmacology for the EMS Provider,
Fourth Edition**
Richard K. Beck, Jill Shelton

Vice President, Career and Professional
Editorial: Dave Garza

Director of Learning Solutions: Sandy Clark

Acquisitions Editor: Janet Maker

Managing Editor: Larry Main

Senior Manager: John Fisher

Editorial Assistant: Amy Wetsel

Vice President, Career and Professional
Marketing: Jennifer Baker

Marketing Director: Deborah Yarnell

Marketing Manager: Kathryn Hall

Marketing Coordinator: Mark Pierro

Production Director: Wendy Troeger

Production Manager: Jim Zayicek

Art Director: Casey Kirchmayer

Cover Images: iStockphoto

For product information and technology assistance, contact us at
Cengage Learning Customer & Sales Support, 1-800-354-9706
For permission to use material from this text or product,
submit all requests online at **www.cengage.com/permissions.**
Further permissions questions can be e-mailed to
permissionrequest@cengage.com

Library of Congress Control Number: 2011926876

ISBN-13: 978-1-111-30769-1

ISBN-10: 1-111-30769-5

Delmar
5 Maxwell Drive
Clifton Park, NY 12065-2919
USA

Cengage Learning is a leading provider of customized learning solutions with
office locations around the globe, including Singapore, the United Kingdom,
Australia, Mexico, Brazil, and Japan. Locate your local office at:
international.cengage.com/region

Cengage Learning products are represented in Canada by Nelson Education, Ltd.

To learn more about Delmar, visit **www.cengage.com/delmar**

Purchase any of our products at your local college store or at our preferred
online store **www.cengagebrain.com**

Notice to the Reader

Publisher does not warrant or guarantee any of the products described herein or perform any independent
analysis in connection with any of the product information contained herein. Publisher does not assume,
and expressly disclaims, any obligation to obtain and include information other than that provided to it by
the manufacturer. The reader is expressly warned to consider and adopt all safety precautions that might be
indicated by the activities described herein and to avoid all potential hazards. By following the instructions
contained herein, the reader willingly assumes all risks in connection with such instructions. The publisher
makes no representations or warranties of any kind, including but not limited to, the warranties of fitness for
particular purpose or merchantability, nor are any such representations implied with respect to the material set
forth herein, and the publisher takes no responsibility with respect to such material. The publisher shall not be
liable for any special, consequential, or exemplary damages resulting, in whole or part, from the readers' use of,
or reliance upon, this material.

Printed in the United States of America
1 2 3 4 5 6 7 15 14 13 12 11

DEDICATION

Working on a project such as this requires time and sacrifice. I am blessed to have a home team who understands and supports. This textbook is dedicated to my team—my wife Suzy, and my children Brian and Amanda. Thank you for your love and support, not only through this project, but for the support you give everyday.

RKB

CONTENTS

PREFACE

Emergency Medical Services (EMS) professionals are routinely placed in positions in which quick decisions can mean the difference between life and death—especially when administering drugs. Administering drugs carries an enormous responsibility, and the knowledge the EMS professional brings to the out-of-hospital setting can make the difference in a successful patient outcome.

Pharmacology for the EMS Provider, 4th edition was revised to fulfill the core module for the pharmacology component of the EMS Educational Standards. The Personnel Licensure Levels. These levels include Emergency Medical Responder (EMR), Emergency Medical Technician (EMT), the Advanced Emergency Medical Technician (AEMT), and Paramedic. All of these EMS licensure levels include some aspect of pharmacology, from the very basic (EMR) to the advanced level (Paramedic). This book also follows the current ACLS and PALS curricula. It can also serve as a comprehensive reference text after graduation for practicing EMS providers.

BACKGROUND

This book was originally written to be a resource for both the EMS student as well as the EMS graduate. There is an old firefighter's adage: it is better to have too much hose on the street than not enough. Admittedly, this book contains too much information for the entry-level paramedic. However, once a student graduates, this book changes from a textbook to a good pharmacology resource text.

ORGANIZATION

Chapters 1 through 8 present basic introductory topics. Chapter 1 introduces the reader to pharmacology. It explains essential drug information about each drug presented. Drug origins, drug preparation, drug testing, and legislation that governs drugs manufactured in the United States are also discussed. Chapter 2 provides a review of how drugs travel and respond once in the body. It is not enough to know

what drugs a patient is taking; EMS professionals may also need to know how the drug(s) works once in the body and how the body may respond to the drug(s). Pharmacokinetics and pharmacodynamics review drug movement including absorption, solubility, distribution, biotransformation, and excretion. Once the drug reaches its destination, pharmacodynamics explains how a drug's mechanism of action affects the patient. Many drugs given in out-of-hospital emergency medicine affect the autonomic nervous system. Chapter 3 gives an overview of the autonomic nervous system and explains how selected drugs interact with its functions. The conditions of the body's pH, fluids, and electrolytes affect the therapeutic effects of drugs. Chapter 4 reviews fluids, electrolytes, and acid-base balance in an attempt to explain the importance of maintaining these factors within normal limits to enable drugs to produce their therapeutic effects. Chapter 5 presents a discussion on blood and blood components. It is becoming more common for EMS professionals to administer blood, or transport patients who are receiving blood or blood products. Therefore, it is important to know the different blood types, who can receive and who can donate the various blood types, and to be able to recognize the signs and symptoms of blood transfusion reactions. Indications for the various kinds of volume expanders, and the indications for the use of antihyperlipidemic drugs used to decrease the lipid levels in the blood, are also included. Some drugs are administered according to body weight, some by a predetermined dosage, and some must be added to intravenous solutions before they are administered. Chapter 6 explains basic mathematics and illustrates how to calculate drug dosages. Chapter 7 presents the various routes by which drugs can be administered and gives step-by-step instruction on the procedures for correct drug administration. Chapter 8 explains the classifications of drugs. Understanding the drug classification makes it easier for the reader to rationalize and understand when to use a drug, and its contraindications and precautions.

Drug monographs in Chapters 9 through 17 are presented by body system affected. Each monograph contains detailed descriptions of the drug's generic and trade names, pregnancy classification, mechanism of action, indications for use, contraindications, precautions, route and dosage, adverse reactions and side effects, and any implications that the EMS providers should be aware of. Chapter 10 incorporates the American Heart Association's new adult and pediatric recommendations concerning the guidelines for cardiopulmonary resuscitation and emergency cardiac care that were presented at the 2000 International Conference.

Appendices for quick reference include (A) Drugs (Generic and Trade Names) and Their Therapeutic Classifications, (B) Pediatric Normal Values, Dosages, and Infusion Rates, (C) Advanced Cardiac Life Support Algorithms, (D) Herbal Remedies, (E) Street Drugs, and (F) Commonly Used Abbreviations and Symbols.

CHAPTER FEATURES

The following features in each chapter help make learning pharmacology less confusing:

■ *Therapeutic Classifications of Drugs* — Each drug discussed in the chapter is listed according to its therapeutic classification(s).

■ *Objectives* — introduce major content areas to be mastered in the chapter.

■ *Key Terms* — alert you to important terms in the chapter. Key terms are in color and defined in the text the first time they are used. A comprehensive glossary at the end of the book includes all key terms and their definitions.

■ *Introduction* — Each chapter includes an introduction to the drugs presented and their relationship to treating emergencies in that specific body system.

■ *Drug Monographs* — Drug monographs in Chapters 9 through 17 are presented in alphabetical order by generic name. The most common brand names are listed immediately below the generic name.

■ *Conclusion* — presents a final statement regarding the drugs contained in the chapter.

■ *Study Questions* — help you review key information presented in the chapter, and understand the drugs more fully.

■ *Case Studies* — Case studies in Chapters 9 through 17 help illustrate how drugs can be used in various emergency situations.

■ *Extended Case Study* — Extended case studies in Chapters 9 through 17 show the progression of an emergency situation.

NEW TO THIS EDITION

■ Updated case studies throughout the book
■ Updated treatment algorithms
■ 20 additional drugs:
  ■ Chapter 9—Albuterol/Ipratropium, Levalbuterol, Furosemide, Milrinone
  ■ Chapter 10—Captopril, Enalapril, Lisinopril, Ramipril, Adenosine, Atenolol, Esinolol
  ■ Chapter 11—Esmolol, Hydrocortisone
  ■ Chapter 12—Dextrose 50% in Water ($D_{50}w$), Acetylsalicylic Acid (Aspirin)
  ■ Chapter 14—Hydralazine
  ■ Chapter 15—Nitroglycerin, Phentolaminme
  ■ Chapter 16—Fluphenazine
  ■ Chapter 17—Midazolam
■ Added websites for reference and research purposes including website with information on:
  ■ American Heart Association
  ■ Drug & awareness & specialist training
  ■ Street drug names around the world
  ■ New instructor resource CD-ROM to accompany the text.

INSTRUCTOR RESOURCES

To assist instructors in classroom preparation and training, Delmar Cengage Learning offers *Instructor Resources on CD-ROM* to accompany this book, which contains the following features:

■ *PowerPoint Presentations®* combine illustrations and photos with an outline of the important concepts in each chapter. The presentations correlate to the *Lesson Plans* and are editable to meet the specific needs of your course.

■ *Lesson Plans* correlate to the accompanying *PowerPoint Presentations®* and prepare the instructor for the classroom. The *Lesson Plans* are also editable to meet the specific needs of your course.

- *Chapter Quizzes* enable you to evaluate student comprehension of the concepts presented in each chapter.
- *Answers to Study Questions and Case Studies* provide feedback on the questions at the end of each chapter and enable instructors to evaluate student knowledge of the content

ACKNOWLEDGMENTS

The author and Delmar Learning wish to thank the following reviewers for their valuable comments:

Mark Branon
Calhoun Community College
Huntsville, Alabama

Tom Fitts
East Central College
Union, Missouri

Janet Gardner
Sinclair Community College
Dayton, Ohio

Thera Granger
Lamar State College
Beaumont, Texas

Matthew Keeler
Palm Beach State
Lake Worth, Florida

We would also like to thank Dr. Gianluca Ghiselli for providing us with a thorough technical review of this text.

I am hopeful that *Pharmacology for the EMS Provider*, 4th edition will be of value in the classroom and an aid for practicing EMS professionals.

Richard K. Beck

PHARMACOLOGY FOR THE
EMS PROVIDER

4TH EDITION

CHAPTER 1

INTRODUCTION TO PHARMACOLOGY

OBJECTIVES

On completion of this chapter and the study questions, you should be able to:

- Differentiate among the laws, regulations, and standards regarding infection control.
- Explain the importance of performing a thorough patient medication assessment.
- Describe historical trends in pharmacology.
- Differentiate among the chemical, generic (nonproprietary), trade (proprietary), and official names of drugs.
- List the five main sources of drugs.
- Describe how drugs are classified.
- Describe the three phases of drug development.
- List and describe the components of a drug profile.
- List the sources of drug information.
- List the legislative acts controlling the use of drugs in the United States.
- Describe the standardization of drugs.
- Describe investigational drugs, including the approval process and the FDA classifications for newly approved drugs.
- Describe special considerations of drugs as they relate to the pregnant, pediatric, and geriatric patient.

KEY TERMS

Assay
Bioassay
Body substance isolation
Chemical name
Drug
Food and Drug
  Administration (FDA)
Generic name
Official name

Parenteral
Pharmacodynamics
Pharmacogenetics
Pharmacokinetics
Pharmacology
Pharmacotherapy
Physicians' Desk
  Reference (PDR)
Standard Precautions

Therapeutic index
Therapeutics
Toxicity
Toxicology
Trade name
United States
  Pharmacopoeia (USP)

INTRODUCTION

If you like solving puzzles, then EMS and especially pharmacology is for you. One of the most important aspects of EMS is a thorough patient assessment. The patient assessment in itself is a puzzle. For example, when you arrive at an emergency scene, you must attempt to determine the following: scene safety, chief complaint, what occurred prior to the chief complaint, airway and circulation status, level of conscious, pain level, and so on.

As a paramedic, a second puzzle must also be put together—the medication assessment. For example, you must attempt to determine medications the patient is currently taking, when was the last time any medications were taken, what conditions are the medications being taken to treat, and so on?

Before you administer any medications to your patient you must know what the patient is currently taking so serious drug-drug interactions do not occur. For example, you do not want to administer nitroglycerin to a patient who has recently taken sildenafil. This combination of drugs may lead to fatal hypotension.

If EMS personnel fail to obtain patient medication information while on scene or during transport, the receiving facility will have to begin their own medication assessment, which may delay treatment and cause serious consequences.

Precautions Against Blood-Borne Pathogens and Infectious Diseases

By just looking at a patient, it is not possible to tell if he or she is infected with a blood-borne infection such as hepatitis, tuberculosis (TB), or human immunodeficiency virus (HIV), which can lead to the fatal acquired immunodeficiency syndrome (AIDS). Therefore, the Centers for Disease Control (CDC) in Atlanta, Georgia, recommend certain body substance isolation precautions. **Body substance isolation** precautions, known as **Standard Precautions**, are infection-control precautions that health-care professionals should apply with *all* patients, in *all* situations. Figure 1–1 provides a comprehensive review of Standard Precautions.

Transmission-based precautions are intended for patients diagnosed with or suspected of specific highly transmissible diseases. These precautions condense the seven existing categories of isolation precautions developed by the CDC in 1970 into three sets of precautions based on routes of infection. Updated in 2007 to complement Standard Precautions, transmission-based precautions (Figures 1–2, 1–3, and 1–4) reduce the risk of airborne, droplet, and contact transmission of pathogens and are always to be used in addition to Standard Precautions.

Health-care professionals should wear gloves whenever touching a patient. This is especially important for health-care professionals in contact with blood or any body fluid. Health-care professionals should also wear gloves when performing procedures such as: starting intravenous lines, drawing blood, giving injections, or inserting an endotracheal tube. After each patient contact, carefully remove the gloves and immediately properly dispose of them. If blood or body fluids come in contact with the skin, thoroughly wash all exposed areas.

If there is a chance that patient blood or body fluids may come in contact with face or clothing, wear protective masks and gowns. Once contact with the patient is completed, carefully remove mask and gown and properly dispose of them.

Whenever possible, health-care professionals should use disposable equipment. Once used, properly dispose of the equipment. Do not re-cap, bend, break, or remove needles from the syringe. Dispose of needles and disposable syringes in designated puncture-resistant containers immediately after use.

To protect yourself against becoming infected with tuberculosis (TB), you should have a National Institute of Occupational Safety and Health approved *High-Efficiency Particulate Air (HEPA) Respirator*. This should be worn whenever coming in contact with a confirmed or suspected TB-infected patient.

All routes for transmission of blood-borne infections have yet to be identified. Therefore, it is extremely important for health-care professionals to take all appropriate precautions against contact with such infections while treating patients. Remember:

- Always wear protective equipment when handling contaminated equipment or coming in contact with the patient.
- Place all contaminated equipment and supplies in properly marked biologic hazard bags, and dispose of properly.

STANDARD PRECAUTIONS

Assume that every person is potentially infected or colonized with
an organism that could be transmitted in the healthcare setting.

Hand Hygiene

Avoid unnecessary touching of surfaces in close proximity to the patient.

When hands are visibly dirty, contaminated with proteinaceous material, or visibly soiled with blood or body fluids, wash hands with soap and water.

If hands are not visibly soiled, or after removing visible material with soap and water, decontaminate hands with an alcohol-based hand rub. Alternatively, hands may be washed with an antimicrobial soap and water.

Perform hand hygiene:
Before having direct contact with patients.
After contact with blood, body fluids or excretions, mucous membranes, nonintact skin, or wound dressings.
After contact with a patient's intact skin (e.g., when taking a pulse or blood pressure or lifting a patient).
If hands will be moving from a contaminated-body site to a clean-body site during patient care.
After contact with inanimate objects (including medical equipment) in the immediate vicinity of the patient.
After removing gloves.

Personal Protective Equipment (PPE)

Wear PPE when the nature of the anticipated patient interaction indicates that contact with blood or body fluids may occur.

Before leaving the patient's room or cubicle, remove and discard PPE.

Gloves

Wear gloves when contact with blood or other potentially infectious materials, mucous membranes, nonintact skin, or potentially contaminated intact skin (e.g., of a patient incontinent of stool or urine) could occur.

Remove gloves after contact with a patient and/or the surrounding environment using proper technique to prevent hand contamination. Do not wear the same pair of gloves for the care of more than one patient.

Change gloves during patient care if the hands will move from a contaminated body-site (e.g., perineal area) to a clean body-site (e.g., face).

Gowns

Wear a gown to protect skin and prevent soiling or contamination of clothing during procedures and patient-care activities when contact with blood, body fluids, secretions, or excretions is anticipated.

Wear a gown for direct patient contact if the patient has uncontained secretions or excretions.

Remove gown and perform hand hygiene before leaving the patient's environment.

Mouth, Nose, Eye Protection

Use PPE to protect the mucous membranes of the eyes, nose and mouth during procedures and patient-care activities that are likely to generate splashes or sprays of blood, body fluids, secretions and excretions.

During aerosol-generating procedures wear one of the following: a face shield that fully covers the front and sides of the face, a mask with attached shield, or a mask and goggles.

Respiratory Hygiene/Cough Etiquette

Educate healthcare personnel to contain respiratory secretions to prevent droplet and fomite transmission of respiratory pathogens, especially during seasonal outbreaks of viral respiratory tract infections.

Offer masks to coughing patients and other symptomatic persons (e.g., persons who accompany ill patients) upon entry into the facility.

Patient-Care Equipment and Instruments/Devices

Wear PPE (e.g., gloves, gown), according to the level of anticipated contamination, when handling patient-care equipment and instruments/devices that are visibly soiled or may have been in contact with blood or body fluids.

Care of the Environment

Include multi-use electronic equipment in policies and procedures for preventing contamination and for cleaning and disinfection, especially those items that are used by patients, those used during delivery of patient care, and mobile devices that are moved in and out of patient rooms frequently (e.g., daily).

Textiles and Laundry

Handle used textiles and fabrics with minimum agitation to avoid contamination of air, surfaces and persons.

Figure 1–1 Standard Precautions for Infection Control. (Courtesy of Brevis Corp)

AIRBORNE PRECAUTIONS
(in addition to Standard Precautions)

 VISITORS: Report to nurse before entering.

Use Airborne Precautions as recommended for patients known or suspected to be infected with infectious agents transmitted person-to-person by the airborne route (e.g., M. tuberculosis, measles, chickenpox, disseminated herpes zoster).

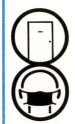 **Patient Placement**
Place patients in an **AIIR** (Airborne infection isolation room).
Monitor air pressure daily with visual indicators (e.g., flutter strips).

Keep door closed when not required for entry and exit.

In ambulatory settings instruct patients with a known or suspected airborne infection to wear a surgical mask and observe Respiratory Hygiene/Cough Etiquette.
Once in an AIIR, the mask may be removed.

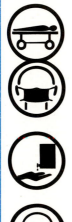 **Patient Transport**
Limit transport and movement of patients to **medically-necessary purposes.**

If transport or movement outside an AIIR is necessary, instruct patients to **wear a surgical mask,** if possible, and observe Respiratory Hygiene/Cough Etiquette.

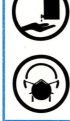 **Hand Hygiene**
according to Standard Precautions.

Personal Protective Equipment (PPE)
Wear a fit-tested NIOSH-approved N_{95} or higher level respirator for respiratory protection when entering the room of a patient when the following diseases are suspected or confirmed.

Figure 1–2 Airborne Precautions. (Courtesy of Brevis Corp)

- Ensure all used sharps are properly secured in a puncture-resistant and clearly marked container.
- Do not re-cap needles after use, or leave them at the scene. Dispose of all sharps properly.
- Properly clean all re-usable equipment as soon after use as possible.
- If exposed to an infectious disease, contact medical control and the receiving hospital immediately.

For complete information on the 2007 Guidelines for Isolation Precautions: Preventing Transmission of Infectious Agents in Healthcare Settings, go to http://www.cdc.gov/hicpac/2007isolationPrecautions.html.

The Patient Medications Assessment

All health-care providers know the importance of a thorough patient assessment. A medication assessment should be part of every patient assessment. Information gained from the medication assessment can provide important information not only for EMS personnel, but for hospital personnel as well.

Information gained from the medication assessment can be used to design a treatment plan for EMS personnel and alerts personnel at the receiving facility what treatment was done and what may need to be done upon arrival. Knowing what medications the patient is taking will aid in preventing drug interactions or overdoses, which might occur from administration of drugs in the out-of-hospital setting, as well as at the receiving facility.

If EMS personnel fail to obtain patient medication information while on scene, the receiving facility will have to begin their own medication assessment, which may delay treatment and cause serious consequences.

Patient medication information may be obtained in several ways. Usually, the patient is the best source. However, in some cases, patients may not know what medications they are taking. They may know why they are taking a medication, but not its name. In other cases, patients may not know what

CONTACT PRECAUTIONS
(in addition to Standard Precautions)

STOP **VISITORS:** Report to nurse before entering.

Gloves
Don gloves upon entry into the room or cubicle.
Wear gloves whenever touching the patient's intact skin or surfaces and articles in close proximity to the patient.
Remove gloves before leaving patient room.

Hand Hygiene
Hand Hygiene according to Standard Precautions.

Gowns
Don gown upon entry into the room or cubicle.
Remove gown and observe hand hygiene before leaving the patient-care environment.

Patient Transport
Limit transport of patients to medically necessary purposes.
Ensure that infected or colonized areas of the patient's body are contained and covered.
Remove and dispose of contaminated PPE and perform hand hygiene prior to transporting patients on Contact Precautions.
Don clean PPE to handle the patient at the transport destination.

Patient-Care Equipment
Use disposable noncritical patient-care equipment or implement patient-dedicated use of such equipment.

Figure 1–3 Contact Precautions. (Courtesy of Brevis Corp)

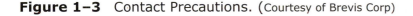

medications they are taking or why. If patients are unable to communicate for a medication assessment, other sources include a family member, friend, Vial of Life, or a home-health aide. Below is an example of a medication assessment:

- *Are you currently taking any medications (drugs) prescribed by a doctor?*
- *What are the names of these medications (drugs)?* Some patients may not know the actual names of the drugs they are taking. If this is the case, EMS personnel should also ask: *Do you have some of the medication(s) to show me? We must take it (them) to the hospital.*
- *Why are you taking the medications (drugs)?* If the patient does not know the name of the medications, they may know the reason for taking the drugs.
- *When did you last take your medications?*
- *Have you been taking your medications according to the prescribed directions? If not, how have you been taking them?*
- *Are you taking any over-the-counter medications (medications purchased without a prescription at the store)? If so, what are these medications, and when did you last take them?*
- *Are you taking any herbal preparations?*
- *Are you taking any medications that were prescribed for someone else?*
- *Have you recently completed taking medications? If so, what were they, and why were you taking them?*
- *Have you experienced any side effects or illness from your medications? If so, have you reported these to your doctor?*

Depending on the circumstances, the medication assessment can be adjusted to address special situations. Additional questions may have to be asked.

It is generally useful to bring any patient medications to the receiving facility with the patient. The most common places patients keep medications include the bathroom, bedroom, and the kitchen (don't forget to look in the refrigerator). To save time, EMS dispatch may have instructed the caller to have any medications ready for EMS when they arrive.

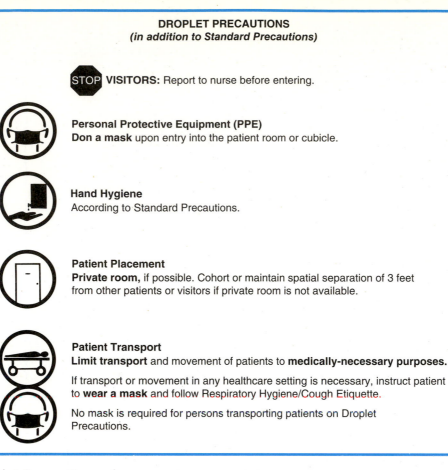

DROPLET PRECAUTIONS
(in addition to Standard Precautions)

STOP **VISITORS:** Report to nurse before entering.

Personal Protective Equipment (PPE)
Don a mask upon entry into the patient room or cubicle.

Hand Hygiene
According to Standard Precautions.

Patient Placement
Private room, if possible. Cohort or maintain spatial separation of 3 feet from other patients or visitors if private room is not available.

Patient Transport
Limit transport and movement of patients to **medically-necessary purposes.**

If transport or movement in any healthcare setting is necessary, instruct patient to **wear a mask** and follow Respiratory Hygiene/Cough Etiquette.

No mask is required for persons transporting patients on Droplet Precautions.

Figure 1–4 Droplet Precautions. (Courtesy of Brevis Corp)

EMS professionals should be familiar with medication labels and the information on them. Figure 1–5 outlines the elements of a prescription.

Also, be aware that many medication containers have additional secondary labels which include additional information, such as: *"swallow whole, DO NOT crush or chew," "take on an empty stomach," "Important: take or use exactly as directed, do not discontinue or skip doses unless directed by your doctor,"* and *"may cause drowsiness."*

Medication Assessment Scenarios

Knowledge of the medications each patient is taking often provides a basis for determining treatment. Medications may be one of your most useful assessment tools, especially if the patient is unresponsive or incoherent. The following three scenarios illustrate the importance of your medication assessment.

Scenario One

You respond to a 72-year-old male who states he has been feeling weak for the past 4 hours. While performing your initial assessment, you notice some medication containers on the kitchen table. These include Lanoxin, Cardizem, and glyburide. What information do these medications tell you about this patient?

- Lanoxin is the trade name for digoxin, an antiarrhythmic. Digoxin increases both the force and velocity of ventricular contractions while simultaneously slowing conduction through the AV node of the heart.
- Cardizem is the trade name for diltiazem, a calcium channel blocker that decreases conduction velocity and ventricular rate.
- Glyburide is an oral antidiabetic agent used to treat type II diabetes.

Therefore, knowledge of the use of these medications, or having access to a resource to research the drug, tells us that this patient is a diabetic with underlying cardiovascular problems.

Scenario Two

You are called to a 59-year-old female patient who is complaining of dizziness and feeling weak. Her pulse rate is 44 beats/minute and regular. Upon questioning her about medications, she tells you that she is on blood pressure medicine, but cannot remember its name. She finds the bottle and the drug name is atenolol. When questioned further, she admits

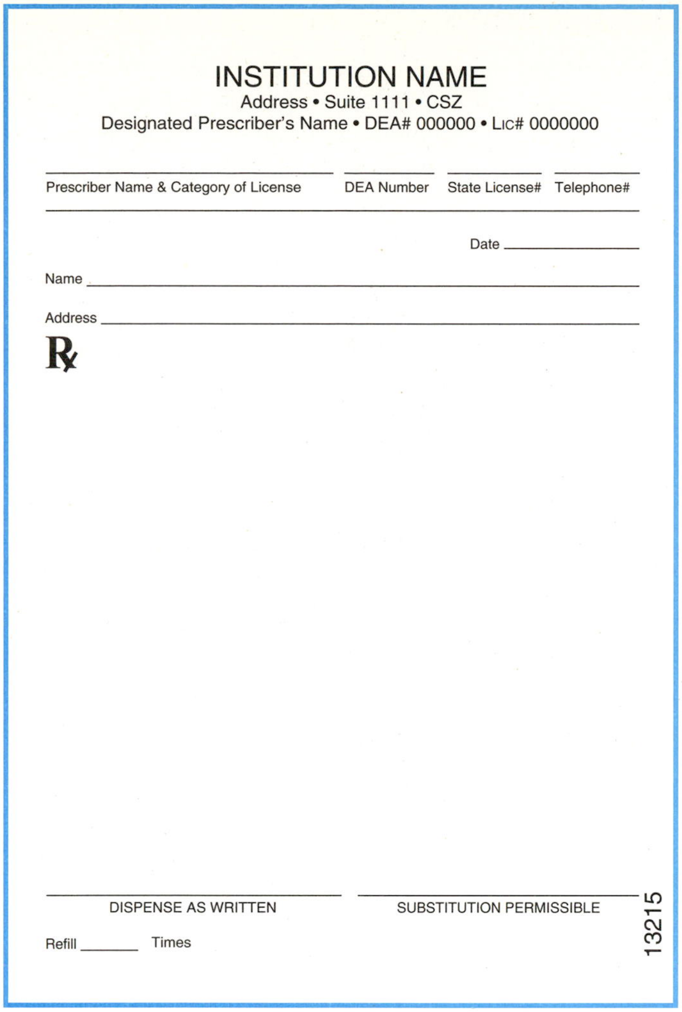

INSTITUTION NAME
Address • Suite 1111 • CSZ
Designated Prescriber's Name • DEA# 000000 • Lic# 0000000

Prescriber Name & Category of License | DEA Number | State License# | Telephone#

Date ______

Name ______

Address ______

℞

DISPENSE AS WRITTEN | SUBSTITUTION PERMISSIBLE

Refill ______ Times

13215

Figure 1–5 Elements of a Prescription.
(© Delmar/Cengage Learning)

not taking her medicine for "about a couple of days." Further questioning reveals that she had taken three tablets today to make up for not taking any over the last couple of days.

- Atenolol is a beta-adrenergic blocking agent used for hypertension and angina pectoris caused by hypertension. It also causes slowing of the heart rate and can mask or hide any other problems that might induce tachycardia.

By taking a multiple dose, this patient most likely is experiencing side effects caused by overdosing. Overdosing on prescribed medications is a common problem with patients who forget to take their medications and try to "catch up," or who just do not understand the instructions on the container.

Scenario Three

You respond to a 69-year-old male who states "my heart feels like a runaway train." His pulse rate is 128 beats/minute and regular. During your assessment, you find out that he has chronic obstructive pulmonary disease (COPD) and has just been prescribed Ventolin. The patient used the Ventolin approximately 30 minutes before he began to feel his heart racing.

- Ventolin is a trade name for albuterol, a bronchodilator used to treat reversible airway obstruction caused by asthma or COPD. Cardiovascular side effects of albuterol include hypertension, chest pain, and arrhythmias, including tachycardia. Unfortunately, the elderly in whom COPD is most common, are more prone to develop adverse reactions and side effects.

It is very important for EMS personnel to perform a thorough patient assessment, including a medication assessment. Medication interactions are sometimes difficult to assess in the out-of-hospital setting. However, any information gathered will benefit the patient when planning a treatment plan, whether in or out of the hospital.

Historical Trends In Pharmacology

Primitive civilizations once believed that evil spirits could inhabit the body and cause disease. This belief continued until 460 B.C. when Hippocrates, known as the Father of Medicine, concluded that disease resulted from natural causes and could only be understood through the study of natural laws. Hippocrates believed that the physician's role in healing was to assist the body's recuperative powers.

The roots of pharmacology go back to the ancient civilizations, which used plants and plant extracts to treat illness and cure disease. For example, opium and morphine were used for pain relief, foxglove extracts (digitalis) for treating symptoms of heart disease. Jesuits' bark was used to treat malaria, willow bark for treating fever, and extracts of the poppy plant (opium) for dysentery. Pharmacology continues to make advances based on knowledge gained from ancient civilizations. The oldest known prescriptions were found around 3000 B.C. on papyrus tablets.

After the fall of the Roman Empire, Christian orders built monasteries. These monasteries became major sites for learning, including the science of pharmacology. Additionally, the monasteries aided the sick with medicinals that were grown in their gardens. In 1240, Emperor Frederic II declared that pharmacy was to be a separate science from medicine. However, it was not until the sixteenth century that Valerius Cordus authored the first pharmacopoeia, or drug reference book.

Some of the most significant pharmacologic discoveries that have taken place throughout history include:

- Seventeenth century: opium, coca, and ipecac, which are still used today.
- 1785: digitalis used as a cardiac medication.
- Nineteenth century: the beginning of large-scale drug manufacturing plants.
- 1815: morphine used to treat severe pain.
- Early 1800s: ether and chloroform used as first general anesthetics, allowing development of surgical treatment of disease.
- 1922: insulin used to treat diabetes mellitus.
- Mid-1940s: the introduction of antibiotics such as penicillin used to treat infections.

- 1955: polio vaccine introduced.
- Mid-1970s: antivirals used to treat viral diseases.
- 1983: Orphan Drug Act signed into law to aid in the research of new treatments to prevent and cure disease.
- 1997: Food and Drug Administration Modernization Act.

Each of these, along with many other advances, significantly advanced the path of medical treatment of disease.

Today, more than ever, modern healthcare is experiencing rapid change. Consumer health education has motivated the public to take more responsibility for their health and disease prevention. For example, more people are now on regular exercise programs and are paying more attention to what they eat. Many people are using the Internet sites such as WebMD and Medline for personal disease self-research. Drug companies are now advertising directly to the consumer encouraging them to "ask your doctor" about specific drugs.

Pharmacology has become multidisciplinary in scope including such subjects as chemistry, genetics, immunology, microbiology, pathology, and physiology.

During the last few decades, there has been remarkable progress in developing new drugs and understanding how they act on the body. However, continuous research will raise endless new questions and challenges that will bring many discoveries in this new century. Research is directed toward new treatments, cures, or methods to prevent disease. For example, the Orphan Drug Act was signed into law January 4, 1983. The term "orphan drug" refers to a product that treats a rare disease affecting fewer than 200,000 Americans. The intent of the act is to stimulate research, development, and approval of products that treat rare diseases. Since the Orphan Drug Act passed, over 190 orphan drugs and biologic products have been brought to market. In contrast, in the decade prior to 1983, fewer than ten such products were brought into market.

There are also social questions to be addressed. Many of the questions involve responsibility issues. For example, keeping basic drugs available to the public. The sudden withdrawal of drugs without warning such as tetanus, and Compazine and the bretylium manufacturing problem caused health concerns for millions of patients. There are also large-scale efforts to retain the South American Amazonian rain forest, which is rich in diversity of plant life and thus is a large source for new medication development.

Modern healthcare continues to change at a rapid pace. One of the many changes is the general public taking more of a responsibility for their healthcare. For example, there is more of an awareness of the importance of regular exercise and a healthy diet. More people are using Internet sites such as WebMD to research topics concerning their healthcare. Communities are regulating where people can and cannot use tobacco products. Pharmaceutical companies are advertising to the consumer encouraging them to ask their physician about specific medications.

Drug Names

A **drug** is any substance that, when taken into the body, changes one or more of the body's functions. Drugs are most commonly used in medicine to diagnose, treat, or prevent disease, which has resulted in an improved quality of life. **Pharmacology** is the science of drugs including the study of their origin, ingredients, uses, and actions on the body. Branches of pharmacology include:

- **Pharmacokinetics:** the movement of a drug in the body with particular emphasis on its distribution, duration of action, and method of excretion.
- **Pharmacodynamics:** the study of drugs and their actions on body tissues.
- **Pharmacotherapy:** the use of drugs in the treatment of disease.
- **Toxicology:** the study of poisons and adverse drug effects.
- **Pharmacogenetics:** the study of the influence of hereditary factors on the response to drugs.

From the time a drug is initially tested in the laboratory until it is approved and marketed, it can acquire up to four names. A drug's **chemical name** is the exact description of the drug's structure and composition. For example, $C_{18}H_{23}NO_3.HCl$, *1,2-benzenediol,4-[2-[[3-(4-hydroxyphenyl)-1-methylpropyl]-,hydrochloride,* ()- is the chemical name for a drug used in treating low cardiac output. This same drug's **generic** (or nonproprietary) **name** is dobutamine hydrochloride. The manufacturer that first formulated the drug usually gives the generic name. Third, the manufacturer registers a drug using a **trade** (or proprietary) **name**. A trade name is often designated in print by its initial capital letter and the raised registered symbol ® following the name. For example, a trade name for dobutamine hydrochloride is Dobutrex®. Finally, the **United States Pharmacopoeia (USP)** and the National Formulary (NF) give a drug its **official name** after it has met specific standards for quality, strength, purity, packaging, and labeling. The letters USP following their name designates drugs meeting these standards. The official name for dobutamine hydrochloride is dobutamine hydrochloride, USP. Table 1–1 illustrates examples of the chemical, generic, trade, and official names of some common EMS drugs as well as some common over-the-counter (OTC) and prescription drugs.

Sources of Drugs

Drugs originate from four main sources: plants, animals/humans, minerals or mineral products, and chemicals made in the laboratory (Figure 1–6).

Plant Sources

Leaves, roots, seeds, and other plant parts may be processed for use as a medicine, and are known as *crude drugs*. Some of the types of pharmacologically active compounds found

Table 1-1 Drug Nomenclature. (© Delmar/Cengage Learning)

Chemical Name	Generic Name	Trade Name*	Official Name
Common Out-of-Hospital Drugs			
2-(diethylamino)-N-(2,6-dimethylphenyl acetamide nomohydrochloride	lidocaine hydrochloride	Xylocaine	lidocaine hydrochloride, USP
1,2-benzenediol, 4-(2-aminoethyl)-, hydrochloride	dopamine hydrochloride	Intropin	dopamine hydrochloride, USP
Common Home Prescription Drugs			
Card-20(22)-enolide, 3-[(0,2,dideoxy-β-D-ribo-hexopyranosyl-(1→4)-0-2, 6-dideoxy-D-ribo-hexopyransoyl) oxy]-12, 14-dihydroxy-, (3β, 5β, 12β)-	digoxin	Lanoxin	digoxin, USP
Benzoic acid, 5-(aminosulfonyl)-4-chloro-2- [(2-furanylmethyl) amino]-	furosemide	Lasix	furosemide, USP
2-propanol, I-[(1-methylethyl) amino]-3-(1-naphthalenyloxy)-, hydrochloride	propranolol hydrochloride	Inderal	propranolol hydrochloride, USP
Common Over-the-Counter Drugs			
Benzoic acid, 2-(acetyloxy)-	aspirin	Ecotrin	aspirin, USP
Ethanamine, 2-(diphenylmethoxy)-N, N-dimethyl-, hydrochloride	diphenhydramine hydrochloride	Benadryl	diphenhydramine hydrochloride, USP
Acetamide, N-(4-hydroxy-phenyl)-	acetaminophen	Tylenol®	acetaminophen, USP

*A single drug may have several different trade names

in plants are alkaloids, glycosides, gums, and oils. *Alkaloids* are a group of organic alkaline substances found in plants that react with acids to form salts. Examples of alkaloids include morphine and atropine. *Glycosides* are plant substances that, on hydrolysis, produce a sugar in addition to one or more other active substances. A common cardiac glycoside used in medicine is digoxin. *Gums* are plant exudates. When water is added, some gums form gelatinous masses, while others remain unchanged in the gastrointestinal tract. Examples of the uses of gums include their use as a natural laxative, or tropical preparations used to soothe irritated skin and mucous membranes. *Oils* are viscous liquids, generally of two kinds, volatile or fixed. A volatile oil puts off a pleasant odor and taste, and is usually used as a flavoring agent, for example, peppermint. Fixed oils are generally greasy. An example of a fixed oil medicine is castor oil.

Animal and Human Sources

Some of the most powerful drugs are extracted from animal and human tissue. These drugs are often used to replace insufficient glandular secretions. Examples of drugs derived from animal and human sources include epinephrine, insulin, and adrenocorticotropic hormone (ACTH).

Minerals or Mineral Products

Materials such as iron and iodine and mineral salts are commonly used to manufacture drugs. Common drugs made from mineral sources include sodium bicarbonate, used to treat metabolic acidosis, and calcium chloride, used to treat acute hyperkalemia and acute hypocalcemia.

Laboratory-Produced Chemicals

Synthetic drugs are produced by chemical processes in the laboratory. Today, most drugs are synthetic. Two common emergency drugs produced in the laboratory are lidocaine, used to treat cardiac dysrhythmias, and diazepam, used to treat seizures, anxiety, and other neurologic disorders.

Deoxyribonucleic acid (DNA)-Produced Drugs

Drugs that are produced through Deoxyribonucleic acid (DNA) engineering have revolutionized medicine. One example of how DNA engineering has developed is in the case of insulin. Insulin controls the metabolism and uptake of sugar in our bodies. It is secreted by the beta cells of the pancreas. In the past, insulin came mainly from beef or pork

Source	Example	Drug name	Classification
Plants	cinchona bark	quinidine	antiarrhythmic
	purple foxglove	digitalis	cardiotonic
Minerals	magnesium	Milk of Magnesia	antacid, laxative
	gold	Solganal; auranofin	anti-inflammatory used to treat rheumatoid arthritis
Animals	pancreas of cow, hog	insulin	antidiabetic hormone
	thyroid gland of animals	thyroid, USP	hormone
Synthetic	meperidine	Demerol	analgesic
	diphenoxylate	Lomotil	antidiarrheal
DNA	oxytocin	Pitocin	hormone
	insulins	Humulin R	antidiabetic

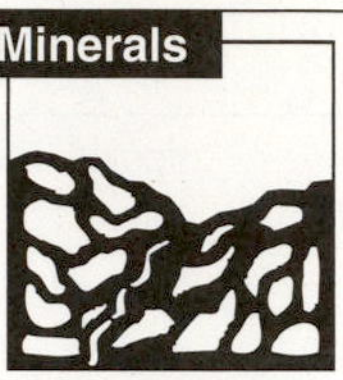

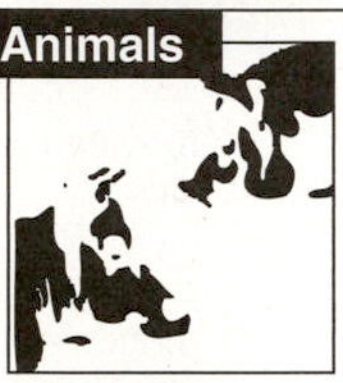

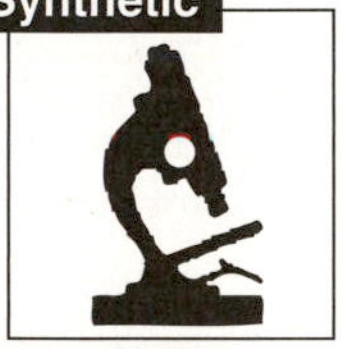

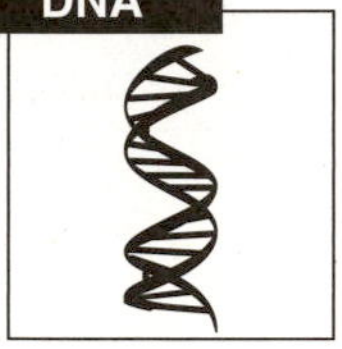

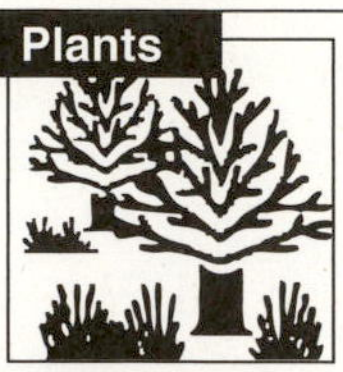

Figure 1–6 Drug Sources. (© Delmar/Cengage Learning)

pancreas. When given to patients, beef or pork insulin occasionally caused drug resistance. Today, insulin for injection made from DNA engineering is equivalent to human insulin.

Drug Classifications

Drugs are generally classified into categories according to the body tissues they affect and their therapeutic and physiologic effects. For example, adenosine is therapeutically classified as an antiarrhythmic, used to slow conduction through the AV node of the heart. It may also interrupt reentry pathways through the AV node. Therapeutically, adenosine can restore normal sinus rhythm (NSR) in patients experiencing paroxysmal supraventricular tachycardia (PSVT). Understanding drug classifications will help you understand why a particular drug is prescribed and how that drug affects the body.

Drugs can have more than one therapeutic classification. For example, epinephrine can be therapeutically classified as

a bronchodilator, cardiac stimulator, or peripheral vasoconstrictor. You should be familiar with the following therapeutic drug classifications.

- Adrenocorticoid: An adrenocorticoid is one of a group of hormones secreted by the adrenal cortex.
- Alkylating agents: Alkylating agents donate an alkyl group to biological macromolecules. They are commonly used to fight cancer.
- Alpha$_1$-adrenergic blocking agents: Alpha$_1$-adrenergic blocking agents selectively block postsynaptic alpha$_1$-adrenergic receptors, resulting in dilation of both arterioles and veins leading to a decrease in B/P.
- Aminoglycosides: Aminoglycosides are broad-spectrum antibiotics believed to inhibit protein synthesis.
- Amphetamines and derivatives: Amphetamines and their derivatives are thought to act on the cerebral cortex and reticular activating system (including the

medullary, respiratory, and vasomotor centers) by releasing norepinephrine from central adrenergic neurons.

- Analgesics: Analgesics include all drugs that relieve pain.
- Angiotensin-converting enzyme (ACE) inhibitors: ACE inhibitors are believed to act by suppressing the renin–angiotensin–aldosterone system, subsequently lowering blood pressure. They are also used to treat congestive heart failure (CHF).
- Antianginal drugs-nitrates/nitrites: An antianginal is a drug that relieves the pain of angina pectoris. Nitrates relax vascular smooth muscle, especially in coronary vessels.
- Antianxiety agent: An antianxiety agent is a drug that prevents or controls anxiety episodes.
- Antiarrhythmic drugs: Antiarrhythmics correct cardiac arrhythmias. Antiarrhythmic drugs are classified as follows:
  1. Group I: Decrease the rate of entry of sodium during cardiac membrane depolarization, and decrease the rate of rise of phase O of the cardiac membrane action potential.
     - Group IA: Depress phase O and prolong the duration of the action potential.
     - Group IB: Slightly depress phase O and are thought to shorten the action potential.
     - Group IC: Slight effect on repolarization but marked depression of phase O of the action potential.

     Examples of drugs classified as Group I include phenytoin, disopyramide, procainamide, and lidocaine.
  2. Group II. Competitively block beta-adrenergic receptors and depress phase 4 depolarization. Examples of some of these beta-blockers include propranolol, metoprolol tartrate, and atenolol.
  3. Group III. Prolong the duration of the membrane action potential (relative refractory period) without changing the phase of depolarization of the resting membrane potential. Examples of Group III drugs include bretylium, and amiodarone.
  4. Group IV. Group IV drugs include calcium channel blockers and cardiac glycosides. A calcium channel blocker inhibits the influx of calcium through the cell membrane, resulting in a depression of automaticity and conduction velocity in both smooth and cardiac muscle. Cardiac glycosides increase the force and velocity of myocardial contraction by increasing the refractory period of the AV node and increasing total peripheral resistance. An example of a calcium channel blocker is verapamil. Verapamil slows conduction velocity and increases the refractoriness of the AV node. An example of a cardiac glycoside is digoxin. Digoxin

causes a decrease in maximal diastolic potential, and increases the slope of phase 4 depolarization. Digoxin is used to treat CHF.

- Anticoagulant agents: Anticoagulants are drugs that affect blood clotting, and can be divided into three classes: (1) *anticoagulants*, drugs that prevent or slow coagulation, (2) *thrombolytic agents*, drugs that increase the rate at which an existing blood clot dissolves; and (3) *hemostatics*, drugs that prevent or stop internal bleeding.
- Anticonvulsants: Anticonvulsants depress abnormal neuronal discharges in the central nervous system that may cause seizures.
- Antidepressants: All antidepressants cause adaptive changes in the serotonin and norepinephrine receptor systems, resulting in changes in the sensitivities of both presynaptic and postsynaptic receptor sites.
- Antidiabetic agents: An antidiabetic agent is a drug that controls diabetes.
- Antidote: An antidote is a drug that neutralizes poisons or alters their effects on the body.
- Antihistamines (H_1 Blockers): An antihistamine is a drug that blocks the effects of histamine, relieving the symptoms associated with allergic reactions, versus H_2 blockers that block production of gastric acid secretion.
- Antihypertensive agents: Antihypertensives lower blood pressure.
- Antipsychotic agent: An antipsychotic is a drug that blocks dopamine receptors in the brain. These drugs help relieve the despondency of the severely depressed, making some patients more accessible to psychotherapy.
- Antitussives: Antitussives are drugs that suppress coughing.
- Beta-adrenergic blocking agents: Beta-adrenergic blocking agents combine reversibly with beta-adrenergic receptors to block the response of sympathetic nerve impulses, circulating catecholamines, or beta-adrenergic drugs.
- Bronchodilators: Bronchodilators are drugs used to treat airway obstruction caused by asthma or chronic obstructive pulmonary disease (COPD). They also reverse bronchospasm.
- Calcium channel blocking agents: Calcium channel blocking agents inhibit the influx of calcium through the cell membrane, resulting in a depression of automaticity and conduction velocity in both smooth and cardiac muscle.
- Calcium salts: Calcium salts return to normal values essential calcium levels for maintaining optimal function of nerves, muscles, the skeletal system, and permeability of cell membranes and capillaries.

- Cardiac glycosides: Cardiac glycosides increase the force and velocity of myocardial contraction (positive inotropic effect) by increasing the refractory period of the AV node and increasing total peripheral resistance.
- Cholinergic agonist: A cholinergic agonist strengthens, prolongs, or prevents the breakdown of the neurotransmitter acetylcholine.
- Cholinergic blocking agents: Cholinergic blocking agents prevent the neurotransmitter acetylcholine from combining with receptors on the postganglionic parasympathetic nerve terminal.
- Coronary vasodilator: A coronary vasodilator is a drug that increases the diameter of the coronary blood vessels.
- Corticosteroids: Corticosteroids basically have two functions, (1) the regulation of metabolic pathways involving protein, carbohydrates, and fat; and (2) electrolyte and water balance.
- Diuretics: Diuretics act to inhibit reabsorption of sodium and chloride in the proximal and distal tubules and the loop of Henle.
- Emetic: An emetic is an agent that causes vomiting.
- Histamine H_2 antagonists: Histamine H_2 antagonists are competitive blockers of histamine.
- Hydrogen ion buffer: A hydrogen ion buffer is used to bring the hydrogen ion concentration of the blood within normal levels.
- Hyperglycemic: A hyperglycemic is a drug used to treat hypoglycemia by restoring blood sugar levels to normal.
- Inotropics: Inotropic drugs increase cardiac output. They are used for short-term management of congestive heart failure (CHF) or poor cardiac output.
- Medicinal gasses: The most common uses for medicinal gasses in the out-of-hospital setting are to increase or maintain the partial pressure of oxygen (PaO_2) in the arterial blood, provide pain relief, and bronchodilation.
- Narcotic analgesics: Narcotic analgesics are classified as agonists, mixed agonist–antagonists, or partial agonist depending on their activity at opiate receptors. They attach to specific receptors located in the CNS (cortex, brain stem, and spinal cord) resulting in various CNS effects.
- Narcotic antagonists: Narcotic antagonists competitively block the action of narcotic analgesics by displacing previously given narcotic from their receptor sites or by preventing narcotics from attaching to the opiate receptors.
- Neuromuscular blocking agents: Neuromuscular blocking agents are categorized as competitive (nondepolarizing) and depolarizing drugs,

both of which act peripherally. These drugs prevent muscle contraction or muscle spasm.
- Skeletal muscle relaxants: Skeletal muscle relaxants decrease muscle tone and involuntary movement. Many of these drugs *may* relieve anxiety and tension as well.
- Succinimide anticonvulsants: Succinimide anticonvulsants act by depressing the motor cortex and by raising the threshold of the CNS to convulsive stimuli.
- Sympathomimetic drugs: Adrenergic drugs act by mimicking the action of norephinephrine or epinephrine by combining with alpha and/or beta receptors, or by causing or regulating the release of the natural neurohormones from their storage sites at the nerve terminals.
- Theophylline derivatives: Theophyllines stimulate the CNS, directly relax the smooth muscles of the bronchi and pulmonary blood vessels, produce diuresis, inhibit uterine contractions, stimulate gastric acid secretion, and increase the rate and force of contraction of the heart.
- Tranquilizers/hypnotics: These drugs are thought to affect the limbic system and reticular formation to reduce anxiety by increasing or facilitating the inhibitory neurotransmitter activity.
- Vasodilator: A vasodilator is a drug that relaxes the blood vessels.
- Vasopressors: A vasopressor is a drug that causes contractions of the muscles of the capillaries and arteries, thus increasing peripheral vascular resistance.

Drug Preparations

Drugs generally come in three types of preparations: solid, liquid, or gas. A drug preparation may produce either local or systemic effects.

Drugs taken orally have the advantage of being easy to take; generally, this is the safest way to take medicines. The disadvantages of oral medications are (1) the drug absorption process generally takes longer, (2) the eventual concentrations of the drug in the bloodstream are often unpredictable, and (3) some drugs may be destroyed or altered by gastric acids.

Drugs administered directly into the bloodstream have the advantage of bypassing the absorption process, which enables the drug to produce its desired therapeutic effect much sooner. However, this type of drug administration has the disadvantage of being more difficult and much more dangerous.

A local drug effect is confined to one specific area of the body. For example, a medicated lotion may be applied to an irritated area of the skin for the relief of a rash. A systemic effect occurs when a drug enters into the bloodstream, affecting

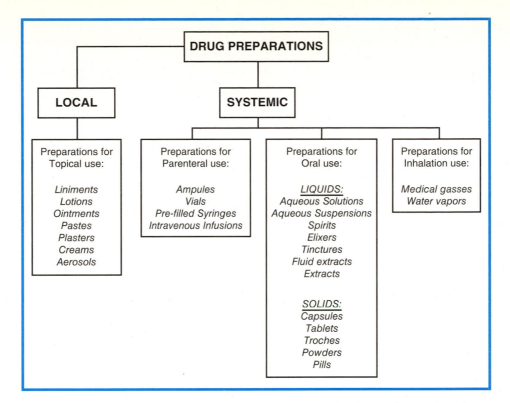

Figure 1–7 The way in which a drug is prepared determines whether it has a local or systemic effect.
(© Delmar/Cengage Learning)

all body tissues. Figure 1–7 categorizes types of drug preparations based on whether they produce local or systemic effects. For example, an antibiotic drug can be absorbed into the bloodstream to systemically fight off infection.

The following are common drug preparations with which you should become familiar.

Drug Preparations for Local Effects

Topical Use

Aerosol. An aerosol is a colloid or glue-like substance finely subdivided into liquid or solid particles that are dispensed in the form of a mist.

Colloid. Glue-like substances, such as a protein or starch, whose particles, when dispersed in a solvent to the greatest possible degree, remain uniformly distributed and fail to form a true solution.

Liniment. A liniment is a liquid containing a medication in oil, alcohol, or water.

Lotion. A lotion is a liquid suspension for external application.

Ointment. An ointment is a semisolid preparation for external application of a drug or medicine.

Paste. A paste is a semisolid gelatinous substance for external application that may contain specific active ingredients or simple materials such as oils, waxes, and starch.

Plaster. Although rarely used, a plaster is an external medicinal preparation formed into a mass harder than an ointment and spread over muslin, linen, skin, or paper.

Cream. A cream is a smooth, thick liquid or a semisolid emulsion for external application.

Drug Preparations for Systemic Effects

Oral Use (Liquids)

Aqueous solution. An aqueous solution is a substance dissolved in water.

Aqueous suspension. An aqueous suspension consists of solid particles mixed with, but not dissolved in, water.

Elixir. An elixir is a sweetened hydroalcoholic liquid used alone or as a vehicle for active drugs.

Extract. An extract is the active ingredient of a vegetable or animal drug obtained by distillation or other chemical process. There are three forms of extracts: semisolid, solid, or powdered.

Fluidextract. A fluidextract is a solution of the dissolved component part of vegetable drugs such that each milliliter equals 1.0 gram of the drug. Fluidextracts contain alcohol as a solvent or preservative or both.

Tincture. A tincture is an alcoholic solution of vegetable or chemical material.

Oral Use (Solid)

Capsule. A capsule is a gelatin container used for single-dose drug administration.

Pill. A pill is a medication in the form of a small solid mass or pellet.

Powder. A powder consists of fine particles of a medicine.

Tablet. A tablet is a small solid mass of medicinal powder. Tablets may be round, oblong, or triangular.

Troche or lozenge. A troche is a solid disk or cylindrical mass of a medication in a flavored base.

Parenteral Use

A **parenteral** route is defined as any route other than the alimentary canal. Intravenous, transtracheal, intraosseous, subcutaneous, or intramuscular routes are all parenteral routes.

Ampule. An ampule is a small, sealed single-dose glass container, containing a liquid injectable drug.

Intravenous infusion. An intravenous infusion is a sterile liquid preparation with or without added drugs.

Prefilled syringe. A prefilled syringe is usually a single-dose glass cartridge containing a liquid drug.

Vial. A vial is a small glass bottle that contains more than one dose of a drug.

Other Preparations for Systemic Effect

Inhalants. An inhalant is a gas, a mixture of gases, or water vapors that transport a drug to the body via the lungs.

Suppositories. A suppository is a semisolid cylinder or cone-shaped mass that provides a drug via the mucous membrane of the rectum, vagina, or urethra.

Investigational Drugs

Before a potential drug comes to market, it must go through a screening process that may take years of research and testing, and require large amounts of financial investment. The **Food and Drug Administration (FDA)** requires the following testing sequence:

1. Animal studies to help determine the following:
   a. **Toxicity**
      - Acute toxicity: The medial lethal dose, that is, the dose that is lethal to 50% of the laboratory animals tested (LD_{50}). Acute toxicity generally develops rapidly.
      - Subacute and chronic toxicity: The terms subacute and chronic refer to the speed at which toxicity develops. For example, chronic shows little change or slow progression over time. Subacute shows moderate change or progression over time.
   b. **Therapeutic index:** The ratio of the LD_{50} to the median effective dose.
   c. Modes of absorption, distribution, biotransformation, and excretion.
2. Human studies:
   a. Initial pharmacologic evaluation (Phase I)
   b. Limited controlled evaluation (Phase II)
   c. Extended clinical evaluation (Phase III)

Drug Development/FDA Approval Process

After the data on the safety and effectiveness of a proposed drug have been reviewed, the FDA will approve an application for an Investigational New Drug (IND). The investigation covered under the IND is divided into three phases:

Phase I: Initial pharmacologic evaluation. Phase I involves small groups of healthy subjects. The goals of phase I are to prove the drug's safety and to identify tolerable dosages. The investigators determine the pharmacokinetics of the drug (absorption, distribution, biotransformation, and excretion). If phase I testing shows that the drug is safe to give in expected therapeutic doses, the studies continue to phase II.

Phase II: Limited controlled evaluation. Phase II consists of controlled evaluations designed to test the drug's effect on the specific illness for which it was designed. Phase II testing also helps to establish dosage and other pharmacokinetic information. Individuals are closely monitored for drug effectiveness and for side effects. After Phase II is complete, investigators submit all collected data to the FDA. At this point, the FDA may approve or reject a New Drug Application (NDA). If the NDA is approved, the drug can be marketed for the selected indication in the dosing schedules as studied, and Phase III is begun.

Phase III: Extended clinical evaluation. Phase III consists of the full-scale or extended clinical evaluations. Phase III evaluations are performed on a large number of subjects to determine therapeutic effect and possible side effects, and to decide if the side effects are low enough to be acceptable. Phase III has three objectives: determine clinical effectiveness, determine safety, and establish tolerable dosage ranges.

Once a drug is placed on the market, it is inevitable that the drug will be reported to produce additional effects. These effects can be both therapeutic or adverse, and may not have been noted during the trial studies. Therefore, *Phase IV* drug testing is a postmarketing evaluation designed to update safety and product results. This phase clarifies incidence of adverse drug reactions and long-term effects. Phases I through III are almost always required. Although phase IV is not required of all drugs, the FDA prefers that all drugs go through all four phases.

Orphan Drugs

The Office of Orphan Products Development (OOPD) was created in 1982. The OOPD is dedicated to promoting the development of products that demonstrate promise for the diagnosis and/or treatment of rare diseases. It administers the major provisions of the Orphan Drug Act (ODA), which provides incentives for sponsors to develop drugs for rare diseases. Approximately 200 drugs for rare diseases have been brought to market since 1983. The OOPD also administers the Orphan Products Grants Program, which provides funding for clinical research in rare diseases.

Components of a Drug Profile

Administering drugs carries an enormous responsibility. Without question, EMS professionals are placed in a position that may save many lives through proper drug administration. Drugs produce a variety of physiologic responses, including raising or lowering blood pressure, increasing or decreasing heart rate, and sedating or stimulating the patient. If the wrong drug or the incorrect dose of the appropriate drug is given, the results could be fatal. Therefore, it is essential that you be thoroughly familiar with the following components of a drug profile:

- *Therapeutic Classification.* Each drug can be placed in a group that indicates how the drug works. A drug can have more than one classification. For example, epinephrine can be classified as a bronchodilator, cardiac stimulator, and peripheral vasoconstrictor.
- *Mechanism of Action.* A drug's mechanism of action describes how the drug produces its desired therapeutic effects (pharmacodynamics).
- *Therapeutic Benefits.* Therapeutic benefits describe the results expected from administering a drug.
- *Pharmacokinetics.* Once given, the drug must move to its site of action before it can produce its therapeutic effects. Drug movement also includes how the drug is absorbed, distributed, and eliminated from the body.
- *Indications.* The indications for a drug's use include the most common uses for that drug in the out-of-hospital setting.
- *Contraindications.* A drug's contraindications are the circumstances under which it should not be used or when alternative drugs should be considered.
- *Precautions.* Precautions describe situations in which drug use may be dangerous to the patient or when dosage or administration techniques may have to be modified.
- *Route and Dosage.* The route of a drug describes how the drug is given. For example, intravenous, endotracheal, intraosseous, intramuscular, and so forth. The dosage is how much of the drug should be given, depending on the route used.
- *Adverse Reactions and Side Effects.* A drug's adverse reactions and side effects are any actions or effects other than those desired. However, some side effects of a drug are predictable and may occur in addition to the expected therapeutic effects.
- *EMS Considerations.* EMS considerations explain special information that may be helpful when giving a specific drug. For example, there may be special considerations EMS professionals need to follow when giving a drug to the pregnant, pediatric, or geriatric patient.
- *How Supplied.* This includes each drug's common concentration and packaging information.

Sources of Drug Information

There are numerous sources where health-care providers can obtain information on drugs. For example, drug manufacturers, package inserts, pharmacists, medical journals, and the Internet are just a few sources where you can obtain information on drugs. Because no one reference is a complete source of drug information, EMS providers should be familiar with the following primary drug reference sources.

- *American Hospital Formulary Service Drug Information* (AHFS) (Bethesda, MD: American Society of Hospital Pharmacists, Inc.)
- *Drug Facts and Comparisons* (St. Louis, MO: Facts and Comparisons, Inc.)
- *Handbook of Nonprescription Drugs* (Washington, DC: American Pharmaceutical Association)
- **Physicians' Desk Reference** (**PDR**) (Oradell, NJ: Medical Economics)
- **United States Pharmacopoeia, (USP)** DI (Rockville, MD: U.S. Pharmacopeial Convention)
- *PDR Nurse's Drug Handbook* (Montvale, NJ: Medical Economics Company)

United States Drug Legislation

At the beginning of the twentieth century, no federal laws controlled drug distribution. During the first ten years of the twentieth century, the use of chemicals in medicine increased rapidly. This increase brought with it an increased use of dangerous ingredients and complex formulas. Some drug companies used poor quality control and made unproven claims for their products. This made it necessary to develop national standards and government regulations to guarantee that drugs sold to the public were accurately identified and of uniform strength and purity. For these reasons, Congress enacted several laws.

Food and Drug Act (Pure Food Act) of 1906

In 1906, Congress enacted the Pure Food Act as the first U.S. law to protect the public from mislabeled, poisonous, or harmful food and drugs. This legislation named the *United States Pharmacopoeia (USP)* and the *National Formulary (NF)* as official drug standards and established the Food and Drug Administration (FDA). The Pure Food Act authorized the FDA to determine if drugs were safe and effective and to enforce these standards.

Harrison Narcotic Act of 1914

The Harrison Narcotic Act was the first federal legislation designed to stop drug addiction or dependence. It established federal control over the importation, manufacture, and sale of the opium and coca plants and all their compounds and derivatives. The Harrison Narcotic Act established the word *narcotic* as a legal term.

Federal Food, Drug, and Cosmetic Act of 1938

The Federal Food, Drug, and Cosmetic Act updated the Pure Food Act. This legislation required that labels list the possible habit-forming properties and side effects of drugs. It also authorized the FDA to determine the safety of drugs before marketing and required that dangerous drugs be issued only by the prescription of a physician, dentist, or veterinarian. This act was amended by the Durham–Humphrey amendment in 1952. The Durham–Humphrey amendment classified certain drugs as "legend" drugs and restricted pharmacists from distributing legend drugs without a prescription. Legend drugs are those that must be labeled "Caution: Federal Law prohibits dispensing without a prescription." In 1962, the Federal Food, Drug, and Cosmetic Act was amended again by the Kefauver–Harris amendment. The Kefauver–Harris amendment authorized the FDA to establish official names for drugs and required drug manufacturers to prove a drug's ability to produce therapeutic results.

Other Drug Laws and Regulations

The Harrison Narcotic Act and all further drug abuse amendments were superseded by the Controlled Substance Act of 1970. The Controlled Substance Act classifies drugs with abuse potential into five schedules by weighing a drug's potential for abuse against its medical usefulness (Table 1–2). For example, a Schedule I drug has a high potential for abuse and no accepted medical usefulness, whereas a Schedule V drug has little potential for abuse and recognized medical use.

The Food and Drug Administration Modernization Act (FDAMA) of 1997, amended the Federal Food, Drug, and Cosmetic Act relating to the regulation of food, drugs, devices, and biologic products for the twenty-first century characterized by increasing technologic, trade, and public health complexities.

Other federal agencies involved in regulating drugs include the Drug Enforcement Administration (DEA), the Public Health Service, and the Federal Trade Commission (FTC). The DEA is empowered to enforce the Controlled Substance Act. The Public Health Service, part of the U.S. Department of Health and Human Services, regulates biologic products such as vaccines. The FTC regulates drug advertising. It has the power to prevent false or misleading advertising of food, drugs, and cosmetics to the public. The FTC also regulates prescription drug advertising to the medical profession for those drugs regulated by the FDA. The FTC relies on the FDA to regulate the claims of nonprescription drug advertisements.

Drug Standardization

The strength and activity of drugs may vary considerably. For example, drugs obtained from plants may vary in strength because of where the plants were grown, and the age the plants were harvested. Additionally, the type of preservation process used after harvesting can affect the potency of the drug. Drugs must be of uniform strength and purity when offered on the market, which means standardization is essential. The federal government establishes and enforces drug standards.

A note of caution about herbal supplements should be observed. Herbal supplements are plant derivatives that the

Table 1–2 Schedule of Controlled Substance. (© Delmar/Cengage Learning)

Drug Schedule	Description	Example Drugs
I	Schedule I drugs are not considered to be legitimate for medical use in the United States. They are used for research only and they cannot be prescribed, having a high risk for abuse.	LSD, Heroin, Marijuana*
II	Schedule II drugs have accepted medical use, but have a high potential for abuse or addiction. These drugs must be ordered by written prescription and cannot be refilled without a new, written prescription.	Morphine, Cocaine, Codeine, Demerol, Dilaudid
III	Schedule III drugs have moderate potential for abuse or addiction, low potential for physical dependence. These drugs may be ordered by written prescription or by telephone order. Prescription expires in 6 months. They may not be refilled more than five times in a 6-month period of time.	Tylenol with Codeine, Butisol, Hycodan
IV	Schedule IV drugs have less potential for abuse or addiction than those of Schedule III, with limited physical dependence. These drugs may be ordered by written prescription or by telephone order. They may be refilled up to five times over a 6-month period of time. Prescription expires in 6 months.	Librium, Valium, Darvon, Equanil
V	Schedule V drugs have a small potential for abuse or addiction. These drugs may be ordered by written prescription or by telephone order and there is no limit on prescription refills. Some of these drugs may not need a prescription.	Robitussin A-C, Donnagel-PG, Lomotil

*Limited special permission has been obtained in some states for MDs to prescribe marijuana for treatment of side effects, such as nausea and vomiting, in patients receiving chemotherapy.

FDA does not have regulatory control, or only limited control, over their potency and purity. Herbal preparations can be of varying quality and have the potential to interact with many drugs.

Drug standardization techniques can either be chemical or biologic. Chemical processing, known as a chemical **assay**, determines the ingredients present in the drug and their amounts. For example, opium contains certain alkaloids, which may vary in different preparations. The U.S. official standard states that opium must contain no less than 9.5% and no more than 10.5% of anhydrous morphine.

In some drugs, either the active ingredients are unknown or there are no methods of chemically analyzing and standardizing them. In these cases, the drug must be standardized by biologic methods. The **bioassay** determines the amount of a preparation required producing a predetermined effect on a laboratory animal. For example, the potency of a sample of insulin is measured by its ability to lower the glucose level of rabbits.

The only official book of drug standards in the United States is the *United States Pharmacopoeia (USP)*. When a drug is added to the USP, it has met high standards of quality, purity, and strength. The letters USP after the official name can identify drugs meeting these high standards.

Special Considerations

Administering drugs can be further complicated by the added factors of patient age, pregnancy, and lactation. For example, the very young and the elderly are generally more susceptible to the adverse effects of drugs. Therefore, drug dosages may have to be modified for these age groups. Additionally, some drugs can cross the placental barrier and reach the fetus, causing adverse effects. Once the baby is born, certain drugs can also be transferred to the child via the breast milk.

Pregnancy and Lactation

There are two potential problems that may occur when giving drugs to pregnant patients. First, drugs have the potential to cross the placental barrier and affect the fetus. When giving drugs to pregnant patients, the potential benefits must always be weighed against the risks. The FDA categorizes drugs based on potential risk during pregnancy (Table 1–3).

Second, pregnancy causes several anatomic and physiologic changes that must be considered prior to administering drugs. These changes include:

- An increase in heart rate
- An increase in cardiac output
- An up to 45% increase in blood volume
- A decrease in blood pressure
- A decrease in protein binding
- A decrease in hepatic biotransformation

Another concern may develop after the baby is born. If the mother must begin to take medications for any reason, and is also breast feeding, many drugs can be excreted into the breast milk and ingested by the baby.

Pediatric Patients

Neonates pose a particular concern during drug administration. The major organ for biotransformation is the liver. However, the neonate's liver is not fully developed, impairing biotransformation. Drug excretion through the neonates' kidney may be impaired as well. Therefore, drug dosages to the neonate have to be modified to account for these factors.

In most cases, drug dosages for the pediatric patient are reduced from that of the adult. Drug dosages for the pediatric patient are generally based on body weight and body surface area (BSA). Therefore, EMS providers must determine body weight of the pediatric patient before administering drugs.

Table 1–3 Pregnancy Categories: FDA Assigned. (© Delmar/Cengage Learning)
The U.S. Food and Drug Administration's use-in-pregnancy rating system weighs the degree to which available information has ruled out risk to the fetus against the drug's potential benefit to the patient. The ratings, and their interpretation, are as follows:

Category	Interpretation
A	**CONTROLLED STUDIES SHOW NO RISK.** Adequate, well-controlled studies in pregnant women have failed to demonstrate a risk to the fetus in any trimester of pregnancy.
B	**NO EVIDENCE OF RISK IN HUMANS.** Adequate, well-controlled studies in pregnant women have not shown increased risk of fetal abnormalities despite adverse findings in animals, or, in the absence of adequate human studies, animal studies show no fetal risk. The chance of fetal harm is remote, but remains a possibility.
C	**RISK CANNOT BE RULED OUT.** Adequate, well-controlled human studies are lacking, and animal studies have shown a risk to the fetus or are lacking as well. There is a chance of fetal harm if the drug is administered during pregnancy; but the potential benefits may outweigh the potential risk.
D	**POSITIVE EVIDENCE OF RISK.** Studies in humans, or investigational or postmarketing data, have demonstrated fetal risk. Nevertheless, potential benefits from the use of the drug may outweigh the potential risk. For example, the drug may be acceptable if needed in a life-threatening situation or serious disease for which safer drugs cannot be used or are ineffective.
X	**CONTRAINDICATED IN PREGNANCY.** Studies in animals or humans, or investigational or postmarketing reports, have demonstrated positive evidence of fetal abnormalities or risk which clearly outweighs any possible benefit to the patient.

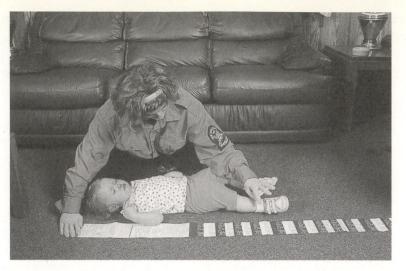

Figure 1–8 The child is being measured with a length-based tape to determine what medications will be appropriate for her age and size. (© Delmar/Cengage Learning)

A device to aid in determining pediatric drug dosages is a length-based resuscitation tape known as the Broselow Tape® (Figure 1–8). This tape is divided into color-coded sections that list such information as drug dosages, endotracheal tube sizes, defibrillator settings, and so forth. EMS providers simply unfold and place the tape alongside the patient to find the required information.

Geriatric Patients

As the baby boomers age, there will be an increased use of the EMS system by this population group. As patients become older, they are more likely to develop more than one disease process at a time. When this occurs, generally an increased use of medications must become a part of their daily lives. Body systems will respond to these medications differently than they would in younger years. Common physiologic effects of aging include a decrease in:

- Cardiac output
- Brain mass
- Renal function
- Respiratory capacity
- Serum albumin
- Body fat
- Total body water
- Biotransformation
- Excretion

The above changes that occur with age may also cause a change in pharmacokinetics and pharmacodynamics. Therefore, the dosages of many drugs may have to be reduced when given to the elderly.

Pharmacologic Abbreviations

Abbreviations are common in medicine. Using abbreviations appropriately can make you more efficient, especially in your never-ending battle with paperwork. Standard pharmacologic and other medical abbreviations and symbols with which you should be familiar are listed in Appendix F in the back of this book.

CONCLUSION

Administering drugs is a part of complete EMS patient care that carries an enormous responsibility. EMS professionals are held responsible for safe and therapeutically effective drug administration. Each EMS provider is personally responsible legally, morally, and ethically for each drug administered.

Understanding pharmacology is more than knowing which drug to administer and when to administer it. Each EMS professional administering drugs must be familiar with the drugs used in the local EMS system. Knowledge of each drug's actions, indications, contraindications, side effects, precautions, and correct dosage; the route in which the drug should be given; and any pertinent drug interactions is essential. Giving the correct drug appropriately can be life-saving. Giving the same drug inappropriately can prove deadly.

▶ STUDY QUESTIONS

1. The *primary* reason for drug legislation (such as the Federal Food, Drug and Cosmetic Act) is to:
a. Keep health-care professionals from abusing drugs
b. Ensure the safety of the drug manufactured
c. Ensure the sterility of manufactured goods
d. Control narcotic drugs

2. The initials "USP" after a drug indicates the drug's _____ name.
a. Chemical
b. Generic (nonproprietary)
c. Trade (proprietary)
d. Official

3. Pharmacodynamics is the study of drugs:
a. Movement
b. Absorption
c. Concentration
d. Mechanism of action

4. _____ effect is the result of repeated doses of drugs that accumulate in the body to produce symptoms of poisoning.
a. Therapeutic
b. Potentiation
c. Depressant
d. Cumulative

5. Name the five major sources of drugs, and give examples of each.

_____

_____

_____

_____

_____

_____

_____

_____

6. The only official book of drug standards in the United States is the:
a. *United States Pharmacopoeia (USP)*
b. *Physicians' Drug Reference (PDR)*
c. *PDR Nurse's Drug Handbook*
d. *Drug Facts and Comparisons*

7. Describe the following components of a drug profile:
a. Mechanism of action
b. Contraindications
c. Precautions
d. Drug interactions

8. The rate of drug absorption depends on all of the following *except*:
a. Circulatory statue
b. Amount given
c. Solubility
d. pH

9. In most cases, drug dosages for the pediatric patient are generally based on patient:
a. Age
b. Height
c. Weight
d. Gender

10. Explain two potential problems that may occur when giving drugs to pregnant patients.

_____

_____

_____

_____

_____

_____

_____

11. Explain the importance of the *patient medication assessment*.

_____

_____

_____

_____

_____

_____

_____

CHAPTER 2

THE BASICS OF PHARMACOKINETICS AND PHARMACODYNAMICS

OBJECTIVES

On completion of this chapter and the study questions, you should be able to:

- Define pharmacokinetics and pharmacodynamics.
- Describe the process of absorption.
- Describe the process of distribution.
- Describe the process of biotransformation.
- Describe the process of excretion.
- Describe the various factors in drug responses.

KEY TERMS

Absorption
Affinity
Agonist
Antagonist
Bioavailability
Biotransformation
Blood-brain barrier
Blood-cerebrospinal fluid
    barrier
Bound drug
Cumulative drug effects

Diffusion
Distribution
Efficacy
Excretion
Filtration
Free drug
Mechanism of action
Metabolite
Minimum therapeutic
    concentration
Onset of drug action

Osmosis
Passive transport
pH
Pharmacodynamics
Pharmacokinetics
Prodrug
Receptor
Solubility
Volatile

INTRODUCTION

Drugs must take a complicated journey through the body before they can produce their desired therapeutic effects. Once a drug is given, it is absorbed into the circulatory system, distributed to its site of action, and finally eliminated from the body. Pharmacokinetics is the study of drug absorption, distribution, biotransformation (metabolism), and elimination, with emphasis on the time it takes for these processes to take place. In other words, pharmacokinetics studies drug movement.

Once a drug reaches its receptors' sites (sites of action), certain biochemical and physiologic actions occur, producing the desired pharmacologic effects. These pharmacologic effects are called the drug's mechanism of action. Pharmacodynamics is the study of drug actions in the body. Drug pharmacokinetics and pharmacodynamics determine the route, frequency, and dosage of drug administration.

Pharmacokinetics

Basic Transport Physiology

Passive Transport

Passive transport depends on three mechanisms: (1) filtration, (2) diffusion, and (3) osmosis.

Filtration is the movement of fluid through a membrane, caused by differences in hydrostatic pressure. Hydrostatic pressure is the force exerted by the weight of a solution; it causes the solution to move from an area of higher pressure to an area of lower pressure. In two compartments separated by a permeable or semipermeable membrane, hydrostatic pressure tends to cause fluid to move from one compartment to the other until the pressure in both compartments is equal.

Diffusion is the tendency of molecules in solution to distribute themselves equally. In diffusion, molecules, atoms, or ions flow from an area of higher concentration to areas of lower concentration, until the concentration (number of molecules of solute per amount of solution) is the same throughout the solution.

Osmosis is the diffusion of solute and/or solvent through a permeable or semipermeable membrane. It is a result of the same force that causes solute molecules or ions within a solution to flow from areas of high concentration to areas of low concentration. With two solutions separated by a semipermeable membrane, a difference in solute concentration creates osmotic pressure, which causes water and (if possible) solute to move across the membrane until the solutions are in equilibrium.

Absorption

Absorption is the passage of a drug from the site of administration (where absorption begins) into the circulatory system. The speed at which a drug is absorbed is very important,

because it determines how quickly the drug reaches its target tissue to produce its therapeutic effects. The rate of absorption depends on the following factors:

- *Nature of the absorbing surface:* The absorbing surface area is a determining factor on how quickly a drug is absorbed. The greater the surface area of the absorption site, the faster a drug becomes absorbed, and the quicker it produces its therapeutic effect.
- *Circulatory status:* Poor circulation results in slow drug absorption and, therefore, delayed or inadequate therapeutic response. However, drugs that can be given via the intravenous (IV) route bypass the absorption process. The IV administration technique permits the drug to go directly into the circulation, thereby permitting a faster therapeutic response.
- *Solubility:* This is the drug's ability to dissolve. The higher a drug's solubility, the faster it enters the bloodstream.
- *Body pH:* Acidosis delays drug absorption in many cases. For example, acidosis can delay the absorption of epinephrine, thus making it inactive. This is why some patients in cardiac arrest do not respond to epinephrine: inadequate ventilations and/or chest compressions may leave them acidotic. However, some drugs can vary significantly in pH. For example, a drug that is acidic will generally absorb better when introduced into the stomach because of the stomach's acidic environment. Also, an alkaline drug will absorb more quickly when introduced into the alkaline environment of the kidneys. Therefore, both a drug's pH and the pH of the body can affect absorption.
- *Concentration:* Generally, the higher the percentage of drug in the preparation administered, the faster the rate of absorption. Approximately 80% of drugs used in medicine are formulated to be taken orally.

Table 2–1 Rates of Drug Absorption.
(© Delmar/Cengage Learning)

Route	Rate of Absorption
Intravenous	Immediate
Endotracheal/Transtracheal	Immediate
Intraosseous	Immediate
Inhalation	Rapid to immediate
Rectal	Rapid
Intramuscular	Moderate
Subcutaneous	Slow
Oral	
Sublingual	Rapid
Intralingual	Rapid
Ingestion	Slow

However, the oral route has two drawbacks. First, it is harder to predict and control the final concentration in the circulatory system of an orally administered drug. This unpredictability results from:

- Changes in the rate of absorption, depending on the presence or absence of food in the digestive system.
- The destruction of some of the drug by gastric enzymes.
- Second, the rate of absorption through the digestive system is slower than the rate from subcutaneous injection and intramuscular injection.
- *Bioavailability:* A sufficient amount of a drug must reach its target site of action in order to produce a therapeutic response. **Bioavailability** is the rate at which a drug enters the general circulation permitting access to the site of action. This is determined by the measurement of the concentration of the drug in body fluids or by the magnitude of the pharmacologic response.

Table 2–1 lists the routes in which drugs can be given and their rates of absorption.

Distribution

Once a drug is administered and absorbed into the circulatory system, it must travel to its site of action before it can be of any benefit. Once in the bloodstream, the entire dose does not travel to its targeted tissues. Instead, the drug travels throughout the entire body. As Figure 2–1 illustrates, a certain amount of the drug may become bound to blood proteins (such as hemoglobin, albumin, and globulin). When this occurs, the drug is unavailable for further **distribution** until it is released from the blood protein. Drugs can also become stored within the body's fatty tissues. The drug must be released from fatty tissue, to be available for distribution. The amount of drug that binds to blood protein, or becomes stored in the body's fatty tissues, is termed **bound drug**. Only the drug not bound, termed **free drug**, can be distributed for metabolism and elimination and is available to targeted tissues.

Because drugs are distributed by way of the circulatory system, they generally concentrate in tissues that are well supplied with blood, such as the heart, liver, kidneys, and brain. The **blood-brain barrier** and the **blood-cerebrospinal fluid barrier**, however, limit delivery of drugs to the brain. These barriers are tightly packed cell membranes that separate the circulating blood from the brain and cerebrospinal fluid. The blood-brain barrier and the blood-cerebrospinal fluid barrier restrict the movement of some damaging drugs and toxins to the brain and cerebrospinal fluid. Only non-protein-bound, highly lipid-soluble drugs can cross these barriers into the central nervous system. Even these drugs generally enter the brain and spinal fluid at a slower rate than other tissues because of this extra barrier.

Biotransformation

There are two ways in which the body eliminates a drug: biotransformation and excretion. **Biotransformation** is the chemical alteration of a drug within the body to an active or inactive water-soluble metabolite. A **metabolite** is

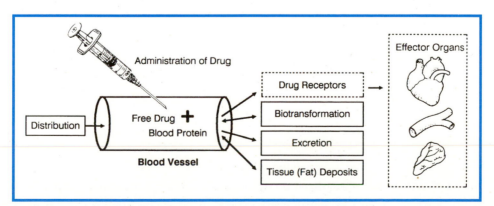

Figure 2–1 The pharmacokinetic phase of drug action. (© Delmar/Cengage Learning)

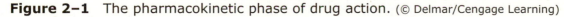

any product that results from biotransformation. Changing a drug to a water-soluble metabolite makes **excretion** from the body easier. Most drugs are inactivated as a result of biotransformation. Some drugs, however, become therapeutically active (**prodrugs**) as a result of biotransformation.

The biotransformation process of a drug to an inactive metabolite begins immediately after drug administration. This actually becomes a race against time. The drug must reach the target site of action at a sufficient therapeutic concentration in the blood before biotransformation converts the drug to an inactive state.

Biotransformation takes place primarily in the liver. It can, however, occur in all body cells and tissues. Biotransformation that takes place in the liver is called *hepatic biotransformation*.

If the rate of drug biotransformation is slowed for any reason, **cumulative drug effects** may occur. Therefore, subsequent doses have more effect. Increasing the rate of biotransformation may produce a state of apparent tolerance, in which the drug effect decreases. Generally, when biotransformation is complete, a drug is no longer able to work therapeutically (unless the drug becomes an active metabolite), and it is excreted.

Excretion

Excretion is the elimination of waste products from the body. Drug excretion takes place through the intestines in the feces, through the kidneys in the urine, through the skin in perspiration, and through the respiratory system in exhaled air.

Volatile (easily evaporated) drugs are excreted from the body through the respiratory system in exhaled air or through the skin in perspiration. Nonvolatile, water-soluble drug metabolites are excreted in the urine. The kidney is the most important site for the excretion of drugs and drug metabolites.

Some drugs are excreted from the body through the alimentary tract. This occurs when the drug passes through the liver, is released into the bile, and is finally eliminated in the feces. Alternatively, the bile enters the small intestine; however, some of the drug travels through the circulatory system until it is finally excreted in the urine. If the reabsorbed drug is in active form, this reabsorption prolongs its actions on the body.

Pharmacodynamics

Unless a drug enters the body via the intravenous, intraosseous, or endotracheal route, some time elapses before the drug reaches its target site of action. The length of time from a drug's first administration, until it reaches a concentration necessary to produce a therapeutic response at its target site of action, is called the **onset of drug action**. Figure 2–2 compares the onset of action for a drug administered intravenously with the onset of action for the same drug given intramuscularly.

Most drugs produce desired effects by inhibiting or increasing the action of targeted **receptors**. A drug receptor is a component of a cell that combines with a drug to initiate a response. In essence, a section of the drug molecule combines with part of the molecular structure on or within a cell to produce a therapeutic effect. Once a drug reaches the site of action, it binds or unites to the receptor so it can cause the desired therapeutic response. This action at the receptor site is also called the drug's mechanism of action.

Drug receptors (target cells) are often referred to as "locks," and drugs that bind to the receptors are generally referred to as the "keys" that fit the locks. A drug's (key) ability to fit a certain

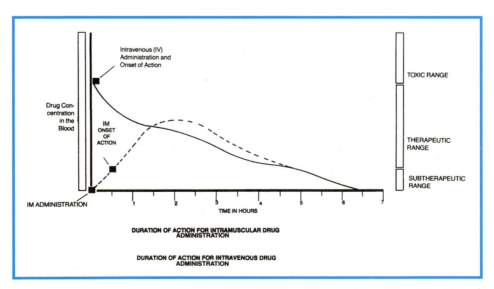

Figure 2–2 The concentration profile (how concentration changes over a period of time) of a drug administered intravenously varies significantly from that of the same drug administered intramuscularly. (© Delmar/Cengage Learning)

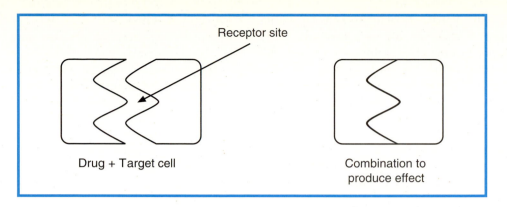

Receptor site

Drug + Target cell

Combination to produce effect

Figure 2–3 Lock-and-Key Union of Drug and Receptor. (© Delmar/Cengage Learning)

receptor (lock) enables a pharmacologic response to occur (Figure 2–3). Such a drug is called an **agonist**. In addition, some drugs bind to receptors, but their effect is to inhibit or counteract a response. These drugs are called **antagonists**.

Affinity and **efficacy** are used to describe the nature of drug-receptor interaction. Affinity means attraction; to say that a drug has an affinity for a receptor means that it tends to combine with that receptor. Efficacy means the power to produce a desired effect. To say a drug has efficacy means that it has the capacity to produce a pharmacologic response when it interacts with its receptor. Drugs that are agonists have both affinity and efficacy, while antagonist drugs have affinity but not efficacy.

Phases of Drug Activity

A drug goes through four phases of activity before it produces a desired pharmacologic effect (Figure 2–4). The administration phase is the introduction of the drug into the body by the appropriate route. Once administered, the drug

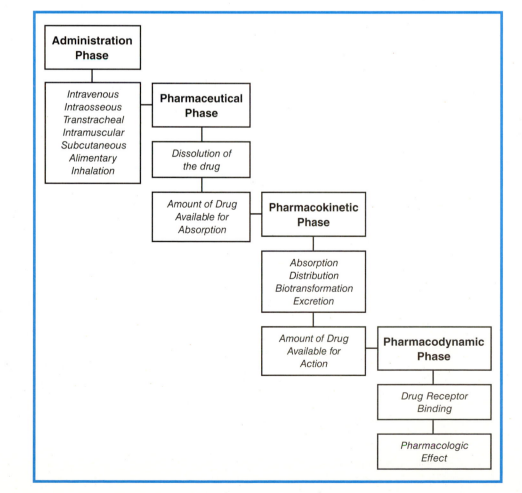

Figure 2–4 The phases of drug activity. (© Delmar/Cengage Learning)

enters the pharmaceutical phase. During this phase, the drug dissolves so it can be made available for absorption. Once dissolved, the drug begins the pharmacokinetic phase. Only free drugs capable of reaching their receptors can be said to exist in the pharmacokinetic phase. Once a drug reaches its receptors, the pharmacodynamic phase of drug activity occurs. It is only when the drug binds to its receptor that the pharmacologic effect occurs.

The minimum concentration necessary for a drug to produce the desired therapeutic response is referred to as the **minimum therapeutic concentration**. A drug concentration below the minimum therapeutic concentration will not produce an effective response, and drug concentrations that are too high may produce toxic effects or may even be fatal.

Most drugs have a predetermined standard dosage or the dosage is determined by body weight. Dosage guidelines are established to achieve minimum therapeutic concentrations. Any deviation from established dosage guidelines might be harmful. Remember that the goal for drug therapy is to give the minimum concentration of a drug necessary to obtain the desired therapeutic response.

Pharmacodynamic Terminology

Drug actions (pharmacodynamics) are described in a variety of ways. EMS professionals should be familiar with the following descriptive terms.

- *Additive.* An additive effect is the effect that one drug contributes to the action of another. For example, a narcotic analgesic such as morphine may have an additive effect on someone who is taking an antihistamine drug like hydroxyzine, because both drugs cause central nervous system (CNS) depression.
- *Antagonistic.* Antagonism is the mutual opposition in effect between two or more drugs. For example, EMS providers may use naloxone to oppose the effects of a morphine overdose, because naloxone and morphine are antagonists.
- *Cumulative.* Cumulative effect is the result of repeated doses of drugs that accumulate in the body to produce symptoms of poisoning.
- *Depressant.* A depressant is a drug that depresses a body function. For example, the drug codeine is a narcotic analgesic that produces generalized CNS depression.
- *Habituation.* Habituation is the act of becoming accustomed. To habituate to a drug is to develop physical tolerance to and dependence on the drug.
- *Hypersensitiveness.* Hypersensitiveness is the excessive susceptibility to the action of a drug.
- *Idiosyncrasy.* Idiosyncrasy is an accelerated, toxic, or uncharacteristic response to the usual therapeutic dose of a drug.
- *Irritation.* An irritation is temporary tissue inflammation caused by drug action.
- *Physiologic action.* Physiologic action is the effect on a body function produced by a drug.
- *Potentiation.* Potentiation is the enhanced action of two drugs, in which the total effects are greater than the sum of each drug's independent effects.
- *Synergism.* Synergism is the joint action of two drugs producing an effect that neither drug could produce alone.
- *Therapeutics.* Therapeutics is the production of favorable results from application of a remedy, such as a drug, in the management of disease.
- *Tolerance.* Tolerance is the progressive decrease in the effectiveness or response of a drug.
- *Untoward reaction.* An untoward reaction is a harmful side effect of a drug treatment.

CONCLUSION

It is not enough for EMS professionals to know when and how much of a drug to give. Understanding basic pharmacokinetics and pharmacodynamics is essential to knowing the desired therapeutic effects and anticipate possible side effects. For each drug administered, you should be aware of such factors as the drug's rate of absorption, minimum therapeutic concentration, and toxic levels, and the possible and anticipated side effects.

▶ STUDY QUESTIONS

1. Pharmacodynamics is the study of drug:
   a. Movement
   b. Absorption
   c. Concentration
   d. Mechanism of action

2. Pharmacokinetics is the study of drug:
   a. Movement
   b. Absorption
   c. Concentration
   d. Mechanism of action

3. The rate of drug absorption depends on all of the following *except*:
   a. Circulatory status
   b. Amount given
   c. Solubility
   d. pH

4. _____ effect is the result of repeated doses of drugs that accumulate in the body to produce symptoms of poisoning.
   a. Therapeutic
   b. Potentiation
   c. Depressant
   d. Cumulative

5. Once dissolved, a drug begins the _____ phase.
   a. Administration
   b. Pharmaceutical
   c. Pharmacokinetic
   d. Pharmacodynamic

6. When a drug tends to combine with its receptor, it is said to have:
   a. Efficacy
   b. Tolerance
   c. Affinity
   d. Cumulative effects

7. The amount of drug that binds to blood protein or becomes stored in the body's fatty tissues is termed:
   a. A volatile drug
   b. A metabolite
   c. Bound drug
   d. Free drug

8. A component of a cell that combines with a drug to initiate a response is called a:
   a. Molecule
   b. Synapse
   c. Receptor
   d. "Key"

9. The speed at which a drug is absorbed determines how quickly the drug reaches its target tissue to produce its therapeutic effects. The rate of drug absorption depends on what four factors?

   _____

   _____

   _____

   _____

   _____

   _____

   _____

10. The goal of drug therapy is to give the minimum therapeutic concentration of a drug to obtain the effective desired therapeutic response. Explain.

   _____

   _____

   _____

   _____

   _____

   _____

   _____

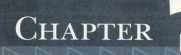
AUTONOMIC PHARMACOLOGY

OBJECTIVES

On completion of this chapter and the study questions, you should be able to:

- Describe an overview of the nervous system.
- Describe the function of neurotransmitters.
- Describe the function of the parasympathetic nervous system.
- Describe the function of the sympathetic nervous system.
- Compare the functions of the adrenergic and cholinergic nervous systems.

KEY TERMS

Acetylcholine
Adrenergic
Alpha$_1$-adrenergic receptor
Alpha$_2$-adrenergic receptor
Autonomic nervous system
Beta$_1$-adrenergic receptor
Beta$_2$-adrenergic receptor
Central nervous system
Cholinergic
Chronotropic

Effector organ
Ganglia
Innervate
Inotropic
Motoneurons
Neurotransmitter
Norepinephrine
Parasympathetic nervous
  system
Parasympatholytic

Parasympathomimetic
Peripheral nervous system
Reflex arc
Somatic nervous system
Sympathetic nervous system
Sympatholytic
Sympathomimetic
Synapse
Vagus nerve

INTRODUCTION

Many of the drugs used by the EMS professional affect tissues that receive their nerve impulses from the autonomic nervous system. Most of these drugs produce effects by imitating or opposing neurotransmitters that are released by fibers that innervate (stimulate) smooth muscle, cardiac muscle, and certain glands. A neurotransmitter is a chemical substance located on a presynaptic neuron. When the neuron is stimulated (excited), the neurotransmitter travels across the synapse to act on the target cell to either excite or inhibit it. The specific tissues stimulated by the autonomic nervous system are called effector organs. The term effector simply means that when a tissue is stimulated, a specific effect should occur.

This chapter presents the general anatomy and physiology of the autonomic nervous system. Included is a discussion of how specific neurotransmitters transmit nerve impulses and how certain drugs can affect the functions of these neurotransmitters. By understanding the basic functions of the autonomic nervous system, health-care professionals can better predict the various effects drugs may produce on the effector organs stimulated by the autonomic nervous system, as these interactions are the basis of much of the treatment in the out-of-hospital setting.

Organization of the Nervous System

The nervous system is divided into two major subdivisions: the central nervous system (CNS) and the peripheral nervous system. The CNS is made up of the brain and spinal cord. The peripheral nervous system is that part of the nervous system outside the CNS. Figure 3–1 illustrates the divisions and subdivisions of the nervous system.

The autonomic nervous system is that portion of the peripheral nervous system that controls the body's automatic or involuntary functions. The autonomic nervous system helps to control arterial blood pressure, cardiac function, gastrointestinal functions, body temperature, bladder emptying, and many other activities. The autonomic nervous system acts on the various tissue effector organs to reduce or slow their activity or to initiate their function.

The autonomic nervous system is capable of causing rapid changes in the body's automatic functions. For example, it can double the heart rate in 3 to 5 seconds or double the arterial blood pressure within 10 to 15 seconds. Conversely, the autonomic nervous system can lower arterial

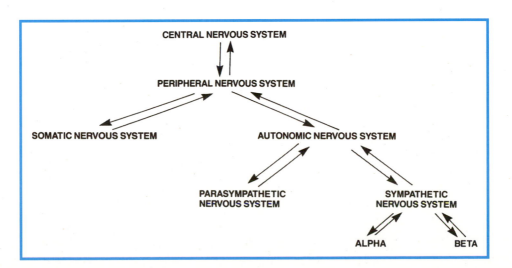

Figure 3–1 Divisions and subdivisions of the nervous system. (© Delmar/Cengage Learning)

blood pressure to the point of fainting within 4 to 5 seconds. In short, the autonomic nervous system maintains rapid and effective control of most internal functions of the body.

The autonomic nervous system contains automatic **motoneurons**. Motoneurons are motor neurons that convey impulses to effector tissues from the central nervous system. In other words, they stimulate effector tissues. Automatic effector tissues include cardiac, smooth muscle, gland, and epithelial tissues.

Neurochemical Transmission

The autonomic nervous system is activated mainly by centers located in the brain and spinal cord. When activated, the autonomic nervous system functions on what is termed the **reflex arc** principle. A reflex arc is the complete circuit of nerves involved in an involuntary movement, from the stimulus to the response: the sensory neuron ending in the spinal cord, the motoneuron from the spinal cord to the effector organ, and connecting neurons within the spinal column. There is not an actual connection between two nerve cells or between a nerve cell and the effector organ it **innervates**. The basic units of the system are its neurons and neuronal synapses (Figure 3–2). A **synapse** is the space between two neurons, or the space between a neuron and an effector organ. An electrical signal travels along the neuron and causes the release of a neurotransmitter (a body-produced chemical) from the *pre*synaptic neuron. The neurotransmitter moves across the synaptic space and combines with receptors on the *post*synaptic neuron. These actions cause an electrical charge in the neuron's membrane ion permeability, which then starts an action impulse

potential in the postsynaptic neuron of the effector organ. The result is a continuation of electrical flow causing contraction of a muscle, the secretion of a gland, the contraction of a pupil, or an alteration of the heart.

The Parasympathetic and Sympathetic Nervous Systems

The autonomic nervous system is composed of two anatomically and physiologically separate divisions: the **parasympathetic** and **sympathetic nervous systems**. The parasympathetic nervous system is connected with the CNS through certain cranial nerves and through the middle three sacral segments of the spinal cord. An alternate name that reminds us of its location is *craniosacral*. The **ganglia** (nervous tissue) of the parasympathetic nervous system are located near the effector organs stimulated. The sympathetic nervous system is connected with the CNS through the thoracic and upper lumbar segments of the spinal cord. An alternate name that reminds us of its location is *thoracolumbar*. Its ganglia are located near the spinal column rather than near the effector organs stimulated (Figure 3–4).

Many effector organs are simultaneously stimulated by both the sympathetic and parasympathetic nervous systems. Physiologically, stimulation by the sympathetic nervous system excites a response, whereas stimulation by the parasympathetic nervous system inhibits a response. The opposition of these two systems works to produce normal automatic body functions. The neural pathways for each system frequently travel together, especially in the thorax, abdomen, and pelvis.

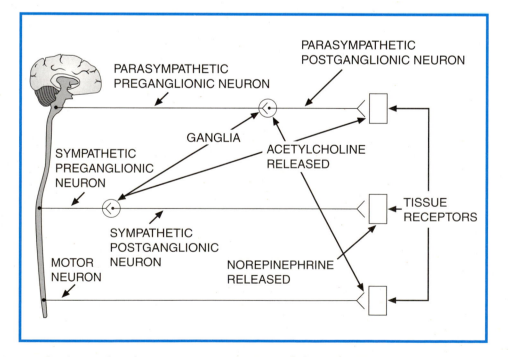

Figure 3–2 Sites of release for the neurotransmitters of the autonomic nervous system.
(© Delmar/Cengage Learning)

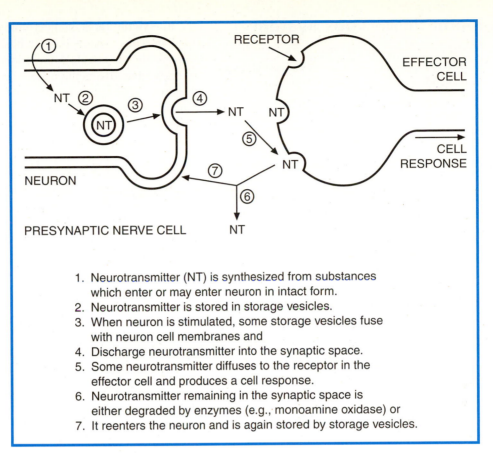

1. Neurotransmitter (NT) is synthesized from substances which enter or may enter neuron in intact form.
2. Neurotransmitter is stored in storage vesicles.
3. When neuron is stimulated, some storage vesicles fuse with neuron cell membranes and
4. Discharge neurotransmitter into the synaptic space.
5. Some neurotransmitter diffuses to the receptor in the effector cell and produces a cell response.
6. Neurotransmitter remaining in the synaptic space is either degraded by enzymes (e.g., monoamine oxidase) or
7. It reenters the neuron and is again stored by storage vesicles.

Figure 3–3 Nerve impulse transmission. (© Delmar/Cengage Learning)

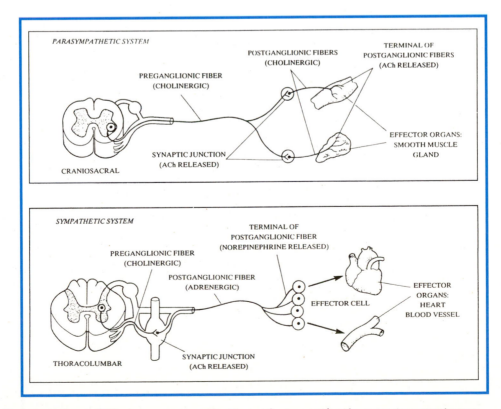

Figure 3–4 Comparision of the parasympathetic and sympathetic nervous systems. (© Delmar/Cengage Learning)

Parasympathetic Nervous System

The major nerves of the parasympathetic nervous system are the two **vagus nerves**. Approximately 75% of all parasympathetic nerve fibers are located in the vagus nerves, which travel the entire thoracic and abdominal region of the body (Figure 3–5).

The parasympathetic nervous system is the main regulator of many automatic effector organs, including: the heart, digestive tract smooth muscle, glands that secrete digestive juices, and endocrine gland cells that secrete insulin. The parasympathetic division of the autonomic nervous system dominates during nonstressful situations with the following effects on the body:

- An increase in secretions of thin saliva
- Heart rate slows to a normal rate (negative **Chronotropic** affect)
- Normal strength of cardiac contractions
- Normal blood pressure
- Increased blood flow to the stomach and intestines
- An increase in glandular secretions of digestive juices
- Pupils constrict to normal
- Bronchioles constrict to a normal diameter

Vagus nerve fibers do not reach the ventricles of the heart. Therefore, vagal stimulation causes decreased heart rate by its effects on atrial muscle, particularly affecting conduction through the atrioventricular (AV) node.

Acetylcholine is the neurotransmitter of the parasympathetic nervous system. Acetylcholine binds to atrial muscle receptor sites to enable vagal nerve stimulation. An example of a drug that affects the parasympathetic nervous system is atropine. Atropine is a parasympathetic blocker. It competes with acetylcholine for receptor sites, blocking its action, thus causing an increase in heart rate. Atropine is used in EMS in cases of symptomatic bradycardia. Drugs such as atropine are referred to as **parasympatholytics** (anticholinergics). A parasympatholytic drug is a drug that has the ability to block parasympathetic nerve fibers. Drugs that stimulate the parasympathetic nervous system are called **parasympathomimetics**. A parasympathomimetic drug is a drug that has the ability to produce effects similar to those resulting from stimulation of the parasympathetic nervous system.

Sympathetic Nervous System

Sympathetic nerves originate in the lateral columns of the thoracic and first three to four lumbar segments of the spinal cord. Stimulation of the sympathetic nervous system prepares the body for emergencies. One of the first steps in the body's reaction to stress is a sudden increase in sympathetic activity, which makes the body ready to use maximum energy and to engage in maximum physical activity. This activity has been historically called the "fight or flight"

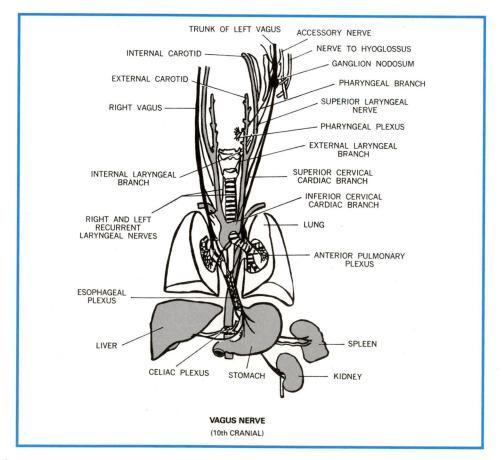

Figure 3–5 The vagus nerve. (© Delmar/Cengage Learning)

response. Table 3–1 compares the fight or flight response of the body to sympathetic nervous system stimulation with the body's response to the parasympathetic nervous system.

The sympathetic division of the autonomic nervous system dominates during stressful situations with the following effects on the body:

- Dry mouth (small amounts of thick saliva are produced)
- Increased heart rate (positive **Chronotropic** affect)
- Increased strength of cardiac contractions (positive **Inotropic** affect)
- Increase in blood pressure
- Dilation of pupils
- Vasoconstriction of the skin, kidneys, and digestive organs
- Vasodilation of the skeletal muscles
- Bronchodilation

The sympathetic nervous system has specific effects on the heart, including:

- Increased firing rate of the sinoatrial (SA) node
- Increased atrial muscle contractility and conduction velocity
- Higher conduction rate of the atrioventricular (AV) node
- Increased contractility and automaticity in the left ventricle
- Increased stroke volume

These effects, caused by stimulation of the sympathetic nervous system, increase cardiac output. The sympathetic nervous system stimulates all blood vessels except the capillaries. Epinephrine and **norepinephrine** are the main neurotransmitters of the sympathetic nervous system.

The Adrenergic and Cholinergic Nervous Systems

The autonomic nervous system can be further described in terms of **adrenergic** (sympathetic) and **cholinergic** (parasympathetic) components. Neurons and effector organs that are activated by epinephrine are called adrenergic. Neurons and effector organs that are activated by acetylcholine are defined as cholinergic. Adrenergic drugs are drugs that imitate the action of epinephrine, and cholinergic drugs are drugs that imitate acetylcholine. Table 3–2 compares the physiologic activities of the adrenergic and cholinergic nervous systems.

Drugs that oppose the action of epinephrine are called *anti*adrenergic drugs, and drugs that oppose the action of acetylcholine are called *anti*cholinergic drugs. For example, isoproterenol is classified as a beta-adrenergic agonist related to epinephrine, which is also a beta-adrenergic agonist. The drug atropine is classified as an anticholinergic agent that competes at receptor sites with acetylcholine.

Adrenergic receptors are classified as either alpha-adrenergic receptors or beta-adrenergic receptors. Sympathetic stimulation of alpha-adrenergic receptors produces constriction of blood vessels, dilation of the pupils, and relaxation of the smooth muscles of the gastrointestinal tract. Stimulation of beta-adrenergic receptors results in an increase in the rate and force of contractions of the heart, relaxation of the smooth muscles of the bronchioles in the lungs and gastrointestinal tract, and vasodilation of blood vessels in the skeletal muscles.

Alpha-adrenergic receptors are identified according to the location of their receptors. **Alpha$_1$-adrenergic-receptor** sites are located on the postsynaptic effector cells, and **alpha$_2$-adrenergic-receptor** sites are located on the presynaptic nerve terminals. Stimulating alpha$_2$-receptors inhibits the release of additional norepinephrine. When alpha$_1$-receptors are stimulated, peripheral and coronary vasoconstriction occurs in part because of the excitatory responses when adrenergic agents such as norepinephrine and epinephrine are released.

Beta-adrenergic receptors are also divided into two categories, beta$_1$ and beta$_2$. Most **beta$_1$-adrenergic receptors** are located in the heart. Stimulation of beta$_1$-adrenergic receptors causes increased heart rate, increased contractility, and an increase in atrioventricular conduction. **Beta$_2$-adrenergic receptors** are located mainly in bronchial and vascular smooth muscle. Stimulation of these receptors causes vasodilation, bronchodilation, and uterine relaxation. Blockage

Table 3–1 Comparison of the Body's Response to Stimulation of the Sympathetic Nervous System vs. the Parasympathetic Nervous System. (© Delmar/Cengage Learning)

Sympathetic (Flight or Fight)	Parasympathetic
The heart beats faster and pumps more efficiently (To aid in flight.)	Heart rate slows to normal
Increase in blood pressure	Normal blood pressure
Vasoconstriction of skin, kidneys, and digestive tract (Urination and digestion are lower priorities during flight.)	Increase in blood flow to the stomach and intestines and an increase in glandular secretions of digestive enzymes
Dry mouth (To assist in keeping the airway clear during flight.)	Salivation
Pupil dilation (For better vision during flight.)	Normal pupil size
Vasodilation of skeletal muscle (To assist in running.)	

Table 3–2 Physiologic Actions of the Adrenergic and Cholinergic Systems. (© Delmar/Cengage Learning)

Effector Organ	Adrenergic Response (Sympathetic)	Cholinergic Response (Parasympathetic)
Heart		
Rate of contractions	Increase	Decrease
Force of contractions	Increase	Decrease
Blood pressure	Increase	Decrease
Blood vessels		
Skin/mucous membrane	Constriction	Dilation
Skeletal muscle	Dilation	Dilation
Coronary	Dilation; constriction	
Renal	Constriction	
Pupils	Dilation	Contraction
Bronchii	Relaxation	Contraction
Adrenal medulla	Secretion of epinephrine and norepinephrine	
Glands		
Sweat	Generalized secretion	Localized secretion
Salivary	Slight secretion	Profuse secretions
Gastrointestinal		Increased secretions
Pancreas (islets)	Inhibit insulin secretion	
Metabolic rate	Increased	

of these receptors opposes the effect of the neurotransmitter. Beta-blocking drugs are either selective for beta$_1$-adrenergic receptors or nonselective. Nonselective blocking drugs block both beta$_1$- and beta$_2$-receptors. Table 3–3 lists the alpha-receptor and beta-receptor sites and their functions.

Drugs that influence the sympathetic nervous system are classified according to the alpha and beta effects they produce. For example, norepinephrine activates all alpha-receptors and some beta-receptors, whereas epinephrine activates all alpha-receptors and all beta-receptors. Isoproterenol is a drug that only activates beta-receptors.

Some drugs block the effects of parasympathetic or sympathetic stimulation. These drugs occupy receptor sites, which prevents parasympathetic or sympathetic neurotransmitters from occupying the sites. For example, atropine blocks the effects of acetylcholine by attaching to the acetylcholine receptor site. Excessive parasympathetic stimulation decreases cardiac output. Atropine increases the heart rate and cardiac output by blocking the parasympathetic effects of acetylcholine on the heart. Drugs that stimulate the sympathetic nervous system are called **sympathomimetics**. Drugs that inhibit the sympathetic nervous system are called **sympatholytics**.

Table 3–3 Alpha-Adrenergic and Beta-Adrenergic Receptor Sites and Functions. (© Delmar/Cengage Learning)

Effector Organ	Alpha	Beta
Heart		
SA Node		Increased rate (beta$_1$)
AV Node		Increased automaticity and conduction velocity (beta$_1$)
Ventricles		Increased force of contraction and conduction velocity (beta$_1$)
Arterioles	Vasoconstriction (alpha$_1$)	Vasodilation (beta$_2$)
Veins	Vasoconstriction (alpha$_1$)	Vasodilation (beta$_2$)
Lungs		Bronchodilation (beta$_2$)
Pupils	Contraction	
Pancreas (Islets)	Decreased secretion	

CONCLUSION

The autonomic nervous system regulates automatic effectors that maintain or quickly restore the state of equilibrium of the body's automatic functions. Doubly stimulated organs receive both sympathetic and parasympathetic impulses, which influence their function in opposing ways. For example, sympathetic impulses make the heart beat faster and parasympathetic impulses slow the heart down. The relationship between the effects of the two opposing systems determines actual heart rate.

The parasympathetic or cholinergic division of the autonomic nervous system regulates the body's involuntary functions. This is mediated through the vagus nerves by the release of acetylcholine. Vagal stimulation slows the heart rate, but this action can be opposed by parasympathetic blocking drugs (anticholinergics).

The sympathetic or adrenergic division enables the body to respond to emergency, or stress. This system is regulated mainly by the release of norepinephrine and epinephrine. The sympathetic division is further subdivided into alpha-adrenergic and beta-adrenergic receptors. Stimulation of alpha-adrenergic receptors causes vasoconstriction of blood vessels, a decrease in gastrointestinal secretion, and dilation of the pupils. Stimulation of beta-adrenergic receptors causes an increase in the rate and force of contraction of the heart, dilation of the arterioles of skeletal muscles, and dilation of the bronchiolar muscles of the lungs.

STUDY QUESTIONS

1. Stimulation of alpha$_1$-receptor sites causes:
   a. Bronchodilation
   b. An increase in heart rate
   c. Peripheral and coronary vasoconstriction
   d. Inhibition of the release of norepinephrine

2. A neurotransmitter is:
   a. An electrical impulse
   b. A body-produced chemical
   c. A postsynaptic neuron
   d. A presynaptic neuron

3. Neurons and effector organs that are activated by epinephrine are called:
   a. Adrenergic
   b. Cholinergic
   c. Antiadrenergic
   d. Anticholinergic

4. The _____ conveys impulses to effector tissues from the CNS.
   a. Synapse
   b. Reflex arc
   c. Motoneurons
   d. Neurotransmitters

5. The space between two neurons, or the space between a neuron and an effector organ, is called the:
   a. Synapse
   b. Reflex arc
   c. Presynaptic space
   d. Postsynaptic space

6. The major nerves of the parasympathetic nervous system are the two:
   a. Preganglionic fibers
   b. Lumbar nerves
   c. Sacral nerves
   d. Vagus nerves

7. The neurotransmitter of the parasympathetic nervous system is:
   a. Atropine
   b. Epinephrine
   c. Acetylcholine
   d. Norepinephrine

8. The main neurotransmitters of the sympathetic nervous system are:
   a. Epinephrine and atropine
   b. Epinephrine and norepinephrine
   c. Norepinephrine and acetylcholine
   d. Epinephrine and acetylcholine

9. Alpha$_1$-receptor sites are located in the:
   a. Heart
   b. Postsynaptic effector cells
   c. Presynaptic nerve terminals
   d. Bronchial and vascular smooth muscle

10. Beta$_2$-receptor sites are located in the:
    a. Heart
    b. Postsynaptic effector cells
    c. Presynaptic nerve terminals
    d. Bronchial and vascular smooth muscle

11. When alpha$_2$-receptors are stimulated:
    a. Release of additional norepinephrine is inhibited
    b. Peripheral and coronary vasoconstriction occurs
    c. Increased atrioventricular conduction occurs
    d. Bronchodilation occurs

12. When beta$_1$-receptors are stimulated, _____ occurs:
    a. Bronchodilation
    b. Increased heart rate
    c. Coronary vasoconstriction
    d. Release of norepinephrine

CHAPTER 4

FLUIDS, ELECTROLYTES, AND INTRAVENOUS THERAPY

OBJECTIVES

On completion of this chapter and the study questions, you should be able to:
- Identify and explain the body water proportions of the major fluid compartments of the body.
- List and describe the roles of the major electrolytes of the body.
- Define and explain the roles of:
  a. Filtration
  b. Diffusion
  c. Osmosis
  d. Passive transport
  e. Active transport
- Define and explain the roles of the following solutions:
  a. Hypotonic
  b. Hypertonic
  c. Isotonic
- List and describe the four clinical situations that result when acid-base balance is disrupted.
- List the various intravenous fluids and describe the major indications for each.

KEY TERMS

Acidosis
Active transport
Alkalosis
Anion
Cation
Colloid
Crystalloid
Diffusion
Electrolyte

Facilitated diffusion
Filtration
Fluid, body
Fluid, extracellular
Fluid, interstitial
Fluid, intracellular
Fluid, intravascular
Homeostasis
Hydrostatic pressure

Hypertonic
Hypotonic
Ion
Isotonic
Nonelectrolytes
Osmosis
pH
Plasma
Semipermeable
   membrane

INTRODUCTION

Maintaining a proper balance of fluids and electrolytes within the body is necessary for life; therefore, it is important to be familiar with the basics of body fluids and electrolytes. If, for instance, you are faced with a patient who is depleted of fluids and electrolytes (such as a person with severe burns or a patient who is severely dehydrated), you must act rapidly to help restore the body's internal balance to increase the patient's chances for survival.

This chapter reviews the basics of fluids, electrolytes, and acid-base balance. The chapter also describes some commonly used intravenous fluids and their roles in the treatment of fluid and electrolyte compromise.

Body Fluids

Total **body fluid** varies from individual to individual depending on both sex and age (Table 4–1). However, the average adult has a total body fluid content of approximately 60% of body weight. This total body fluid is divided into **intracellular** and **extracellular fluid** compartments (Figure 4–1). Intracellular fluid (ICF) is the fluid contained inside the body's cells. It accounts for approximately 45% of total body weight. Extracellular fluid (ECF) is body fluid outside the cells. It accounts for approximately 15% of body weight. Extracellular fluid is further divided into two separate fluid types: **interstitial fluid** and

intravascular fluid or **plasma**. Interstitial fluid is extracellular fluid located in the spaces between the body's cells. It accounts for approximately 10.5% of body weight. Intravascular fluid is the noncellular, fluid portion of blood. It accounts for approximately 4.5% of body weight.

To illustrate, a person who weighs 176 pounds (80 kilograms) has approximately 48 liters (1 liter weighs approximately 1 kg) of body fluid (80 × 0.60 = 48). This amount is broken down as follows:

- *Intracellular fluid:* 36 liters (80 × 0.45 = 36)
- *Extracellular fluid:* 12 liters (80 × 0.15 = 12)

Table 4–1 Approximate Body Water Content as Percentage of Body Weight. (© Delmar/Cengage Learning)

Body Water			
Age	Total	ECF	ICF
Children			
Newborn	79%	45%	34%
2–30 d	74%	40%	34%
1–12 m	63%	30%	33%
1–2 yr	59%	24%	35%
2–8 yr	62%	25%	37%
Men			
9–16 yr	59%	26%	33%
17–35 yr	60%	28%	32%
36–69 yr	55%	25%	30%
70+ yr	51%	25%	26%
Women			
9–15 yr	56%	25%	31%
16–35 yr	50%	25%	25%
36–59 yr	48%	23%	25%

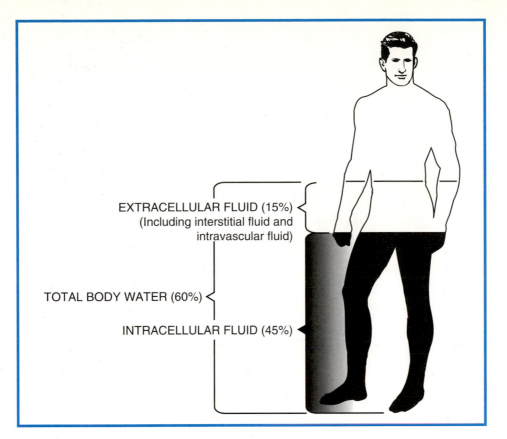

Figure 4–1 Distribution of body fluids. (© Delmar/Cengage Learning)

- *Interstitial fluid:* 8.4 liters ($80 \times 0.105 = 8.4$)
- *Intravascular fluid:* 3.6 liters ($80 \times 0.045 = 3.6$)

It is the extracellular fluid that aids in controlling the body's internal environment by bathing the cells. The internal environment of the body must be kept within a dynamic state of equilibrium. This state of equilibrium is called **homeostasis**. The body's regulation mechanisms to maintain homeostasis control body temperature, osmotic pressure of the blood and its hydrogen ion concentration (pH), nutrients supplied to the cells, and remove waste products before they accumulate and reach toxic levels.

Electrolytes

An **electrolyte** is a substance, that when placed in water, separates into electrically charged particles called **ions**. A **cation** is a positively charged ion, and an **anion** is a negatively charged ion (Figure 4–2). The major cations of the body include:

- *Calcium (Ca^{2+}):* Calcium is the most abundant cation in the body. It is required for bone growth, metabolism, blood clotting, normal cardiac function, and the initiation of neuromuscular contractions.
- *Magnesium (Mg^{2+}):* Magnesium is required for body temperature regulation, protein and carbohydrate metabolism, and neuromuscular contraction.
- *Potassium (K^+):* Potassium is the major intracellular cation. It is responsible for acid-base regulation, muscle excitability, and nerve impulse conduction.

- *Sodium (Na^+):* Sodium is the major extracellular cation. It is responsible for fluid balance. When the body eliminates sodium, water is lost also. Conversely, when sodium levels in the body rise, water is retained. Sodium also preserves the balance between calcium and potassium.

The major anions of the body include:

- *Bicarbonate (HCO_3^-):* Bicarbonate is the major buffer of the body. Its main function is to maintain acid-base balance.
- *Chloride (Cl^-):* Chloride is the major extracellular anion. Its main function is to maintain fluid balance.
- *Phosphate (HPO_4^{2-}):* Phosphate is the major intracellular anion. It helps maintain acid-base balance.

Electrolytes are measured in milliequivalents (mEq). A milliequivalent is the concentration of electrolytes in a certain volume of solution, based on the number of available ionic charges. One milliequivalent of a cation will completely react with 1 milliequivalent of an anion forming a new compound.

For example,

Na^+ (1 mEq of sodium) and

Cl^- (1 mEq of chloride) combine to form NaCl

or

Ca^{2+} (2 mEq of calcium) and

Cl^- (1 mEq of chloride) + Cl^- (1 mEq of chloride) combine to form $CaCl_2$

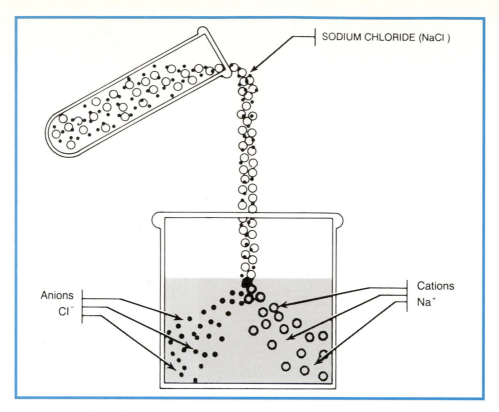

Figure 4–2 Dissociation of electrolytes. When sodium chloride (NaCl) is dissolved in water, the ions dissociate, resulting in atoms of chloride with a negative charge (anions) and atoms of sodium with a positive charge (cations). (© Delmar/Cengage Learning)

Note that Ca^{2+} has two positive charges, or 2 milliequivalents. Therefore, it must have 2 milliequivalents of a singly charged anion (Cl^- + Cl^-) to combine to form calcium chloride. In practice, electrolytes are given as milliequivalents per liter (mEq/L), as in intravenous solution.

Body fluid also contains compounds with no electrical charges. These substances are called **nonelectrolytes**. Nonelectrolytes are normally measured in milligrams (mg). Nonelectrolytes include:

- *Glucose:* Glucose is a carbohydrate or sugar formed during digestion. It is the most important carbohydrate in metabolism.
- *Urea:* Urea is the major nitrogen end product of protein metabolism. It is formed in the liver.

Fluid Transport

Pharmacologists think of intracellular and extracellular fluid as occupying two separate compartments—the intracellular compartment and the extracellular compartment. For normal metabolism to occur, water, electrolytes, and other substances must pass between these two compartments. To do this, they must cross a **semipermeable membrane** that allows only some molecules to pass through. There are two ways in which this movement occurs: (1) passive transport and (2) active transport.

Passive Transport

Passive transport depends on three mechanisms: (1) filtration, (2) diffusion, and (3) osmosis.

Filtration

Filtration is the movement of fluid through a membrane caused by differences in **hydrostatic pressure**. Hydrostatic pressure is the force exerted by the weight of a solution; it causes the solution to move from an area of higher pressure to an area of lower pressure. In two compartments separated by a permeable or semipermeable membrane, hydrostatic pressure causes fluid to move from one compartment to the other until the pressure in both compartments is equal.

Diffusion

Diffusion is the tendency of molecules in solution to distribute themselves equally. You can see diffusion at work by adding a drop of ink to a container of water (Figure 4–3). Soon, without stirring, the ink (solute) spreads itself evenly throughout the water. In diffusion, molecules, atoms, or ions flow from an area of higher concentration to areas of lower concentration, until the concentration (the number of molecules of solute per amount of solution) is the same everywhere in the solution. Diffusion is generally considered a passive process. However, there are instances where active transport (energy) may be required for the diffusion process to take place. This is referred to as **facilitated diffusion**.

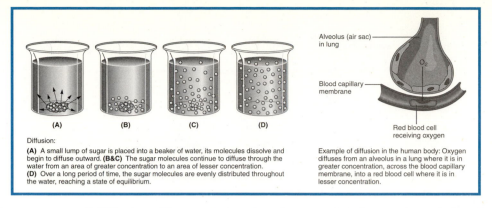

Diffusion:

(A) A small lump of sugar is placed into a beaker of water, its molecules dissolve and begin to diffuse outward. **(B&C)** The sugar molecules continue to diffuse through the water from an area of greater concentration to an area of lesser concentration.
(D) Over a long period of time, the sugar molecules are evenly distributed throughout the water, reaching a state of equilibrium.

Example of diffusion in the human body: Oxygen diffuses from an alveolus in a lung where it is in greater concentration, across the blood capillary membrane, into a red blood cell where it is in lesser concentration.

Figure 4–3 The process of diffusion. The sugar molecules eventually reach a state of equilibrium.
(© Delmar/Cengage Learning)

Osmosis

Osmosis is the diffusion of solute and/or solvent through a permeable or semipermeable membrane. It is a result of the same force that causes solute molecules or ions within a solution to flow from areas of high concentration to areas of low concentration. With two solutions separated by a semipermeable membrane, a difference in solute concentration creates osmotic pressure, which causes water and (if possible) solute to move across the membrane until the solutions are in equilibrium (Figure 4–4).

Whether both solute and water cross the membrane, or just water, depends on the nature of the solution. There are two kinds of solutions, with opposite reactions to osmotic pressure: **crystalloid** and **colloid** solutions.

A crystalloid is a substance that truly dissolves—that is, its molecules or atoms separate and disperse completely and equally throughout the solvent. Such a solution is called a *true solution* or a *crystalloid solution*. In a crystalloid solution, the small, individual molecules or atoms of solute easily pass through (diffuse across) a semipermeable membrane. When two crystalloid solutions of unequal concentration are separated by a semipermeable membrane, the osmotic pressure will cause the dissolved molecules or ions to cross the membrane, from the concentrated solution to the solution with lower concentration, until the solute concentration is equal on both sides of the membrane.

Colloids are the physical opposites of crystalloids. When mixed with water, colloids do not truly dissolve. Instead,

they form a suspension (sometimes called a *colloid solution*), in which groups of colloid molecules are dispersed throughout the liquid. Unlike crystalloids, colloids do not pass through semipermeable membranes. Therefore, when two colloid solutions of unequal concentration are separated by a semipermeable membrane, osmotic pressure causes the flow of *water* across the membrane, from lower concentration to higher, until the concentration of solute is equal on both sides of the membrane.

In pharmacology, the difference in behavior of the two kinds of solutions allows for different applications. When a crystalloid solution (such as lactated Ringer's, normal saline, or dextrose 5% in water) is injected into the bloodstream, both solute and water can travel across the cell membrane. Crystalloid solutions, therefore, are effective ways of getting water *and* the dissolved substance into the cells. On the other hand, when a colloid solution (such as Dextran or Plasmanate) is injected into the bloodstream, the colloid cannot enter the cells, so osmotic pressure causes water to flow from the cellular compartment into the bloodstream. The flow of water from cell to bloodstream helps maintain vascular volume.

Two solutions may contain different substances but have the same milliequivalence, or ionic potential. Separated by a semipermeable membrane, each has the same osmotic pressure. Such solutions are said to be **isotonic**. For instance, normal saline solution, a common intravenous (IV) solution, is isotonic. Because osmotic pressure on both sides of cell membranes are equal, normal saline solution tends to stay

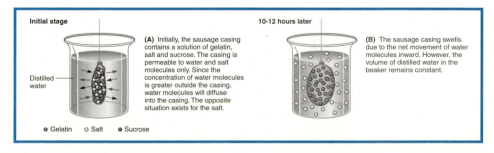

Initial stage

(A) Initially, the sausage casing contains a solution of gelatin, salt and sucrose. The casing is permeable to water and salt molecules only. Since the concentration of water molecules is greater outside the casing, water molecules will diffuse into the casing. The opposite situation exists for the salt.

Distilled water

● Gelatin   ○ Salt   ● Sucrose

10-12 hours later

(B) The sausage casing swells due to the net movement of water molecules inward. However, the volume of distilled water in the beaker remains constant.

Figure 4–4 Osmosis: the diffusion of water through a semipermeable membrane. (A sausage casing is an example of a semipermeable membrane). (© Delmar/Cengage Learning)

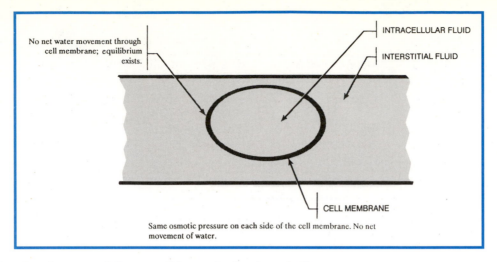

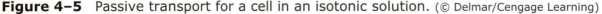

Figure 4–5   Passive transport for a cell in an isotonic solution. (© Delmar/Cengage Learning)

in the extracellular space (primarily the bloodstream) longer than **hypotonic** or **hypertonic** solutions, thus maintaining and increasing vascular volume. Figure 4–5 illustrates the situation when intracellular and extracellular solutions are isotonic.

A hypotonic solution has a lower ionic potential than the solution to which it is compared. A solution of one-half normal saline, for instance, is hypotonic to normal body fluid. For a normal body cell surrounded by hypotonic fluid, the osmotic pressure on the inside of the cell is greater than on the outside. Water will tend to flow from outside the cell to inside the cell to lower the solute concentration (and therefore the ionic potential). Figure 4–6 illustrates the situation when extracellular solution is hypotonic to intracellular solution.

A hypertonic solution has a higher solute concentration and ionic potential than the solution to which it is compared. For instance, a solution of dextrose 50% in water is hypertonic to normal body fluid. For a cell in a hypertonic solution, the osmotic pressure inside the cell is lower than outside. The higher osmotic pressure outside the cell pulls water out of

the cell to lower the solute concentration in the extracellular fluid. Figure 4–7 illustrates this situation.

Active Transport

As we have seen, passive transport allows some solutes to travel across cell membranes, but only from the concentrated solution to the less concentrated solution. Cell metabolism, however, requires substances to travel "upstream," that is, from the less concentrated solution to the more concentrated one (Figure 4–8). Cell health also requires that the concentration of some substances be higher inside the cell than outside, and vice versa. For instance, under normal conditions, the cellular fluid has more potassium ions than does the extracellular fluid. The process of moving substances across the cell wall from the less concentrated to the more concentrated solution, and keeping the concentration of solutes higher on one side of the cell wall than on the other, is called **active transport**. Active transport requires metabolic energy. Substances that require active transport across cell membranes include potassium, sodium, calcium, hydrogen, chloride, and several sugars and amino acids.

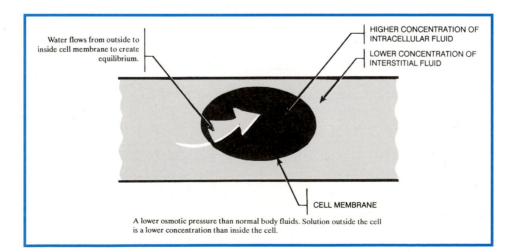

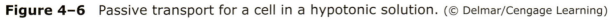

Figure 4–6   Passive transport for a cell in a hypotonic solution. (© Delmar/Cengage Learning)

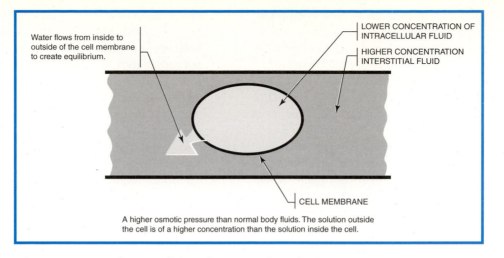

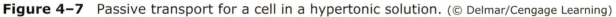

Figure 4–7   Passive transport for a cell in a hypertonic solution. (© Delmar/Cengage Learning)

Acid-Base Balance

We have discussed how body chemistry and metabolism work to maintain equilibrium between fluid compartments. A state of equilibrium must also be maintained between the acidity and alkalinity of body fluid. Acid-base balance is the body's way of maintaining this equilibrium.

Body fluid *potential of hydrogen* **(pH)** is the most frequently used measurement of acid-base balance. The pH measurement is inversely related to the body's hydrogen ion concentration. The higher the hydrogen ion concentration in a fluid, the lower the pH. Conversely, the lower the hydrogen ion concentration, the higher the pH. The pH scale ranges from 1 to 14. A pH reading of 1 means that a substance consists of only hydrogen ions. A pH of 14 means that there are no hydrogen ions present. A pH of 7 is neutral.

Arterial blood gases are measured to determine acid-base imbalance using three values; (1) pH, (2) $PaCO_2$, and (3) HCO_3. The normal pH of the body ranges from 7.35 to 7.45. When body fluid's pH is greater than 7.45, the body is in a state of **alkalosis**. Body fluid pH of less than 7.35 indicates a state of **acidosis**. Increases or decreases in body pH can be

potentially harmful. For example, a significant decrease in the body's pH can cause diminished heart contractions, reduce the body's response to catecholamine release, and inhibit the therapeutic action of drugs. An increase in the body's pH can inhibit the release of oxygen from the red blood cells. A body fluid pH above 7.8 or below 7.0 indicates a serious, usually fatal condition. Slight changes in H^+ ion concentration can markedly affect rates of chemical reactions in cells. Therefore, regulating the H^+ ion concentration is one of the most important facets of homeostasis and is critical to maintaining life.

The buffer system is the body's primary mechanism for adjusting and maintaining acid-base balance. The buffer system can act within a fraction of a second to prevent excessive changes in hydrogen ion concentration. This system's effect on acid-base balance is almost instantaneous. Two components of the buffer system include bicarbonate ion (HCO_3^-) and carbonic acid (H_2CO_3), which maintain an equilibrium with the hydrogen ion (H^+):

$$\begin{array}{ccccc} & & 20 & : & 1 \\ H^+ & + & HCO_3^- & \longleftrightarrow & H_2CO_3 \\ \text{Hydrogen ion} & & \text{Bicarbonate ion} & & \text{Carbonic acid} \end{array}$$

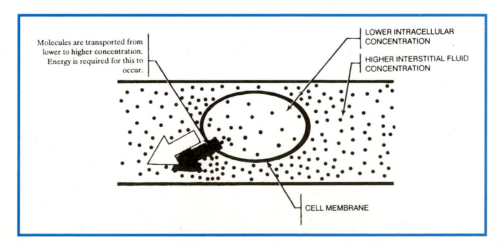

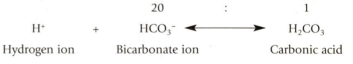

Figure 4–8   Active transport. (© Delmar/Cengage Learning)

This reaction requires 20 molecules of bicarbonate ion for every molecule of carbonic acid. For the buffer system to maintain body fluid pH, any change in this 20:1 ratio must be immediately corrected.

The respiratory system is the second mechanism for acid-base regulation. If the $PaCO_2$ is greater than 45 mm Hg, respiratory acidosis occurs; if $PaCO_2$ is less than 35 mm Hg, respiratory alkalosis is present. It takes approximately 1 to 3 minutes for the respiratory system to be effective. The respiratory system works to regulate acid-base balance by altering the carbon dioxide (CO_2) level in the bloodstream. When the respiration rate increases, the lungs excrete more carbon dioxide, which causes a decrease in hydrogen ions and an increase in the pH. Conversely, when respirations are decreased, more carbon dioxide remains in the blood, causing hydrogen ions to increase and pH to decrease.

The renal system is the third and slowest mechanism for acid-base regulation. If the HCO_3^- is less than 24 mEq/L, metabolic acidosis occurs; if it is greater than 28 mEq/L, metabolic alkalosis is present. It takes from several hours to days for this system to correct acid-base imbalance. The kidneys regulate acid-base balance by eliminating excess hydrogen or bicarbonate ions from the bloodstream. For example, if the hydrogen ion concentration of the body increases, the body's pH falls and the kidneys eliminate more hydrogen ions to restore equilibrium. On the other hand, if the hydrogen ion concentration falls, body pH increases and the kidneys eliminate bicarbonate ions to restore equilibrium.

There are four clinical situations that result when acid-base balance is disrupted: respiratory acidosis, respiratory alkalosis, metabolic acidosis, and metabolic alkalosis.

- *Respiratory acidosis (pH < 7.35 and $PaCO_2$ > 45 mm Hg):* This condition results from inadequate ventilations, resulting in the retention of carbon dioxide and an increased level of carbonic acid in the blood. The pH of a person in respiratory acidosis falls as the carbon dioxide level increases. To reverse respiratory acidosis, improve ventilation, using 100% oxygen. This removes carbon dioxide from the circulation via the lungs.
- *Respiratory alkalosis (pH > 7.45 and $PaCO_2$ < 35 mm Hg):* This condition occurs when excessive amounts of carbon dioxide have been eliminated from the patient. In emergency situations, respiratory alkalosis often occurs when a patient hyperventilates, blowing off more carbon dioxide than normal. When more carbon dioxide than normal is blown off, body pH increases. Treatment of respiratory alkalosis should include having the patient take deep breaths and breathe slowly. EMS personnel can demonstrate a slow, relaxed breathing pattern for the patient. Medications may have to be given to relax the patient and restore a normal breathing pattern.
- *Metabolic acidosis (pH > 7.35 and HCO_3^- < 24 mEq/L):* This condition occurs when the body produces an excessive amount of metabolic acids. This increase

in acid consumes some of the bicarbonate buffer, causing a further acid buildup and a decrease in base. Metabolic acidosis causes a decrease in pH and bicarbonate, but carbon dioxide levels remain within normal limits. In emergency situations, treat metabolic acidosis by attempting to improve ventilation by using 100% oxygen. This removes carbon dioxide and, subsequently, hydrogen ions. When the diagnosis of metabolic acidosis is documented, treatment may also include giving the patient sodium bicarbonate.
- *Metabolic alkalosis (pH > 7.45 and HCO_3^- > 28 mEq/L):* During metabolic alkalosis, excitability of the CNS occurs. Symptoms may include irritability, mental confusion, and hyperactive reflexes. Hypoventilation may occur as a compensatory mechanism for metabolic alkalosis to conserve the hydrogen ions and carbonic acid. During metabolic alkalosis, the buffer, renal, and respiratory systems try to reestablish balance. In the buffer system, the excess bicarbonate reacts with buffer acid salts to decrease the number of bicarbonate ions and increase the concentration of carbonic acid. The renal system conserves the hydrogen ions and excretes the sodium, potassium, and bicarbonate ions. The respiratory system maintains balance through hypoventilation. This retains carbon dioxide and increases the concentration of carbonic acid. To treat metabolic alkalosis, EMS personnel need to determine and treat the underlying cause.

Intravenous Therapy

There are two basic reasons for starting an intravenous (IV) line in the out-of-hospital setting: (1) as a route for fluid replacement such as for hemorrhage, severe diarrhea, vomiting, heat exposure, or burns, and (2) as a route for drug administration. Five basic classifications of IV infusions include: crystalloids, colloids, hydrating solutions, hypertonic solutions, and blood or blood components (see Chapter 5).

Crystalloids

Crystalloids are solutes that, when placed in a solvent, mix with and dissolve into a solution, and cannot be distinguished from the resultant solution. Crystalloids are considered to be true solutions. They are able to diffuse through cell membranes. Crystalloids may be isotonic, hypotonic, or hypertonic solutions.

Colloids

Colloids are substances whose particles do not form a true solution because their molecules, when dispersed in a solvent, do not dissolve. Instead, the molecules remain uniformly suspended and distributed throughout the fluid. The particles of colloid solutions are too large to pass through cell membranes, thus, they stay in the bloodstream. Colloid infusions raise colloid osmotic pressure, thus, they are often called plasma or volume expanders. Common colloid infusions are: albumin, dextran, plasmanate, and the artificial blood substitute, hetastarch.

Hydrating Solutions

Various IV solutions are given by EMS personnel to patients to supplement caloric intake, supply nutrients, provide water for maintenance or rehydration, or promote effective renal output. Their rate of administration is adjusted so the equilibrium of body fluids are not disturbed. In most cases, glucose solutions are used. When glucose and other nutrients are given in water, they are rapidly metabolized, leaving an excess of water. This is why glucose solutions are often called hydrating solutions. Any water that is not needed by the body is excreted by the kidneys.

Isotonic Solutions

Isotonic solutions have the same tonicity as body fluids. Once infused, isotonic solutions remain within the intravascular space because osmotic pressure is equal between the intracellular and extracellular compartments. For this reason, isotonic solutions are used to treat hypotension resulting from hypovolemia. Table 4–2 lists the indications for use and precautions for isotonic solutions. An example of an isotonic crystalloid solution is lactated Ringer's solution.

Hypotonic Solutions

Hypotonic solutions cause fluid to shift out of the blood and into the cells and interstitial spaces. The rate of administration must be carefully controlled to prevent water from rupturing the red blood cells. As hypotonic solutions hydrate the intracellular compartment, care must be taken to prevent circulatory depletion as fluid moves from the bloodstream into the intracellular compartment. These solutions should not be given to hypotensive patients, as this can further lower blood pressure. Table 4–2 lists the indications for use and precautions for hypotonic solutions. An example of a hypotonic dextrose-containing solution is 5% dextrose in water (D_5W).

Hypertonic Solutions

Hypertonic solutions pull fluids from the intracellular and interstitial compartments into the blood vessels. They act to expand the intravascular compartment and are given when there is a serious saline depletion. Caution must be taken when giving hypertonic solutions, as they can cause circulatory overload. They also can cause irritation to the intima of the veins. Table 4–2 lists the indications for use and precautions for hypertonic solutions. An example of a hypertonic dextrose-containing solution is 10% dextrose in water ($D_{10}W$).

Table 4–2 Indications and Contraindications for Commonly Used Intravenous Solutions.
(© Delmar/Cengage Learning)

Solution	Indications	Contraindications
Colloids		
Plasma Protein Fraction	Hypovolemic shock	None
Dextran	Hypovolemic shock	Known hypersensitivity Patient is receiving anticoagulants
Hetastarch	Hypovolemic shock	None
Crystalloids		
Lactated Ringer's (LR)	Hypovolemic shock	CHF Renal Failure
Dextrose 5% in water (D_5W)	Intravenous drug route Dilution of concentrated drugs for intravenous infusion	Volume replacement
Dextrose 10% in water ($D_{10}W$)	Hypoglycemia	Volume replacement
Normal saline (NS; 0.9% sodium chloride)	Hypovolemia Heat-related emergencies Freshwater drowning Diabetic ketoacidosis (DKA)	CHF
1/2 Normal saline (1/2NS; 0.45% sodium chloride)	Compromised cardiac function	Emergency rehydration
Dextrose 5% in 1/2 normal saline ($D_5$1/2NS)	Heat emergencies Diabetic emergencies	Emergency rehydration
Dextrose 5% in normal saline (D_5NS)	Heat emergencies Volume replacement Freshwater drowning	Compromised cardiac function/renal function
Dextrose 5% in lactated Ringer's (D_5LR)	Volume replacement	Compromised cardiac function/renal function

CONCLUSION

EMS personnel must be able to recognize and rapidly treat fluid, electrolyte, and acid-base abnormalities. The major key to treatment is rapid fluid-aggressive therapy. To replenish fluids and electrolytes, the proper intravenous fluids must be chosen and given at the appropriate rate. To maintain appropriate acid-base limits or correct acid-base abnormalities, you must maintain a patent airway and improve ventilation (using 100% oxygen as needed). The most important drug in correcting acid-base abnormalities is oxygen. Appropriate airway support, coupled with correct cardiopulmonary resuscitation, if needed, can maintain pH levels within or very close to normal limits within the lungs, heart, and brain.

STUDY QUESTIONS

1. Fluid located in the spaces between the body's cells, accounting for approximately 10.5% of body weight, is called _____ fluid.
   a. Interstitial
   b. Intravascular
   c. Extracellular
   d. Intracellular

2. Two major cations of the body are:
   a. Calcium and chloride
   b. Sodium and bicarbonate
   c. Potassium and phosphate
   d. Magnesium and potassium

3. A solution equal in milliequivalents to normal body fluid is called a[n] _____ solution.
   a. Hypotonic
   b. Isotonic
   c. Hypertonic
   d. Colloid

4. The body's primary mechanism for adjusting and maintaining acid-base balance is the _____ system.
   a. Buffer
   b. Renal
   c. Respiratory
   d. Circulatory

5. Body fluid pH is the most frequently used measurement of acid-base balance.
   a. True
   b. False (if false, explain why)
   _____
   _____

6. There are four clinical situations that result when acid-base balance is disrupted. Briefly explain the mechanism of each situation, and the out-of-hospital treatment.
   _____
   _____
   _____
   _____
   _____
   _____
   _____

7. The process of moving substances across the cell wall from the less concentrated to the more concentrated solution, and keeping the concentration of solutes higher on one side of the cell wall than the other, is called:
   a. Filtration
   b. Passive transport
   c. Diffusion
   d. Active transport

8. The normal pH of the body ranges from 7.35–7.45. When the body fluid's pH is greater than 7.45, the body is in a state of :
   a. Alkalosis
   b. Equilibrium
   c. Acidosis
   d. Metabolisis

9. When the body's pH is less than 7.35, the body is in a state of:
   a. Alkalosis
   b. Equilibrium
   c. Acidosis
   d. Metabolisis

10. Two components of the buffer system include bicarbonate ion (HCO_3^-) and carbonic acid (H_2CO_3), which maintain an equilibrium with the hydrogen ion (H^+). This reaction requires _____ molecule(s) of bicarbonate ion for every _____ molecule(s) of carbonic acid.
   a. 1:10
   b. 10:1
   c. 1:20
   d. 20:1

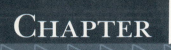

CHAPTER 5

BLOOD AND BLOOD PRODUCT ADMINISTRATION

OBJECTIVES

On completion of this chapter and the study questions, you should be able to:

- Describe the basic concepts of immunology to include antigens, antibodies, and immune response.
- Describe the basic concepts of blood grouping.
- Describe the basic concepts of blood typing and crossmatching.
- Describe the signs and symptoms of transfusion reactions.
- Describe the volume expanders and their indications for use.
- Describe the antihyperlipidemic drugs and their indications for use.

KEY TERMS

Agglutination	Blood typing	Immune response
Agglutinins	Colloid	Immunity
Agglutinogens	Crossmatching	Isoantigen
Antibody	Epitope	Universal donor
Antigen	Genotype	Universal recipient

INTRODUCTION

It is becoming more and more common for EMS professionals to give and/or transport patients who are being administered blood or blood products. Therefore, it is important to have a solid understanding on the blood forms that can be administered, the therapeutic results expected, and the side effects administering these products can create. For example, red blood cells carry oxygen; white blood cells aid in the immune response to infection; platelets are important in blood clotting, and plasma transports nutrients, waste products, hormones, carbon dioxide, and other substances, and helps regulate electrolyte balance and thermal regulation. Adverse reactions and side effects of the cardiovascular system that can occur while administering blood products include chest pain, hypotension, and arrhythmias.

Basic Immunology

The human immune system protects the body from harm by invading organisms. It accomplishes this through all the body cells, tissues, organs, and physiologic processes. **Immunity** is the condition in which a person is protected from disease. The **immune response** is the ability of the immune system to recognize and respond to foreign invaders. Once an invader has been recognized, the immune system neutralizes or eliminates it, so the invader cannot cause damage to the body. An **antigen** is an agent that combines with an antibody to elicit an immune response. An **antibody** is an immunoglobulin (Ig) molecule. The antibody develops in response to an antigen that enters the body and combines with it. When an immune response occurs, the antibody combines with just a portion of the antigen called an **epitope**.

Basic Immunohematology

Within each of us, there is a special combination of genes called a **genotype**. The genotype determines our characteristics for certain traits. Our genetic differences occur because of the variations in cell surface composition. These variations in cell surface composition form the basis for blood compatibility.

Red Blood Cells

Red blood cells, erythrocytes, have an important protein called hemoglobin. Hemoglobin is responsible for the transportation of oxygen and carbon dioxide. Approximately 45% of our blood is composed of red blood cells.

An **isoantigen** is a substance that can stimulate the production of antibodies when introduced into the body. Blood groups are based on the isoantigens that are present on the surface of red blood cells (RBCs). There have been hundreds of isoantigen groups identified. However, the two most significant isoantigen groups are the ABO system and the Rh system. These two groups are likely to cause blood transfusion reactions because of their cell surface composition.

Blood Groups

A significant segment of the population has two related antigens on the surface of their red blood cells, A and B. However, over 40% of the population has neither A nor B antigens on the RBC surface. These people are said to have blood type "O." Every person has two genotypes that decide blood type. These pairs are what determine one of the four blood types; A, B, AB, or O. This pairing of genotypes may be AA, AO, BB, BO, AB, or OO. AA and AO genotypes produce blood type A. BB and BO produce blood type B. AB produces blood type AB, and genotype OO produces blood type O (Table 5–1).

Rh Factor (Type D)

The Rh (D) antigen is a component of the Rh blood groups. When a person has the Rh factor on the surface of their RBCs, they are Rh positive (Rh$^+$). When the Rh factor is

Table 5-1 Blood Types Determined by Genotypes. (© Delmar/Cengage Learning)

Genotype	Blood Type
AA	A
AO	A
BB	B
BO	B
AB	AB
OO	O

not on the surface of the RBCs, the person is Rh negative (Rh⁻). Approximately 95% of all African-Americans are Rh⁺, approximately 85% of Caucasians are Rh⁺, and virtually all Native Americans are Rh⁺. Antibodies are not present in the plasma in either Rh⁺ (in patients not previously exposed to an Rh⁺ patient) or Rh⁻ blood. A patient who is Rh⁺ may receive either Rh⁺ or Rh⁻ blood. However, a patient who is Rh⁻ can only receive Rh⁻ blood to avoid the formation of antibodies to Rh⁺ blood. The first time an Rh⁻ patient receives Rh⁺ blood, a reaction will generally not occur. However, antibodies will slowly develop over a 2-week to 4-month period. If the patient receives another transfusion of Rh⁺ blood, the Rh antibodies will clump with the Rh antigens (**agglutinogens**) of the blood being transfused.

Blood Typing and Crossmatching

Before blood can be administered to a patient, there must be compatibility between the blood types of the donor and the recipient. The process to determine this compatibility is called blood typing and crossmatching. **Blood typing** is the test run to determine the patient's blood type. **Crossmatching** is the process that determines the compatibility between the blood donor and the patient (recipient). If the blood donor and the recipient are incompatible, **agglutination** occurs, obstructing circulatory flow, and ultimately causing death.

Patients who have blood type A should only receive blood type A, and those patients who have blood type B should only receive blood type B. However, in emergency situations, blood type O can be administered to any of the four blood types, because it does not contain either A or B antigens. A person who has blood type O is considered the **universal donor**. In emergency situations, persons who have type AB blood are able to receive all four types of blood, because they have no A or B antibodies. People who have type AB blood are considered a **universal recipient**. However, unless there is an emergency, blood typing and crossmatching should be done to avoid any type of transfusion reaction. Table 5–2 illustrates blood types and their compatibilities with other blood types.

Blood and Blood Components

The EMS professional may find it necessary to administer and/or transport a patient receiving whole blood or blood components in an emergency situation. A thorough understanding of blood products will assist in the understanding of assisting with these types of patients.

Whole Blood

There may be occasion when the EMS professional will be called upon to administer and/or transport a patient who is receiving whole blood. Whole blood consists of red and white blood cells, platelets, electrolytes, plasma, and stable clotting factors. One unit of blood equals 500 mL. In emergencies, whole blood is indicated for massive blood loss equal to or exceeding 25% of a patient's total blood volume.

Many times it is difficult and impractical to administer whole blood during an emergency. Therefore, protocols have largely been replaced with the use of blood components, which supply the patient with specific blood components. This has allowed one unit of blood to be separated into RBCs, plasma, and platelets, which in turn can be used to treat several different patients. Another advantage of separating whole blood into components is that the ABO incompatibility between blood groups is eliminated. Also, colloidal and crystalloid infusions can often be used when up to one-third of an adult's blood volume is lost.

Whole blood should be administered as rapidly as the patient can tolerate. The loss of potassium from the RBCs into the plasma increases proportionately to the length of time the blood is stored. Therefore, the administration of whole blood to cardiac patients may be contraindicated. The only thing that can be mixed with whole blood is 0.9% normal saline.

Packed Red Blood Cells

Packed RBCs have 80% of the plasma removed, but provide the same amount of RBCs as whole blood. Packed RBCs are indicated for patients who are anemic, do not need fluid volume expansion, but do need increased oxygen-carrying ability of their blood.

The major advantage of packed RBCs over whole blood is the reduction of anti-A or anti-B **agglutinins** with the removal of the plasma. During an emergency, when typing and crossmatching are not feasible, packed type O RBCs can be given.

Table 5–2 Blood Compatibilities. (© Delmar/Cengage Learning)

Type	RBC Antigen	Plasma Antibody	Recipient Status	Donor Status
A	A	B	A or O	A or AB
B	B	A	B or O	B or AB
AB	A & B	None	A, B, AB, O	AB
O	None	A & B	O	A, B, AB, O

Plasma

Plasma is the liquid portion of the blood and lymph. It carries nutrients to body tissues and wastes are transported for excretion. Rh crossmatching is not necessary before administering plasma, as plasma contains no RBCs. However, ABO compatibility must be determined. In emergency situations, AB plasma can be given to all ABO patients. This is because plasma does not have anti-A or anti-B agglutinins. During an emergency, if only volume expansion is needed, the patient should be given a crystalloid solution to avoid disease transmission and/or adverse side effects and reactions.

Blood Transfusion Reactions

The administration of blood or any of its components can cause a transfusion reaction, which may be fatal if not recognized and treated appropriately. As an EMS professional, it is important for you to recognize the signs and symptoms associated with a transfusion reaction, and carry out interventions necessary to reverse its effects. The best way to recognize the signs and symptoms of a transfusion reaction is to assess the patient by body system:

Respiratory:
- Apnea
- Cough
- Dyspnea
- Rales
- Tachypnea
- Wheezing

Cardiovascular:
- Shock
- Chest pain
- Hyper- or Hypotension
- Bradycardia or tachycardia
- Weak pulse

Nervous system:
- Apprehension
- Fever
- Headache
- Numbness
- Tingling
- Sense of impending doom

Renal:
- Flank pain
- Concentrated, dark urine
- Renal failure

Musculoskeletal:
- Back pain
- Abdominal cramping

Gastrointestinal:
- Abdominal cramping or pain
- Diarrhea (may be bloody)
- Nausea/vomiting

Integumentary:
- Diaphoresis
- Urticaria (hives)
- Itching/rash
- Edema
- Cyanosis
- Facial flushing
- Cool/clammy or dry/flushed/hot

General:
- Chest pain
- Back pain
- Chills
- Headache
- Muscle aches
- Heat at infusion site

It is important to understand that reactions from blood or blood product transfusions can occur within 5 minutes of the start of the transfusion, or as late as 48 hours after the transfusion is discontinued. Some patients have been known to experience a transfusion reaction up to 6 months after the transfusion.

Fluid Replacement

There are two major indications for intravenous (IV) therapy: 1) replace fluid loss, and 2) provide a route for medication administration. The basic classifications of IV infusions are crystalloids, colloids, hydrating solutions, and blood or blood components.

Crystalloids

Crystalloids have the ability to form crystals. Crystals when placed in a solvent, homogeneously mix and dissolve into a solution. Since crystalloids are considered true solutions, they are able to diffuse through membranes. Crystalloid infusions are electrolyte solutions that can be isotonic, hypotonic, or hypertonic in nature.

Colloids

Colloids are substances whose particles, when placed into a solvent, cannot form a true solution. This is because their molecules do not dissolve, but remain uniformly suspended and distributed throughout the fluid. Colloidal particles are too large to pass through cell membranes.

Colloid intravenous infusions raise osmotic pressure. Therefore, colloids are called volume expanders. The colloid infusions that are commonly used consist of: albumin, dextran, plasmanate, and the artificial blood substitute, hetastarch.

Hydrating Solutions

Many times intravenous infusions are given to patients to supplement caloric intake, supply nutrients, provide free water for rehydration, or promote adequate renal output. The chemical makeup of these infusions or the rate of administration is adjusted, so that the equilibrium of current body fluids is not changed. Glucose solutions are the hydrating solutions most often used. When glucose or other nutrients are given in water, they are rapidly metabolized, leaving an excess of water. Any excess water not needed by the body is excreted by the renal system.

Dextrose Solutions

Dextrose solutions are manufactured as percentage concentrations in water or sodium chloride. Solutions manufactured on a percentage basis express the number of grams of solute per 100 g of solvent. One mL of water equals one gram as solvent. For example, dextrose 5% in water (D_5W) contains 5 g of dextrose in 100 mL of water.

Isotonic Solutions

Isotonic solutions have a similar electrolyte composition as body fluids. Because of this, they remain within the intravascular space because the osmotic pressure is equal between the intracellular and extracellular compartments. Because of their electrolyte composition, isotonic solutions can be administered at a more rapid rate than either hypo- or hypertonic solutions. A common use for isotonic solutions is to treat hypotension resulting from hypovolemia.

Hypotonic Solutions

Hypotonic solutions cause fluid to shift out of the blood and into the cells and interstitial spaces. If administered too rapidly, hypotonic solutions can cause the red blood cells to rupture. Hypotonic solutions are used to hydrate the intracellular and interstitial compartments and lower sodium levels. They should not be given to hypotensive patients, as this can further lower blood pressure.

Hypertonic Solutions

Hypertonic solutions pull fluids from the intracellular and interstitial compartments into the blood vessels. They act to expand the intravascular compartment. Extreme cautions must be used when administering hypertonic solutions, as they can cause circulatory overload. Hypertonic solutions are also irritating to the intima of the veins.

Fluid replacement is based on patient need and the patient's underlying condition. The following IV fluids are most frequently used in the out-of-hospital setting:

PLASMA PROTEIN (ALBUMIN)

Classification: Protein-containing colloid

Mechanism of Action
Remains in circulating blood volume. Aids in maintaining adequate blood volume and blood pressure.

Indications
Used to replace protein and to treat hypovolemic shock.

Contraindications
None.

Adverse Reactions
Monitor the patient for hives, chills, fever, headache, urticaria, nausea and vomiting.

DEXTRAN

Classification: Sugar-containing colloid

Mechanism of Action
Remains in the circulating blood volume for up to 12 hours. Thus, dextran is used as an intravascular volume expander.

Indications
Hypovolemic shock.

Contraindications
Known hypersensitivity, bleeding disorders, Congestive Heart Failure (CHF), and renal failure.

Adverse Reactions
Though generally mild, monitor the patient for rash, itching, dyspnea, chest tightness, and hypotension.

HETASTARCH (HES)

Classification: Starch-containing colloid

Mechanism of Action
Increases intravascular volume caused by the colloid osmotic pressure.

Indications
Hypovolemic shock and septic shock.

Contraindications
Bleeding disorders, CHF, and renal failure.

Adverse Reactions
Though generally mild, monitor the patient for chills, itching, urticaria, nausea and vomiting.

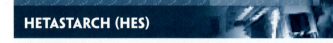

MANNITOL

Classification: Osmotic diuretic

Mechanism of Action
Inhibits the reabsorption of water and electrolytes.

Indications
Used to relieve excessive intracranial pressure.

Contraindications
Pulmonary edema, cellular dehydration.

Adverse Reactions
May cause fluid overload or may cause electrolyte imbalance.

LACTATED RINGER'S (HARTMANN'S SOLUTION)

Classification: Isotonic crystalloid

Mechanism of Action

Contains 28 mEq of lactic acid that acts as a buffer, also the following electrolytes: Sodium (Na^+) = 130 mEq/L, Chloride (Cl^-) = 109 mEq/L, Calcium (Ca^{2+}) = 3 mEq/L, and Potassium (K^+) = 4 mEq/L. Lactated Ringer's replaces water and electrolytes.

Indications

Rehydration, restores fluid volume, and treats mild metabolic acidosis associated with renal insufficiency because lactic acid is converted to bicarbonate.

Contraindications

Hyperkalemia, CHF, edema, sodium retention, and renal failure.

Adverse Reactions

Monitor patient for fluid overload.

DEXTROSE 5% IN WATER (D_5W)

Classification: Dextrose-containing hypotonic solution

Mechanism of Action

While in the container, D_5W is isotonic. However, when administered, the dextrose is rapidly metabolized and the infusion becomes hypotonic. D_5W provides dextrose and free water.

Indications

Provides IV access for drugs that are directly injected into the vein, and used as a diluent for concentrated drugs given as an IV infusion.

Contraindications

Do not use for volume replacement in hypovolemic states.

Adverse Reactions

Rare.

NORMAL SALINE (NS, 0.9% SODIUM CHLORIDE)

Classification: Isotonic crystalloid solution

Mechanism of Action

Replaces electrolytes and water.

Indications

Hypovolemia, heat-related emergencies, diabetic ketoacidosis, keep-open IV, and diluent for concentrated drugs to be given as an IV infusion.

Contraindications

CHF and edema with sodium retention.

Adverse Reactions

Rare.

ONE-HALF SODIUM CHLORIDE (1/2NS; 0.45% SODIUM CHLORIDE)

Classification: Hypotonic crystalloid solution

Mechanism of Action

1/2NS has about half the sodium and chloride concentration as NS. It replaces electrolytes and free water.

Indications

Compromised cardiac or renal function where rapid rehydration is not needed.

Contraindications

In patients who require rapid rehydration.

Adverse Reactions

Rare.

DEXTROSE 5% IN 0.9% SODIUM CHLORIDE (D_5NS)

Classification: Dextrose-containing hypertonic crystalloid solution

Mechanism of Action

Provides nutrient in the form of dextrose, and replaces electrolytes and free water.

Indications

Volume replacement, heat-related emergencies, and freshwater near-drowning.

Contraindications

Do not administer to patients with impaired renal or cardiac function.

Adverse Reactions

Rare.

DEXTROSE 5% IN 0.45% SODIUM CHLORIDE ($D_51/2NS$)

Classification: Dextrose-containing hypertonic crystalloid solution

Mechanism of Action

Replaces electrolytes, free water, and provides nutrients from dextrose.

Indications

Heat-related emergencies, diabetic disorders, and can be used as a keep-open IV solution for patients with impaired cardiac or renal function.

Contraindications

Do not use in patients who require rapid fluid resuscitation.

Adverse Reactions

Rare.

DEXTROSE 5% IN LACTATED RINGER'S SOLUTION (D₅LR)

Classification: Dextrose-containing hypertonic crystalloid solution

Mechanism of Action
Replaces electrolytes, free water, and provides nutrients using dextrose.

Indications
Volume replacement.

Contraindications
Do not administer to patients with decreased renal or cardiovascular function.

Adverse Reactions
Rare.

Antihyperlipidemic Agents—HMG–CoA Reductase Inhibitors

The National Cholesterol Education Program Expert Panel on Detection, Evaluation, and Treatment of High Cholesterol in Adults has developed guidelines for the treatment of high cholesterol and LDL in adults. The following lists the adult recommendations for both LDL and HDL levels of cholesterol.

Status and Total Cholesterol

- Desirable: (<200 mg/dL)
- Borderline high: (200–239 mg/dL)
- High: (>240 mg/dL)

Status and LDL Cholesterol

- Optimal: (<100 mg/dL)
- Near optimal: (100–129 mg/dL)
- High-risk: (160–189 mg/dL)
- Very high-risk: (190 mg/dL or higher)

Status of HDL Cholesterol

- High-risk: (<40 mg/dL)
- Average: (40–50 mg/dL)
- Low-risk: (>60 mg/dL)

An antihyperlipidemic drug prevents or counteracts the accumulation of fatty substances in the blood. These drugs are used as an adjunct to diet to decrease elevated total LDL and cholesterol in patients when the response to diet and other nondrug approaches has been unsuccessful.

ATORVASTATIN (AH-TORE-VAH-STAH-TIN) CALCIUM

Pregnancy Class: X

Lipitor (Rx)

Classification: Antihyperlipidemic, HMG–CoA reductase inhibitor

Mechanism of Action
HMG–CoA reductase inhibitors increase HDL cholesterol, decrease LDL cholesterol, and plasma triglycerides. It takes approximately 4-6 weeks for a maximum therapeutic response.

Indications
An adjunct to diet in the reduction of total and LDL cholesterol levels. Also can be used in patients with changes in diet who have high triglyceride levels.

Contraindications
Active liver disease, pregnancy, and lactation.

Precautions
The safety and efficacy have not been determined in children.

Route and Dosage
Tablets orally, beginning with 10 mg/day. May be necessary to increase dosage to 10-80 mg/day.

Adverse Reactions and Side Effects
CNS: Headache.

Musculoskeletal: Myalgia.

Miscellaneous: Infection, rash, allergy.

EMS Considerations
None.

CERIVISTATIN (SEH-RIHV-AH-STAT-IN) SODIUM

Pregnancy Class: X

Baycol (Rx)

Classifications: Antihyperlipidemic, HMG–CoA reductase inhibitor

Mechanism of Action
Inhibition of cholesterol synthesis and decrease in plasma cholesterol levels.

Indications
An adjunct to diet to reduce elevated total and LDL cholesterol levels.

Contraindications
Active liver disease, pregnancy, and lactation.

Precautions
Renal or hepatic insufficiency. Safety and efficacy have not been determined in children.

Route and Dosage
Oral tablets at 0.3 mg each evening.

Adverse Reactions and Side Effects
CNS: Headache, dizziness, tremor, vertigo, memory loss, insomnia, depression.

Respiratory: URI, cough.

Musculoskeletal: Rarely.

GI: Nausea and vomiting, abdominal cramps or pain.

EMS Considerations
None.

FLUVASTATIN (FLU-VAH-STAH-TIN) SODIUM

Pregnancy Class: X

Lescol (Rx)

Classification: Antihyperlipidemic drug

Mechanism of Action

Reduces elevated total and LDL cholesterol levels.

Indications

An adjunct to diet for the reduction of elevated total and LDL cholesterol levels. Also slows the progression of coronary atherosclerosis in coronary artery disease (CAD).

Contraindications

Pregnancy and lactation.

Precautions

Severe renal impairment.

Route and Dosage

Oral capsules at 20 mg, daily at bedtime. Dosage range is 20-40 mg/day at bedtime.

Adverse Reactions and Side Effects

Respiratory: URI, cough, pharyngitis.

CNS: Headache, dizziness, insomnia.

Musculoskeletal: Myalgia, back pain, arthritis.

Miscellaneous: Rash, fatigue, influenza, allergy.

EMS Considerations

None.

LOVASTATIN (LOW-VAH-STAT-TIN)

Pregnancy Class: X

Mevacor (Rx)

Classification: Antihyperlipidemic drug

Mechanism of Action

HMG—CoA reductase inhibitors increase HDL cholesterol and decrease LDL cholesterol. This also slows the progression of coronary atherosclerosis in patients with CAD.

Indications

Used as an adjunct to diet to lower total and LDL cholesterol. Slows the progression of coronary atherosclerosis in patients with CAD.

Contraindications

Active liver disease, pregnancy, lactation, and use in children.

Precautions

Patients with impaired renal function, and patients who consume heavy amounts of alcohol.

Route and Dosage

Tablets orally, 20 mg once daily with evening meal.

Adverse Reactions and Side Effects

CNS: Headache, dizziness, and insomnia.

Musculoskeletal: Muscle cramps, leg pain, shoulder pain, and localized pain.

GI: Abdominal pain, cramps, diarrhea, heartburn, and nausea and vomiting.

Miscellaneous: Blurred vision, rash, eye irritation.

EMS Considerations

None.

PRAVASTATIN (PRAH-VAH-STAH-TIN) SODIUM

Pregnancy Class: X

Pravachol (Rx)

Classification: Antihyperlipidemic drug

Mechanism of Action

Inhibits LDL production and lowers elevated levels of total cholesterol. Increases the survival rate in heart transplant patients.

Indications

Adjunct to diet for reducing elevated total and LDL cholesterol levels.

Contraindications

Active liver disease, pregnancy, lactation, and children.

Precautions

Renal insufficiency, or heavy alcohol use.

Route and Dosage

Tablets orally. Initial dose is 10-20 mg once daily at bedtime. Maintenance dose is 10-40 mg once daily at bedtime.

Adverse Reactions and Side Effects

Respiratory: Common cold, cough.

CV: Chest pain, palpitation, postural hypotension, arrhythmia.

CNS: Headache, dizziness, vertigo, memory loss, psychic disturbances.

GI: Nausea and vomiting, abdominal pain, cramps, dry mouth.

EMS Considerations

None.

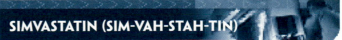

SIMVASTATIN (SIM-VAH-STAH-TIN)

Pregnancy Class: X

Zocor (Rx)

Classification: Antihyperlipidemic drug

Mechanism of Action

Inhibits HMG—CoA reductase, reducing levels of LDL cholesterol and plasma triglycerides, and increasing levels of HDL cholesterol.

Indications

An adjunct to diet for the reduction of elevated total and LDL cholesterol. Reduces the risk of non-fatal MI, and the risks of stroke or TIAs.

Contraindications

Active liver disease, pregnancy, lactation, and use in children.

Precautions

Use with caution in patients who consume large amounts of alcohol.

Route and Dosage

Tablets orally. Begin at 20 mg once daily in the evening. Maintenance dose of 5-80 mg daily in the evening.

Adverse Reactions and Side Effects

CNS: Headache, tremor, vertigo, memory loss, anxiety, and insomnia.

GI: Diarrhea, abdominal pain, anorexia, and constipation.

EMS Considerations

None.

Table 5-3 lists some common statin-combination drugs that are also used to help control high cholesterol levels.

Table 5-3 Common Statin-combination Drugs. (© Delmar/Cengage Learning)

Generic Name	Trade Name	Mechanism of Action
niacin with lovastatin	Advicor	Lowers LDL cholesterol and raises HDL cholesterol
atorvastatin with amlodipine	Caduet	Lowers how much cholesterol the body makes, plus lowers blood pressure.
gemfibrozil	Tricor	Lowers triglycerides and raises HDL cholesterol. May slightly increase LDL cholesterol.
ezetimibe with simvastatin	Vytorin	Lowers how much cholesterol the body makes. Also affects how the body absorbs cholesterol.
ezetimibe	Zetia	Lowers how much cholesterol the body can absorb.

CONCLUSION

Administering blood and blood products can be lifesaving; however, if done improperly, it can also become deadly. It is imperative that once blood or a blood product is given, the EMS professional knows the signs and symptoms of an adverse reaction to a transfusion, and reports and treats the patient accordingly. Heightened awareness of the pertinent signs and symptoms of a reaction enable the caregiver to report and treat the patient accordingly.

It is very important that the EMS professional understands the rationale behind giving a particular IV solution. Each solution has been developed to treat a particular emergency situation. Using the incorrect IV fluid can have a serious impact on the outcome of the patient.

Finally, there are many individuals taking medications to help in lowering their cholesterol levels. EMS professionals should become familiar with each of these drugs so they can better understand the disease process of coronary artery disease (CAD) and hypercholesterolemia. Antihyperlipidemic drugs have helped greatly to combat these disease processes.

STUDY QUESTIONS

1. Within each human being, there is a unique combination of genes called a(n):
   a. Antigen
   b. Genotype
   c. Antibody
   d. Epitope

2. A significant segment of the population has two related antigens on the surface of their red blood cells. They are _____ and _____.

3. List the four different blood types and indicate both the donor and recipient status of each.
   _____
   _____
   _____
   _____
   _____
   _____
   _____

4. Upon completing the chart in question 3, who is considered the universal recipient, and who is considered the universal donor?
   _____
   _____
   _____

   _____
   _____
   _____
   _____

5. Explain what might occur if a hypotonic solution is infused into a patient too rapidly.
   _____
   _____
   _____
   _____
   _____
   _____
   _____
   _____
   _____

6. Normal saline (0.9% sodium chloride solution) is a common out-of-hospital IV solution. List the classification, mechanism of action, indications, and contraindications for normal saline.
   _____
   _____
   _____
   _____
   _____

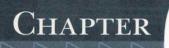

CHAPTER 6

DRUG–DOSAGE CALCULATIONS

OBJECTIVES

On completion of this chapter and the study questions, you should be able to:

- Interpret a medication order accurately.
- Convert quantities from the U.S. system to the metric system.
- Convert quantities within the metric system.
- Calculate drug solutions, including rates of infusion.
- Calculate drug dosages for adults and children.
- Convert temperature measurements from Fahrenheit to Celsius.

KEY TERMS

Apothecaries' system	Liter	Unit
Celsius	Mass	U.S. system
Concentration	Meter	U.S.P. unit
Fahrenheit	Metric system	Volume
Gram	Proportion	
Length	Ratio	

INTRODUCTION

Administering drugs would be much easier if they all came in the same forms, same concentrations, and were packaged in the same way. However, drugs come in a variety of forms, packages, and concentrations (Figures 6-1 and 6-2). Everyone with the responsibility for administering drugs must (1) be familiar with their various forms and concentrations, (2) know how to prepare the drug for administration, and (3) be able to calculate the dosage and rate of administration. The following list illustrates the bewildering variety of forms in which drugs often used in EMS are packaged:

- *Lidocaine:* 2 grams (2 g) in solution in a 10-milliliter (10 mL) syringe. In this case, the drug concentration is 200 milligrams per milliliter (200 mg/mL). The EMS professional dilutes this in an appropriate intravenous fluid before administration. Lidocaine is also commonly available, for direct intravenous bolus injection, as 100 milligrams of a 20 milligrams per milliliter solution in a prefilled 5-milliliter syringe.

- *$D_{50}W$ (50% dextrose in water):* This widely used EMS drug is commonly available in a 50-milliliter prefilled syringe, which contains 25 grams of dextrose.

- *Furosemide:* 20 milligrams in a 2-milliliter prefilled syringe. Furosemide is also packaged in ampules of different sizes (e.g., 20 milligrams in a 2-milliliter ampule, 100 milligrams in a 10-milliliter ampule).

- *Nitroglycerin tablets:* Commonly available in 1/150 grain (1/150 gr), which equals 0.4 milligram, or 1/200 grain, which equals 0.3 milligram. (One grain, in apothecaries' measure, equals about 60 milligrams.)

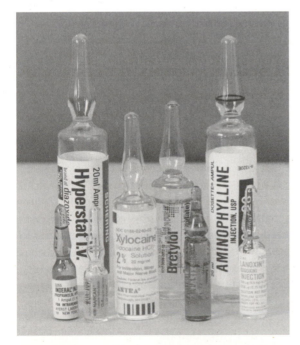

Figure 6-1 A common type of drug preparation is the liquid solution in a glass ampule. (© Delmar/Cengage Learning)

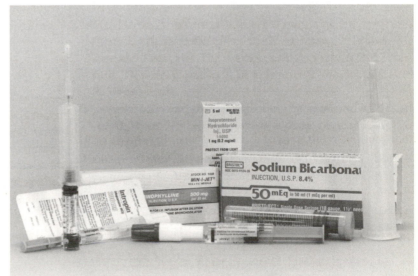

Figure 6-2 Drugs come in many forms, some of which are shown above. (© Delmar/Cengage Learning)

- *Oxytocin:* Commonly packaged as 10 U.S.P. units in a 1-milliliter ampule. A unit is defined as one of anything. It is a specific amount adopted as a standard of measurement. A U.S.P. unit is any unit specified in the *United States Pharmacopeia.*
- *Dopamine:* One of the forms in which you may encounter this drug is as 200 milligrams in solution in a 5-milliliter prefilled syringe.
- *Sodium bicarbonate:* Sodium bicarbonate is usually packaged in prefilled 50-milliliter syringes, containing either 44.4 or 50 milliequivalents (mEq). A *milliequivalent* is the concentration of electrolytes (see Chapter 4) in a certain volume of solution, usually expressed as milliequivalent per liter (mEq/L).

As the preceding list shows, drugs come in a bewildering variety of forms, concentrations, and packages. EMS professionals who administer drugs must be able to use mathematical calculations to determine the correct dosages. This chapter reviews the necessary calculations involved in the safe administration of drugs to the patient.

Weights and Measures

Throughout history, humans have developed various systems of weights and measures—ways of describing the size and/or amount of physical objects or substances. Each system has units of measure for three physical characteristics:

1. **Length:** The distance between two points.
2. **Mass:** How much matter is in an object or a substance; this is commonly expressed as its weight.
3. **Volume:** How much space is occupied by an object or a substance.

Some systems use different measures for dry and liquid volume. For instance, in the system used in the United States (called the **United States system** or household system), the units of dry measure are pint, quart, peck, and bushel, and the units of liquid measure include fluid ounce, pint, quart, and gallon.

Because of the historic roots of pharmacology, drug dosages in the United States are expressed in any one of three systems:

1. *The* metric system: (discussed in the next section).
2. *The United States system*: The United States system is based on the traditional English system. This system, derived from the English, has been almost completely replaced by the metric system.
3. *The* **apothecaries' system**: Apothecary is the old name for pharmacist. The apothecaries' system has units of measure for weight (mass) and liquid weight (capacity).

Table 6–1 lists the various units of measure in each system. Table 6–2 shows the equivalents between various units in the English and metric systems.

To administer drugs safely, EMS professionals must be able to convert various units of measure:

- You will need to convert an amount expressed in one unit of measure into its equivalent in another unit of measure in the same system. For example, if a physician tells you to administer 1500 milligrams of a drug and the drug is packaged in tablets, each containing 0.5 grams of the drug, you must convert 0.5 grams to its equivalent in milligrams in order to calculate how many tablets are required. (You will learn how to do this in the "Decimal Review" section.)
- You must also know how to convert an amount expressed in one unit of measure into its equivalent in another system. For example, many drug orders are based on body weight. If the order tells you to administer 0.5 milligrams per kilogram of body weight, and your patient weighs 165 pounds, you must convert pounds to kilograms. (The "U.S.-to-Metric Conversions" section shows you how.)

The Metric System

The **metric system** is used in many countries of the world and in all scientific disciplines, including medicine and pharmacology. It is a decimal system, meaning it is based on the number 10. Every unit of length is ten times larger than the next smaller unit and ten times smaller than the next larger unit. The basic unit of length is the **meter**; the basic unit of mass (weight) is the **gram**; and the basic unit of volume is the **liter**. The names of all the other units of measure in the metric system are formed by adding prefixes to the names of

Table 6–1 Systems of Weights and Measures. (© Delmar/Cengage Learning)

United States (English)	Metric	Apothecaries'
Mass (Weight)		
Pound (lb)	Kilogram (kg)	Pound* (lb ap)
Ounce (oz)	Hectogram (hg)	Ounce (ox ap)
Dram (dr)	Dekagram (dag)	Dram (dr ap)
Grain (gr)	Gram (g)	Scruple (s)
	Decigram (dg)	Grain*
	Centigram (cg)	
	Milligram (mg)	
	Microgram (mcg)	
Volume (Liquid Measure)		
Gallon (gal)	Kiloliter (kL)	Gallon (gal)
Quart (qt)	Hectoliter (hL)	Quart (qt)
Pint (pt)	Dekaliter (daL)	Pint (pt)
Gill (gi)	Liter (L)	Gill (gi)
Fluidounce (fl oz)	Deciliter (dL)	Fluidounce (fl oz)
Fluidram (fl dr)	Centiliter (cL)	Fluidram (fl dr)
Minim (min)	Milliliter (mL)	Minim (min)
	Microliter (μL)	
Length		
Mile (mi)	Kilometer (km)	
Yard (yd)	Hectometer (hm)	
Foot (ft or ')	Dekameter (dam)	
Inch (in or ")	Meter (m)	
	Decimeter (dm)	
	Centimeter (cm)	
	Millimeter (mm)	
	Micrometer (μm)	

*Although the English pound and apothecaries' pound are not equivalent, the English grain and apothecaries' grain are—each is equal to approximately 60 milligrams.

Table 6–2 Commonly Used Equivalents. (© Delmar/Cengage Learning)

Metric–English	English–Metric
1 kilogram (k) = 2.2 pounds (lb)	1 pound (lb) = 0.454 kilograms (k)
1 gram (g) = 0.035 ounces (oz)	1 ounce (oz) = 28.35 grams (g)
1 milligram (mg) = 0.015 grains (gr)	1 grain (gr) = 0.0645 grams (gr) or 64.5 milligrams (mg)
1 liter (L) = 1.057 quarts (qt)	1 fluidounce (fl oz) = 29.57 milligrams (mg)
1 deciliter (dL) = 3.38 fluidounce (fl oz)	
1 milliliter (mL) = 0.27 fluidram (fl dr)	

Table 6–3 Metric Prefixes. (© Delmar/Cengage Learning)

Prefix	Multiple of Base
Mega-	1,000,000
Kilo-	1000
Hecto-	100
Deka-	10
Base	1
Deci-	1/10
Centi-	1/100
Milli-	1/1,000
Micro-	1/1,000,000

the basic units. The prefix indicates how many times larger or smaller than the basic unit the new unit will be. For example, a kilometer equals 1000 meters; a millimeter equals one thousandth of a meter. Table 6–3 illustrates the progression of prefixes used in the metric system.

Review of Mathematical Principles

Decimals

Converting dosages within the metric system is easy because it is a decimal system. A review of decimal arithmetic will show how simple calculating metric dosages can be.

Each amount in the metric system consists of a whole number (in many cases, the whole number is 0) and a decimal fraction separated by the decimal point (e.g., 1.5). The whole number is on the left of the decimal point, and the decimal fraction is expressed by the numbers on the right of the decimal point. The position of a number in relation to the decimal point gives that number its name and its value (Figure 6–3). For example, the first place to the left of the decimal point is the unit place, the second is the ten place, and so on. A 2 in the second place to the left of the decimal point (e.g., 20.00) indicates that there are two tens in the ten's place. A zero in the first place to the left of the decimal point indicates that there is nothing in the units place, which means, so far, that the number is twenty. A 2 in the second place to the right of the decimal point (e.g., 0.02) indicates two one-hundredths. The number 20.02, then, means "twenty and two-hundredths."

For amounts less than 1, it is a good idea to place a 0 in the unit place (the first place to the left of the decimal point). For example, the best way to express the fraction 1/2 in decimals is 0.5.

Adding and Subtracting Decimals

When adding decimal numbers, place the second number below the first number, the third below the second, and so on, just as with whole numbers—but remember to line the numbers up on the decimal point.

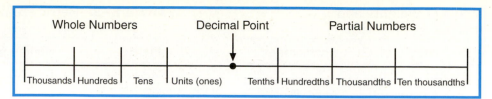

Figure 6–3 In the decimal system, the position of a number in relation to the decimal place determines the name and value of the number. (© Delmar/Cengage Learning)

Example:

Add: 3.3 + 29.75 + 4

Solution:

```
      3.30
  + 29.75
  +  4.00      [Add 0s to the right of the decimal
    37.05      point as needed]
```

Subtracting one decimal number from another number also requires lining the two numbers up, one below the other, on the decimal point.

Example:

Subtract: 17.20 − 6.25

Solution:

```
    17.20      [Add 0s to the right of the decimal
  −  6.25      point as needed]
    10.95
```

Example:

Subtract: 33.02 − 17

Solution:

```
    33.02
  − 17.00
    16.02      [Add 0s to the right of the decimal
               point as needed]
```

Rounding Decimals

For many decimal calculations, it is necessary or convenient to "round" the answer up or down. Round down to the nearest whole number if the decimal fraction is below 0.5 (change 6.4 to 6). If the decimal fraction is 0.5 or higher, round up to the next larger whole number (change 6.5 to 7). You can also round down or up to the next decimal place (change 6.43 to 6.4; change 6.68 to 6.7).

There are other systems for rounding numbers that you may prefer to use and that will work efficiently.

Multiplying Decimals

First, multiply decimal numbers together as if they were whole numbers, without regard to the decimal point. Then add the number of decimal places (places to the right of the decimal point) in both of the multipliers. That total is the number of decimal places in the product of the two numbers; the decimal point goes that number of places to the left of the last number in the product.

Example:

Multiply: 12.5 × 3.7

Solution:

```
     12.5      [1 decimal place]
  ×   3.7      [+1 decimal place]
      875
  + 375
    46.25      [2 decimal places in the product]
```

Example:

Multiply: 25.75 × 6.04

Solution:

```
       25.75      [2 decimal places]
  ×     6.04      [+2 decimal places]
      10300
  +    0000
  + 15450
     155.5300     [4 decimal places in the product]
```

[After determining where the decimal point goes, drop any final zeros at the right of the decimal point.]

Whenever you multiply by any multiple of 10, a shorter method is to move the decimal point to the right by the number of zeros in the multiple. For example, when multiplying by 10, move the decimal point one place to the right:

$$15.75 \times 10 = 157.50$$

When multiplying by 100, move the decimal point two places to the right:

$$15.75 \times 100 = 1575.0$$

When multiplying by 1000, move the decimal point three places to the right:

$$15.75 \times 1000 = 15,750.0$$

Dividing Decimals

When dividing by a decimal number, place a caret (c) as many places to the right of the decimal point in both the divisor and the dividend as there are places in the divisor. Then place the decimal point in the quotient above the caret in the dividend.

Example:

Divide: $253.680 \div 10.5$

Solution:

```
           24.16
    10.5 ) 253.680
           210
           ___
           436
           420
           ___
           168
           105
           ___
           630
           630
           ___
```

Example:

Divide: $50.2990 \div 0.125$

Solution:

```
            402.4
    0.125 ) 50.2990
            500
            ___
            299
            250
            ___
            490
            490
            ___
```

There is a shorter method for dividing a decimal number by any multiple of 10. Move the decimal point in the dividend to the left by the number of zeros in the divisor.

Example:

When dividing by 10, move the dividend's decimal point one place to the left:

$$15.0 \div 10 = 1.5$$

Example:

When dividing a decimal number by a multiple of 100, move the decimal point two places to the left:

$$6.0 \div 100 = 0.06$$

Ratio and Proportion

Nearly every medication problem can be broken down to simple ratio and proportion. Developing skill in setting up ratios and proportions will be an invaluable aid to every EMS professional in solving drug-dosage problems quickly and accurately.

Ratio

A **ratio** is the relationship of two quantities. It may be expressed in the form 1:10 or 1:3300, or it may be expressed as a fraction—1/10 or 1/3300. The ratio expression 1:10 or 1/10 can be read as one in ten, or one-tenth, or one part in ten parts.

Example:

For every 15 students, there is 1 instructor.

The ratio of instructors to students is 1 in 15 or 1:15 or 1/15.

Proportion

A **proportion** is formed by using two ratios that are equal. For example, $1/2 = 5/10$.

When two ratios or fractions are equal, their cross product is also equal. The cross product is obtained by multiplying the denominator of one ratio by the numerator of the other.

Example:

$1/2 = 5/10 = 2 \times 5 = 10 \times 1$

The cross products are equal: $10 = 10$.

Therefore, the ratio 1/2 is equal to the ratio 5/10.

Does $1/4 = 3/12$?

The cross products are equal: $12 = 12$.

Therefore, 1/4 is equal to 3/12.

Practice Problem:

The physician orders you to give 20 mg of a drug to your patient. The drug comes packaged in a 10 mL vial containing 50 mg of the drug. How many milliliters will be needed to give the dose of 20 mg?

Solution:

There are three knowns:

1. 10 mL vial of the drug on hand
2. 50 mg of the drug in the 10 mL vial
3. 20 mg is the ordered dose

A ratio can be stated for the drug on hand:

$$\frac{10 \text{ mL}}{50 \text{ mg}} \text{ reduced to the lowest terms } = \frac{1 \text{ mL}}{50 \text{ mg}}$$

A ratio can also be stated for the required dosage:

$$\frac{X \text{ mL}}{20 \text{ mg}}$$

Thus, the proportion is:

$$\frac{1 \text{ mL}}{5 \text{ mg}} = \frac{X \text{ mL}}{20 \text{ mg}}$$

Note in the proportion that the units are labeled and like units are located in the same position in each fraction or ratio (1 mL is opposite X mL and 5 mg is opposite 20 mg). It is important to label the parts of the proportion correctly. Note that the answer label is always the label with "X."

Three conditions must be met when using ratio and proportion:

1. The numerators must have the same units.
2. The denominators must have the same units.
3. Three of the four parts must be known.

To solve the last example, simply find the cross product and solve for the unknown (X).

$$\frac{1 \text{ mL}}{5 \text{ mg}} = \frac{X \text{ mL}}{20 \text{ mg}}$$
$$5 \times X = 1 \times 20$$
$$5X = 20$$
$$X = 4 \text{ mL} \ (20 \div 5)$$

Therefore, 4 mL of the solution contains 20 mg of the drug.

Metric-to-Metric Conversions

Because the metric system is a decimal system, it is easy to convert from one metric unit to another. For example, to convert grams to milligrams, all you have to do is multiply by 1000. As a shortcut, move the decimal point three places to the right.

Example:

Convert 3 grams to milligrams

Solution:

$3.0 \text{ g} \times 1000 = 3000 \text{ mg}$ [Multiply by 1000]

or simply move the decimal point three places to the right.

$3.0 \text{ g} = 3000 \text{ mg}$ [Add zeros as needed to move the decimal point]

Example:

Convert 5.25 grams to milligrams

Solution:

$$5.25 \text{ g} \times 1000 = 5250 \text{ mg}$$

or

$$5.25 \text{ g} = 5250 \text{ mg}$$

To convert milligrams to grams, divide by 1000—move the decimal point three places to the left.

Example:

Convert 4000 milligrams to grams

Solution:

$$4 \text{ g}$$
$$4000 \text{ mg} \div 1000$$
or
$$4000 \text{ mg} = 4.000 \text{ g}$$

Problem:

You are a paramedic student in the emergency department. A physician orders you to administer 1500 milligrams of a drug. The drug comes in 0.5-gram tablets. You must convert within the metric system to find out how many milligrams are in each tablet. Then, you must calculate to find out how many tablets are required.

Solution:

To find the number of milligrams in each tablet, move the decimal point three places to the right.

1. Step 1 (Convert): Convert grams to milligrams.

   0.5 g = 500.0 mg [Move the decimal point three places to the right]
   Answer = each tablet contains 500 mg.

2. Step 2 (Calculate): Divide the required dosage by the amount of drug per tablet.

   $$1500 \times 500 = 3$$

Three tablets are required for the prescribed dose.

When converting liters to milliliters (larger unit to smaller unit), you must multiply by 1000 (or just move the decimal point three places to the right). For example:

6 L = 6000 mL (6 × 1000 or 6000)
4.5 L = 4500 mL (4.5 × 1000 or 4500)

To convert milliliters to liters (smaller unit to larger unit), you must divide by 1000 (or just move the decimal point three places to the left). For example:

5000 mL = 5 L (5000 ÷ 1000 or 5.000)
2500 mL = 2.5 L (2500 ÷ 1000 or 2.500)

The cubic centimeter (cc) is a once-common unit of measure whose use is decreasing. Both a milliliter and cubic centimeter are equal to one-thousandth of a liter. Even though milliliter and cubic centimeter are equivalent expressions, milliliter is the preferred term.

U.S.-to-Metric Conversions

For many drugs administered in EMS, the drug order is expressed as a volume of drug based on body weight. For example, an order for lidocaine might call for administering 1 milligram per kilogram of body weight (1 mg/kg). Most patients do not know their body weight in kilograms, so you must be able to convert pounds (U.S.) to kilograms (metric).

If 2.2 pounds equals 1 kilogram (Table 6–2), 1 pound equals 0.454 kilograms (kg). To convert pounds to kilograms, simply divide the number of pounds by 2.2.

Example:

100 lb = 100 ÷ 2.2 = 45 kg.

150 lb = 150 ÷ 2.2 = 68 kg [68.18 is rounded down to 68]

235 lb = 235 ÷ 2.2 = 107 kg [106.82 is rounded up to 107]

The Apothecaries' System

The apothecaries' system of measurement is rarely used by physicians when ordering drugs in EMS. However, some drugs are available only in (apothecary) grains. For this reason, EMS professionals should be able to use the apothecaries' system. The apothecaries' system measures solids in units of grains, drams, ounces, and pounds. It measures liquids in minims, fluidrams, fluidounces, pints, and gallons.

Apothecary System of Weights

The apothecary system of weights is based on the grain (gr), which is the smallest unit in the system. You will seldom see apothecary units in EMS with the exception of the grain, which is commonly used in ordering drugs such as nitroglycerin (1/150 gr, 1/200 gr), codeine sulfate (1/8 gr, 1/4 gr, 1/2 gr, 1 gr), and morphine sulfate (1/6 gr, 1/8 gr, 1/2 gr). To convert grains to metric units, the following approximate equivalent is used:

Example:

Convert 4 grains to grams.

Solution:

$$\frac{15 \text{ gr}}{1 \text{ g}} = \frac{4 \text{ gr}}{X \text{ g}}$$
$$X = 0.27 \text{ g}$$

Calculating Drug Solutions

Many drugs are given in solution—that is, pure drug in powder or liquid form is dissolved in a liquid. To administer a prescribed amount of a drug in solution, you must know the drug concentration of the solution. Drug **concentration** is the amount of drug per unit of volume; it is usually expressed in milligrams per milliliter (mg/mL). The formula for determining concentration is:

$$\text{Concentration} = \frac{\text{Amount of Drug (mg)}}{\text{Volume of Solution (mL)}}$$

For example, a common preparation of furosemide is a prefilled 4 milliliter (4 mL) syringe containing 40 milligrams (40 mg) of furosemide. In this case, the drug concentration is 10 milligrams per milliliter (10 mg/mL).

$$\text{Concentration} = \frac{40 \text{ mg [Total mg]}}{4 \text{ mL [Total mL]}} = 10 \text{ mg/mL}$$

When you know the drug concentration, you know how much drug is in one milliliter of solution. From that, you can determine how much solution is required to deliver the amount of drug ordered. Divide the amount of drug ordered by the drug concentration:

$$\begin{array}{l}\text{Required Volume of} \\ \text{Solution (mL)}\end{array} = \frac{\text{Required Drug Amount (mg)}}{\text{Drug Concentration (mg/mL)}}$$

Problem:

The physician orders a patient to receive 200 milligrams (200 mg) of a drug. The preparation on hand is a 10 milliliter (10 mL) syringe containing 500 milligrams (500 mg) of the drug. How much of the preparation do you administer?

Solution:

First, find the drug concentration (amount of drug per milliliter of solution) in the syringe by dividing the amount of drug in the syringe by the total volume of the solution:

$$\frac{500 \text{ mg}}{10 \text{ mL}} = 50 \text{ mg/mL}$$

Next, find the volume of solution required (mL) to deliver the required drug amount (mg) by dividing the required drug amount by the drug concentration (mg/mL).

$$\frac{200 \text{ mg}}{50 \text{ mg/mL}} = 4 \text{ mL} \text{ [The answer will be in mL.]}$$

Give the patient 4 milliliters (4 mL) of the solution in the 10 milliliter (10 mL) syringe.

Sometimes drug concentration is expressed as a percentage. For example, a common preparation of lidocaine is a 2% concentration in a 5 milliliter syringe. To find out how much lidocaine is in the syringe, multiply the percentage of drug (expressed as a decimal fraction) in solution by the total volume of the syringe.

0.02 [Concentration] × 5 mL [Volume] = 0.1 g

What is the concentration in milligrams per milliliter? Convert grams to milligrams and divide by the number of milliliters in the preparation.

$$0.1 \text{ g} \times 1000 = 100 \text{ mg}$$
$$\frac{100 \text{ mg}}{5 \text{ mL}} = 20 \text{ mg/mL}$$

Sometimes, as with epinephrine, the drug concentration is expressed as a ratio. For example, two often-used preparations are epinephrine in a 1:1000 solution and epinephrine 1:10,000 solution. The ratio of 1:1000 indicates that

1 milliliter of solution contains 1 milligram of the drug. The 1:10,000 ratio indicates that there is 1 milligram of drug in 10 milliliters of solution.

Remember, in the metric system the cubic centimeter, milliliter, and gram are equivalent. One cubic centimeter holds one milliliter of water, and one milliliter of water (or most other liquids) weighs one gram.

Calculating Rates of Infusion

Intravenous tubing is packaged in macrodrop or microdrop sets. Macrodrop intravenous tubing is available in both 10- and 15-drop sets. With a 10-drop intravenous set, 10 drops equals 1.0 milliliter. With a 15-drop set, 15 drops equals 1.0 milliliter. A microdrop intravenous set takes 60 drops to deliver 1.0 milliliter.

To calculate the drip rate for an intravenous infusion, health-care professionals need to know three values: (1) the volume of fluid required, (2) the intravenous set size, and (3) the total time of the infusion in minutes. For example: How many drops per minute will it take to infuse 500 milliliters of fluid using a 15-drop-per-minute (gtt/min) intravenous set for 45 minutes?

$$\text{Infusion Rate (drops/minute)} = \frac{\text{Volume Required (mL)} \times \text{Set Size (drops/min)}}{\text{Infusion Time (min)}}$$

$$\text{Infusion Rate (gtt/min)} = \frac{500 \text{ mL} \times 15 \text{ gtt/mL}}{45 \text{ min}}$$

$$= \frac{7500 \text{ gtt}}{45 \text{ min}} = 167 \text{ gtt/min}$$

Example:

How many drops per minute will it take to infuse 250 milliliters of fluid using a microdrop intravenous (60 drops per milliliter) set for 1 hour?

Solution:

$$\text{Infusion rate} = \frac{250 \text{ mL} \times 60 \text{ gtt/mL}}{60 \text{ min}} = \frac{15000}{60} = 250 \text{ gtt/min}$$

Example:

The paramedic is ordered to prepare a lidocaine infusion by adding 2 grams of lidocaine to 500 milliliters of dextrose 5% in water. Once the infusion is prepared, it is to run at 3 milligrams per minute, using a microdrip IV set. What is the concentration (milligrams per milliliter) of the lidocaine infusion, and at what rate (drops per minute) should the infusion run to deliver 3 milligrams of lidocaine per minute?

Solution:

Step 1: Determine the lidocaine concentration.

$$\text{Concentration} = \frac{\text{Amount of Drug}}{\text{Volume of Solution}}$$

$$= \frac{2 \text{ g}}{500 \text{ mL}} \quad \text{[Convert to mgs]}$$

$$= \frac{2000 \text{ mg}}{500 \text{ mL}} = 4 \text{ mg/mL}$$

Step 2: Determine the volume of solution needed to deliver 3 milligrams of lidocaine.

$$\text{Required Volume of Solution} = \frac{\text{Required Drug Amount}}{\text{Drug Concentration}}$$

$$= \frac{3 \text{ mg}}{4 \text{ mg/mL}} = 0.75 \text{ mL}$$

Step 3: Determine the infusion rate required.

$$\text{Infusion Rate} = \frac{\text{Volume of Solution Required} \times \text{Set Size}}{\text{Infusion Time}}$$

$$= \frac{0.75 \text{ mL} \times 60 \text{ gtt/mL}}{1 \text{ min}}$$

$$= 45 \text{ gtt/min}$$

Converting Temperature Measurements

EMS professionals must understand the **Celsius** system of temperature measurement as well as the metric system of weights and measures. They need to be able to convert temperatures expressed in Celsius to **Fahrenheit**, and vice versa.

Figure 6–4 compares the Fahrenheit and Celsius systems of temperature measurement. The freezing point of Celsius is 0 degrees, and the freezing point for Fahrenheit is 32 degrees. On the Celsius scale, the boiling point of water is 100 degrees; it is 212 degrees on the Fahrenheit scale. Normal body temperature on the Celsius scale is 37 degrees, and normal body temperature on the Fahrenheit scale is 98.6 degrees.

Two formulas will assist conversion between the two systems. To convert Fahrenheit to Celsius, use the following formula:

$$\text{Degrees Celsius} = (\text{Degrees Fahrenheit} - 32) \times 0.556$$

Example:

Convert 212 degrees F to Celsius

Solution:

$$C = (212 - 32) \times 0.556 = 100 \text{ degrees}$$

To convert Celsius to Fahrenheit, use this formula:

$$\text{Degrees Fahrenheit} = \text{Degrees Celsius} \times 1.8 + 32$$

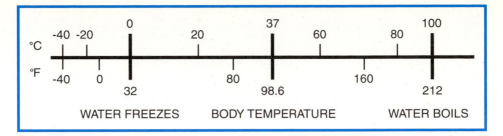

Figure 6–4 How the Fahrenheit and Celsius temperature scales compare. (© Delmar/Cengage Learning)

Example:

Convert 37 degrees C to Fahrenheit

Solution:

$$F = 37 \times 1.8 = 66.6 + 32 = 98.6 \text{ degrees}$$

Pediatric Dosage Calculations

On occasion, a manufacturer's recommended dosage for children is not available. When this occurs, the nomogram is the most accurate method for determining pediatric drug dosages. The nomogram (Figure 6–5) is a chart that uses the weight and height of a child to estimate body surface area (BSA) in square meters (m^2). This body surface area is then placed in a ratio with the body surface area of an average adult (1.73 m^2). The formula used with the nomogram method is:

$$\frac{\text{Pediatric}}{\text{dose}} = \frac{\text{Pediatric BSA in } m^2}{1.73 \ m^2 \ (\text{BSA of average adult})} \times \frac{\text{Adult}}{\text{dose}}$$

To determine the BSA of a pediatric patient, the weight and height of the child must be known. The nomogram scales contain both metric (kg, cm) and U.S. (lb, inches) values for height and weight. Therefore, the BSA can be determined for pounds and inches or kilograms and centimeters without making conversions.

Using the nomogram "Pediatric Nomogram," note the three columns labeled height, body surface area, and weight. To determine BSA, a ruler or straightedge is needed. The following steps illustrate the use of the nomogram.

1. Determine the height and weight of the patient. Remember, this information can be metric, U.S., or a combination of both systems.
2. Place a straightedge on the nomogram connecting the two points on the height and weight scales that represent the patient's values. For example, suppose your patient weighs 26.5 pounds and is 33.5 inches tall. Then, 26.5 pounds on the weight scale and 33.5 inches on the height scale are connected with a straightedge.

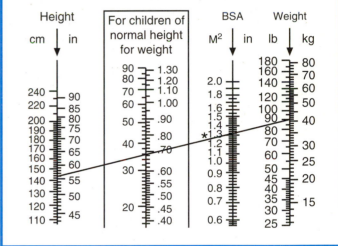

Figure 6–5 Pediatric nomogram.
(© Delmar/Cengage Learning)

3. Where the straightedge crosses the center column (BSA), a reading is taken. In this example, BSA = 0.52 m^2.
4. Substitute the BSA value in the formula to calculate the dosage for the patient. For example, the adult dosage of a particular drug is 500 mg. What is the dose for our patient with a calculated BSA of 0.52 m^2?

$$\begin{aligned}\frac{\text{Pediatric}}{\text{dose}} &= \frac{\text{BSA of child in } m^2}{1.73 \ m^2 \ (\text{BSA of average adult})} \times \frac{\text{Adult}}{\text{dose}} \\ &= \frac{0.52 \ m^2}{1.73 \ m^2} \times 500 \text{ mg} \\ &= 0.3 \times 500 \text{ mg} \\ &= 150 \text{ mg of the drug}\end{aligned}$$

As with anything else, using the nomogram takes practice. But once proficient using the nomogram, it is a useful tool for calculating pediatric drug dosages.

CONCLUSION

When many of us hear the word "math," we immediately have a catecholamine release, sending our stress levels through the roof. The key to feeling comfortable with math is patience and practice.

This chapter presents basic information on which to build. As with any skill, math requires frequent practice to maintain acceptable proficiency levels.

▶ PROBLEM SET A

1. A physician has ordered the administration of 1 mg/kg of a drug to a patient in cardiac arrest. The paramedic estimates that the patient weighs 175 pounds. The drug is packaged as 100 mg in a 5-mL prefilled syringe.
   a. How many milligrams of the drug are required?

   _____

   b. How many milliliters of solution are needed for the required dose?

   _____

2. A paramedic is ordered to administer 0.5 mg of a drug by IV bolus. The drug comes packaged as 1 mg in a 10-mL prefilled syringe. How many milliliters will be given?

   _____

3. A physician orders the administration of a drug infusion. The paramedic is to begin the infusion at 2 mcg/min using a microdrip (60 gtt/min) IV set. The infusion is prepared by adding 1 mg of the drug to 500 mL of normal saline.
   a. What is the concentration of the drug when it is added to the normal saline (mcg/mL)?

   _____

   b. What infusion rate is needed to administer 2 mcg/min?

   _____

4. A physician orders the addition of 800 mg of a drug to 500 mL of normal saline solution. What will be the resulting concentration in mcg/mL?

   _____

5. The paramedic receives an order to administer 20 mg of a drug. The drug comes packaged as 40 mg in a 4-mL prefilled syringe. How many milliliters will be administered?

   _____

6. A physician orders the administration of 5 mg/kg of a drug. The patient weighs 175 pounds. The drug is packaged as 500 mg in a 10-mL vial.
   a. How many milligrams will be administered?

   _____

   b. How many milliliters will be administered?

   _____

▶ PROBLEM SET B

1. The health-care professional has diluted 2 g of a drug in 500 mL of normal saline solution.
   a. What is the resulting concentration (mg/mL)?

   _____

   b. What infusion rate is needed when using a minidrip (60 gtt/min) IV set to deliver 2 mg/min?

   _____

2. The paramedic has a 20% solution of a drug in 500 mL of IV fluid. The physician orders the administration of 1.5 g/kg of the drug to the patient over 1 hour. The patient weighs 120 pounds. Supplied is a 15 gtt/min IV set.
   a. What is the concentration (g/mL) of the solution?

   _____

   b. How many gtt/min will be administered to your patient?

   _____

3. The health-care professional has been ordered to administer 2 L of IV solution over a 3-hour period. How many gtt/min will be administered if the standard IV set yields 10 gtt/min?

_____

4. The paramedic has a patient in severe anaphylactic shock. The physician orders 0.5 mg of a 1:10,000 solution of epinephrine by IV bolus. The epinephrine comes packaged as 1 mg in a 10-mL solution. How many milliliters will be administered?

_____

5. After the administration of the dose in question 4, the paramedic is requested to start an epinephrine infusion. The physician orders 1 mcg/min. Two milligrams of 1:1000 epinephrine are added to 500 mL of IV solution.

a. What is the resulting concentration (mcg/mL)?

_____

b. What infusion rate is needed with a microdrip (60 gtt/min) IV set?

_____

6. The physician orders an IV infusion at a rate of 2 mcg/min. The paramedic prepares the infusion by adding 4 mg of drug to 500 mL of IV solution.

a. What is the resulting concentration (mcg/mL)?

_____

b. What infusion rate is needed with a minidrip (60 gtt/min) IV set?

_____

PRACTICE PROBLEMS

Conversions

1. 50 kg = _____ lb

2. 180 lb = _____ kg

3. 0.2 mg = _____ mcg

4. 3.0 L = _____ mL

5. 0.3 g = _____ mg

6. 10 mL = _____ cc

7. 3.0 g = _____ mg

8. 0.06 g = _____ mg

9. 200 lb = _____ kg

10. 4.0 g = _____ mg

11. 0.03 g = _____ mg

12. 8000 mg = _____ g

13. 200 mL = _____ cc

14. 2.0 mg = _____ mcg

15. 0.1 L = _____ mL

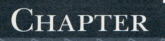

CHAPTER 7

DRUG ADMINISTRATION

OBJECTIVES

On completion of this chapter and the study questions, you should be able to:

- Describe the seven rights of drug administration.
- Describe the advantages and disadvantages of alimentary and parenteral drug administration.
- List and describe the alimentary drug routes.
- List and describe the parenteral drug routes.
- Describe the methods of administering drugs through inhalation.
- Describe the pediatric drug routes.
- Describe special considerations in administering drugs to the pediatric patient.

KEY TERMS

Alimentary route
Bolus
Endotracheal (ET)
Inhalation
Inhaler
Intradermal
Intramuscular (IM)

Intraosseous (IO)
Intravenous (IV)
Intravenous infusion (IV infusion)
Intravenous bolus injection
Local
Piggyback

Prophylactic
Rectal
Small-volume nebulizer
Subcutaneous (SQ or SC)
Sublingual (SL)
Systemic

INTRODUCTION

Drug administration is one of the most important, demanding, and risky functions the EMS professional will perform. He/she is responsible for the interpretation, evaluation of appropriateness, and administration of the drug order. Drug administration requires training, a solid knowledge base, and well-developed decision-making abilities.

To have its intended therapeutic effect, a drug must reach its site of action. To do this, the drug must enter the body, be absorbed into the circulation, and then be transported to the targeted tissues. All these events vary according to the route of administration, which is determined by the amount of drug needed, the rapidity of action desired, and the patient's condition.

There are two ways to introduce drugs into the body: by alimentary routes and *parenteral* routes. In EMS, drugs are most often given by parenteral routes, as these are much more rapid and generally more predictable.

The Drug Order

EMS professionals are required to select, prepare, and give many different medications. Before a drug is given, a thorough patient assessment, including the medication assessment, must be performed. Depending on the type of EMS system, drugs are given by written treatment protocols, standing orders, or by direct contact with medical control. EMS professionals should be familiar with the written protocols and standing orders of their facility. A copy of these documents should be kept with you in case they may be needed for reference. If your patient assessment is not complete or is inaccurate, the wrong drug could be given.

If an EMS professional receives an order from medical control that is different from the protocols, medical control should be contacted to have the order clarified. If the physician at medical control insists on the order, give the drug at the dose ordered, documenting carefully. However, if at any time the drug order will harm the patient, do not give the drug. Instead, tell medical control the rationale for not giving the drug, and thoroughly document the situation.

Seven Rights of Drug Administration

Before administering drugs, EMS professionals must adhere to the *seven rights of drug administration:*

1. The Right drug
2. The Right drug amount
3. The Right patient
4. The Right time
5. The Right route
6. The Right documentation
7. The Rights of the patient

The Right Drug

One of the most common EMS drug administration errors is selecting the incorrect drug. If there are any questions concerning a drug, do not administer it until it has been confirmed. Verify the order with medical control and/or your partner if there is any doubt about the drug to be given.

EMS professionals must be very careful not to inadvertently pick up the wrong drug. Most EMS drugs come packaged as ampules, vials, or prefilled syringes, and many of these look very much alike. After selecting a drug, read the label and inspect the drug three times, verifying the drug name, concentration, expiration date, and the drug's clarity. The first time the drug is checked is when it is selected from its box or cabinet. Check the drug again when preparing the drug. And third, check the drug just prior to administration.

The Right Drug Amount

Another common mistake made by health-care professionals is giving the incorrect dosage of a drug. Most of these errors occur because of calculation or preparation errors. It is very important that EMS professionals are familiar with all the drugs that they may be called upon to use. When preparing to give a drug, be certain to calculate and prepare the drug accurately. If appropriate, have a colleague check your accuracy before the drug is given. Remember, in many cases, accuracy may save more lives than speed.

The Right Patient

Most emergency responses will only involve one patient. However, there will be times when multiple patients are at the scene. It is very important that each patient be distinguished by assigning each a label. For example, you can label numerically (e.g., patient 1, patient 2, etc.) or alphabetically (e.g., patient A, patient B, etc.).

When multiple patients are involved at a scene, not only is it important to correctly identify each patient, but also identify the ambulances as well. Treatment errors will be kept at a minimum by an organized scene management system. Each patient and each ambulance should be identified; this will give medical control a better picture of the scene, and the types of patient treatments given before arrival to the emergency department.

The Right Time

Time is a critical factor when giving drugs. Some drugs may only have to be given one time. However, other drugs, such as epinephrine, are given by **intravenous (IV)** bolus every 3–5 minutes during a cardiac arrest. There also are drugs that are given by IV infusion over a specific period of time. For example, lidocaine may be ordered at 2 mg/min, or aminophylline can be given at 250 mg over 20 minutes. Some drugs should be given by rapid IV bolus, such as adenosine, and some drugs should be given by slow IV bolus, such as morphine. Knowledge of the time factors for each drug to be given will affect the success of the drug therapy. It is a good idea to have a drug reference text available for questions that may arise.

The Right Route

Depending on the emergency, different drugs will be given through different routes. For example, during a cardiac arrest, epinephrine is generally given by IV bolus every 3–5 minutes. However, if an IV cannot be started or is delayed, epinephrine can be given down the endotracheal tube. The initial dose of lidocaine is generally given by IV bolus, and followed with an IV infusion.

There are some drugs that are administered by inhalation, others are given intramuscularly, subcutaneously, or sublingually. A strong knowledge base of each drug's routes of administration is invaluable for EMS personnel.

The Right Documentation

All health-care professionals who come in contact with each patient must know what treatment has already been done, including medications. There is an old saying in EMS; "if it was not written down, it did not happen." All documentation should be completed as soon after treatment as possible. Do not try to rely on your memory when the call is complete. Attempting to provide all documentation after the completion of a call can be detrimental for the patient. The longer the wait to complete documentation, the more likely vital information may be left out or entered incorrectly.

The Rights of the Patient

Do not forget the rights of each patient. Patients have the right to refuse some or all treatment. Also, if a patient elects to accept treatment, he/she has the right to be informed as to what a medication is for, how it works, side effects, and

so forth. Therefore, when appropriate, explain which drug(s) you are giving, why you are giving the drug, and possible side effects the patient may experience.

Venous Access

It is common practice in the management of most injured or ill patients for the EMS professional to establish an IV line. The IV line provides a route for fluid replacement in the injured patient, and provides a route for medications for the patient with a medical disorder. The type of medical emergency will determine the size of the catheter to be used when establishing the IV line. For example, the patient involved in trauma may require a large-bore, 14- or 16-gauge, catheter. On the other hand, the medical patient will only require a smaller, 18- or 20-gauge, catheter. It is important for EMS personnel to try to plan for the future. For example, if a patient may require the infusion of whole blood, a larger catheter must be initially inserted.

Not only is the IV catheter size important, but so is the type of IV administration set to be used. There are two types of IV administration sets, macro- and minidrip sets. The macrodrip set is generally used for the injured patient, while the minidrip set is generally used for medical patients. Macrodrip IV sets can deliver anywhere from 10 to 20 gtt/mL, while the minidrip set delivers 50–60 gtt/mL, depending on the manufacturer.

The IV should be started in a large vein, generally above the wrist. Avoid starting an IV in the hand, as it can be more painful than one in the arm. If, for some reason, an IV cannot be started in the arm, other sites include the leg, and the external jugular in the neck, which are both considered peripheral veins. However, the best vein for IV insertion in the traumatic or cardiac arrest patient is the antecubital vein.

Procedure for Starting an Intravenous Line

1. Observe body substance isolation precautions.
2. Receive, confirm, and write down the order.
3. Prepare the equipment:
   - IV fluid
   - Administration set (macro- or minidrip)
   - Appropriate size indwelling catheter
   - IV extension tubing (some protocols do not use extension tubing for trauma patients)
   - Tourniquet
   - Antibiotic swab
   - 2 × 2 or 4 × 4 sterile gauze pads
   - 1/2- or 1-inch tape
   - Antibiotic ointment
   - Short arm board, if appropriate
4. Remove IV fluid from package. Inspect the fluid for clarity and particulate matter. Do not use if discolored or any presence of particles.
5. Open and inspect the IV tubing.

6. Attach extension tubing if appropriate.
7. Remove the sterile cover from the IV bag and the administration set. Insert the administration set into the IV fluid port.
8. Squeeze the IV tubing drip chamber to fill with fluid, and then bleed the air out of the IV tubing.
9. Close the clamp on the IV tubing.
10. Hang the IV bag or have it held at the appropriate height.
11. If appropriate, attach the tourniquet, occluding the patient's venous blood flow.
12. Select an appropriate vein.
13. Clean the selected site using an antibiotic swab.
14. Make the puncture, observe flashback, and advance the catheter while removing the needle.
15. Connect the IV tubing and remove the tourniquet.
16. Open the IV tubing, confirming fluid is flowing with no evidence of infiltration.
17. Apply antibiotic ointment over the puncture site and cover with sterile gauze or adhesive bandage.
18. Tape the IV catheter and tubing in place.
19. Adjust fluid flow rate.
20. If appropriate, attach short arm board.
21. Label the IV bag with patient name, date, time the IV was started, gauge of the catheter, and your initials.
22. Call medical control to confirm successful completion of the IV.
23. Monitor the patient and report any changes.

Some protocols may require EMS personnel to collect a blood sample when starting the IV. Blood is taken before the IV line is attached to the IV catheter by using a 10-mL syringe. Once the blood has been taken, the syringe is removed and the IV line attached. Blood collection should be done, if at all possible, before the administration of any medicine.

Once the blood has been withdrawn, it is placed into an evacuated blood collection tube. Most of these tubes contain chemicals to prevent the blood from clotting. Each tube has a specific colored rubber top which determines the use of the contents. After the evacuated blood tube is filled, it should be inverted several times in order to mix thoroughly with the chemical. The patient's name, date, time sampled, and EMS personnel name should be noted on the tube. If necessary, the tubes may be taped to the IV bag for transport.

Drug Administration Routes

Alimentary Tract Routes

Oral

As explained in Chapter 1, oral (PO) administration of drugs provides the most convenient, safe, and economic way to get drugs into the body. Although some orally administered drugs are absorbed from the stomach and colon, most are absorbed from the small intestines. Because they must travel through the mouth, throat, and stomach before entering the bloodstream, the onset of action of oral drugs is slower. The delay in onset sometimes means a decrease in, or a lack of, therapeutic effects. Therefore, when a rapid therapeutic effect is required, such as in life-threatening emergencies, parenteral drug administration is preferred.

Rectal

Rectal drug administration can have either local or systemic effects. Systemic drug absorption from rectal administration, however, can be incomplete and unpredictable, especially if the patient is unable to retain the drug. For two reasons, rectal drug administration quickly results in a high concentration of the drug in the circulation. First, the rectum contains a rich network of capillaries. Second, because venous blood from the lower part of the rectum does not pass through the liver, drugs absorbed in the rectum are not biotransformed in the liver before reaching other body sites.

Rectal drug administration may be necessary when oral administration is unsuitable, for example, unconscious or nauseated patients or small children who are unable to swallow drugs. An example of a drug administered rectally is promethazine (Phenergan), used in the treatment of motion sickness, as a sedative, and as an antiemetic.

Rectal drug administration is usually not performed in the out-of-hospital setting.

Parenteral Routes

Sublingual

To administer a drug sublingually (SL), place it under the patient's tongue and give instructions to keep it there until it is dissolved and absorbed into the capillaries.

The underside of the tongue is rich in capillaries, which permits rapid absorption, and therefore, quick drug action. Sublingual drug administration permits the drug to enter the general circulation without passing through the liver or being affected by gastric and intestinal enzymes. This yields a higher concentration of the drug in the circulation than does oral administration.

Obviously the tongue is in the mouth, which is the beginning of the alimentary tract. However, because the drug is absorbed through the mucosa of the tongue, and directly into the circulation without interference from gastric enzymes and other material found in the alimentary tract, the sublingual drug route is considered a parenteral route. An example of an EMS drug administered sublingually, is nitroglycerin, used to treat anginal attacks and for the long-term prophylactic management of angina pectoris. (*Prophylactics* are designed to prevent illness or disease.)

Transdermal Infusion

Transdermal infusion is a method of administering drugs by placing the drug in a special gel-like matrix that is applied to the skin. The drug is absorbed through the skin into the bloodstream at a fixed rate. Each application can provide medicine for one to several days. Nitroglycerin and analgesics are commonly administered through transdermal infusion.

Intradermal

Intradermal administration is the injection of a drug into the upper layers of the skin, with the needle almost parallel to the skin surface. These injections are usually done with a fine, short (5/8-inch by 26- to 27-gauge) needle and a small-barrel (1-mL) syringe. Intradermal drug administration is used to provide local effects for the treatment of allergies or to perform allergy skin testing. The amount of drug that can be injected intradermally is small; the rate of absorption is slow because absorption is limited to the capillaries of the dermis.

Subcutaneous

A **subcutaneous (SC/SQ)** injection is performed by inserting a small needle (1/2 to 5/8 inches long, with a gauge of 25 or less) into the fatty tissue above the muscle. Usually, the largest dose that can be injected by this method is 2 mL. Subcutaneous injection causes minimal tissue trauma and avoids damage to large blood vessels and nerves. Figure 7–1 illustrates the common subcutaneous injection sites.

Drug absorption after a subcutaneous injection largely depends on the physical condition of the patient. For example, subcutaneous injection is undesirable for patients with compromised circulatory perfusion, for instance, patients in shock or patients with peripheral vascular disease.

An example of an EMS drug administered by subcutaneous injection is epinephrine (1:1000 solution) used in treating bronchoconstriction associated with anaphylaxis (see Chapter 9).

Intramuscular

Intramuscular (IM) injection is the most common method of administering parenteral drugs. However, it is not common in the out-of-hospital setting. The drug is injected deep into the muscle tissue, where it is absorbed into the capillaries and enters the bloodstream. Drug doses of up to 5 mL can be given via the intramuscular route; this requires needles of 21- to 23-gauge and 1 to 1 1/2 inches in length. If larger amounts of a drug are to be given, it is better to use two injection sites. Figure 7–2 illustrates common sites for intramuscular drug administration.

The rate of absorption of a drug administered by intramuscular injection depends on the physical condition of the patient. For example, intramuscular injection may be contraindicated for patients with decreased peripheral perfusion or inadequate muscle mass. On the other hand, intramuscular drug administration usually yields a predictable absorption rate.

In emergencies in which an intravenous line cannot be established, intramuscular injection is sometimes the answer. For example, EMS personnel can use intramuscular injection to administer thiamine to patients in a coma of unknown origin or a coma caused by alcohol, and to patients suffering delerium tremens. There is also the option of sedating the patient before an IV is started in difficult situations.

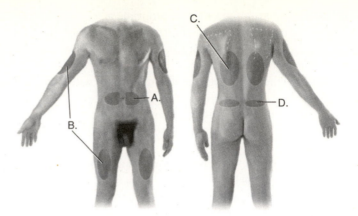

Figure 7–1 Subcutaneous injection sites.
(© Delmar/Cengage Learning)

Intravenous

When the situation calls for a rapid therapeutic effect, intravenous (IV) injection allows direct administration of a drug directly into the bloodstream, either as a **bolus** or as an infusion. A bolus is one dose of a drug injected into the vein all at once. Continuous infusion is the controlled introduction (at a specific rate) of a drug into the bloodstream over a period of time. Continuous infusion is a way to keep the amount of drug available to body tissues at a constant level. Most out-of-hospital emergency drugs are administered by intravenous injection.

Drug administration by intravenous bolus yields quick, predictable therapeutic concentrations, which makes it the route of choice in most emergency situations. However, the rapidity of absorption of an intravenous bolus carries the risk of producing immediate adverse reactions and side effects.

The rate of an intravenous infusion can be set to maintain therapeutic levels of a drug. In some emergency situations, the physician or paramedic first gives an intravenous bolus to achieve therapeutic levels quickly, then uses an **intravenous infusion** to maintain those established levels. For instance, lidocaine is administered in this way to treat ventricular fibrillation. The bolus of lidocaine is used to produce therapeutic levels as quickly as possible. Once circulation has been restored, an infusion maintains the established therapeutic level of lidocaine in the bloodstream.

Transtracheal

Some emergency drugs can be administered down an **endotracheal (ET)** tube when an intravenous line cannot be started or cannot be established quickly enough. Drugs given down the endotracheal tube are absorbed into the capillaries of the lungs. When endotracheal administration is done correctly, the rate of absorption of the drug is just as rapid as when the drug is given by intravenous injection. Drugs that can be administered down the endotracheal tube

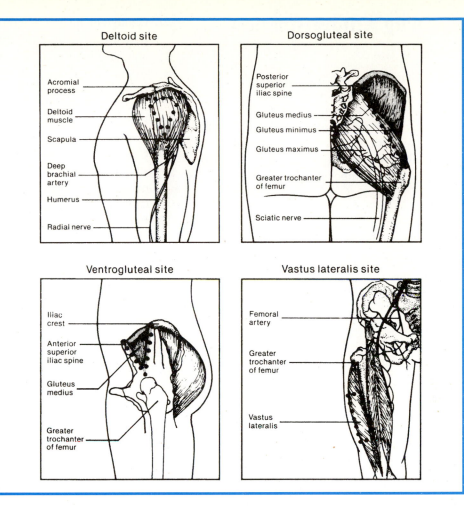

Figure 7–2 Intramuscular injection sites. (© Delmar/Cengage Learning)

include: epinephrine, lidocaine, atropine, and naloxone. When giving these drugs down the endotracheal tube, the dosages are 2–2.5 times the intravenous dosages.

Intraosseous

Intraosseous (IO) administration is a safe, rapid, and effective way to introduce fluids and drugs into the bloodstream via the highly vascular bone marrow. The paramedic can establish an intraosseous line at the proximal tibia (the preferred site), distal femur, or distal tibia of a pediatric patient with circulatory failure or cardiac arrest. Currently in EMS, this procedure is generally performed on patients 5 years of age or younger, who are unconscious, unresponsive, and in immediate danger of dying. In most cases, the intraosseous line should not be attempted until at least two attempts at establishing a peripheral intravenous line have failed.

Currently, there are studies in place that are using the intraosseous route on adult patients. The intraosseous line is established at the midsternum of the adult patient who is unresponsive, and when an intravenous line has failed to be established.

Inhalation

Inhalation administration may involve giving drugs, water vapors, and gases into the lungs. An inhaler may be used to administer drugs to the lungs. An **inhaler** is a small hand-held device, usually an aerosol unit, that contains a microcrystalline suspension of a drug. When used, the inhaler produces a fine mist or spray containing the drug. This suspension is drawn into the respiratory tract and down into the alveoli.

Drugs that utilize an inhaler include: bronchodilators, mucolytic (expectorants) agents, and steroids. Inhalers are useful for treating chronic obstructive pulmonary disease (COPD) and reversible obstructive airway disease.

Another inhalation device used during emergencies to administer drugs is called a **small-volume nebulizer**. The small-volume nebulizer has a chamber where the drug is placed, usually with 2 to 3 mL of sterile saline solution. As oxygen is blown past the chamber, the drug is aerosolized and the patient inhales the drug with each breath. This system allows both the drug and oxygen to be inhaled simultaneously.

Common Drug Administration Techniques

Most emergency drugs are given parenterally, by the intravenous, transtracheal, intraosseous, intramuscular, or subcutaneous route. Because of the advances in protocols and the increase in medical facilities employing EMS professionals as health-care providers, it is becoming more important to be familiar with all common drug routes and administration techniques. Always remember the seven rights of drug administration.

Subcutaneous Injection

1. Perform a thorough patient assessment and history, confirming: that the drug is needed, and that the patient does not have any allergies that contraindicate the use of the drug.
2. Receive, write down, and confirm the order.
3. Calculate the required dosage.
4. Prepare the appropriate equipment:
   - Drug
   - 1- to 2-mL syringe
   - 5/8-inch by 25-gauge needle
   - Antibacterial swab and ointment and alcohol prep
   - 2 × 2 or 4 × 4 gauze pads
   - Adhesive bandage strip
   - Sharps container
5. Explain the procedure to the patient.
6. Examine the drug, reconfirming that:
   - It is the correct medication.
   - It has not expired.
   - It is not discolored.
   - There are no visible particles in the solution.
7. Gently tap the upper part of the ampule or shake the ampule down, forcing the drug to the lower portion of the ampule.* Figure 7–3 illustrates the withdrawal of a drug from an ampule.
8. Using a gauze pad or alcohol prep to protect your hand, break off the top of the ampule.
9. Draw the drug into the syringe and expel any excess air from it.
10. Choose a suitable administration site. A commonly used site is the subcutaneous tissue over the triceps brachii muscle on the back of the arm.
11. Cleanse the site with an antibacterial swab.
12. Pinch the skin and insert the needle at a 45-degree angle (Figure 7–4).
13. Aspirate the syringe (gently pull the plunger back to create suction) to make sure that the needle is not in a blood vessel. If blood enters the syringe, withdraw the needle and prepare another site for another attempt, *using a new needle.*
14. Inject the drug slowly.
15. Remove and properly dispose of the needle.
16. Gently massage the injection site. (This aids in drug absorption, as well as patient comfort.)
17. Cover the site with an adhesive bandage strip.
18. Confirm and document administration of the drug.
19. Closely monitor the patient and report any changes.

*Some drugs come in a vial instead of an ampule. Figure 7–5 illustrates the procedure for withdrawing a drug from a vial. When withdrawing a drug from a vial, first clean the rubber stopper with an antibacterial swab. Insert the needle and inject a volume of air into the vial equal to the volume of drug you need to withdraw. For example, if you need 4 mL of a drug, inject 4 mL of air into the vial. Doing so makes it easier to draw the drug into the syringe.

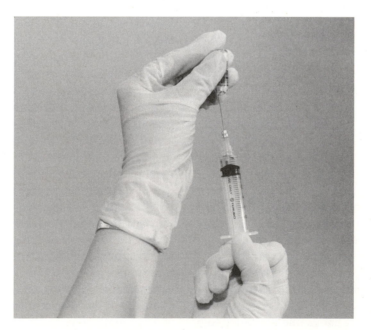

Figure 7–3 Withdrawing a drug from an ampule. (© Delmar/Cengage Learning)

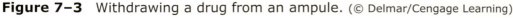

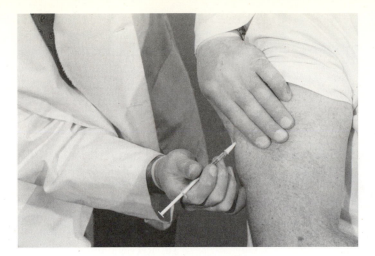

Figure 7–4 Subcutaneous injection. (© Delmar/Cengage Learning)

Intramuscular Injection

In most cases, intramuscular injections should be avoided when the patient's chief complaint is chest pain. An intramuscular injection may cause a rise in the amount of certain muscle enzymes circulating within the bloodstream. The level of these enzymes can help the physician determine if a myocardial infarction (MI) is the cause of the patient's chest pain. An intramuscular injection in the out-of-hospital setting may confuse the picture when measurements of muscle enzymes are evaluated at the hospital. The procedure for intramuscular administration of drugs is as follows:

1. Perform a thorough patient assessment and history, confirming that the drug is needed, and that the patient does not have any allergies that contraindicate the use of the drug.
2. Receive, write down, and confirm the order.
3. Calculate the required dosage.
4. Prepare the appropriate equipment:
   - Drug
   - Appropriate size syringe (1- to 3-mL)
   - 1- to 1 1/2-inch by 21- to 23-gauge needle
   - Antibacterial swab and ointment and alcohol prep
   - 2 × 2 or 4 × 4 inch gauze pads
   - Adhesive bandage strip
   - Sharps container
5. Explain the procedure to the patient.
6. Examine the drug, reconfirming that:
   - It is the correct drug
   - It has not expired
   - It is not discolored
   - There are no visible particles in the solution
7. Gently tap the upper part of the ampule or shake the ampule down, forcing the drug to the lower part of the ampule.

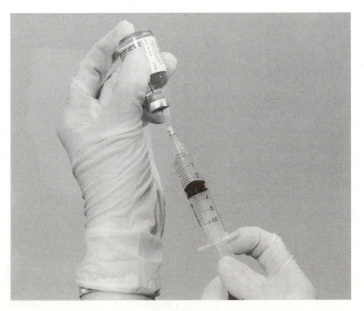

Figure 7–5 Withdrawing a drug from a vial. (© Delmar/Cengage Learning)

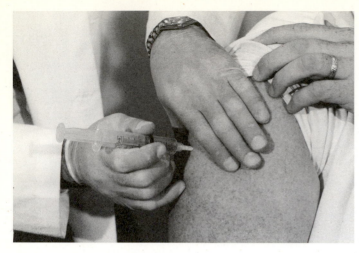

Figure 7–6 Intramuscular injection.
(© Delmar/Cengage Learning)

8. Using a gauze pad or an alcohol prep to protect your hand, break off the top of the ampule.
9. Draw the drug into the syringe and expel any excess air from it.
10. Choose a suitable administration site. A commonly used site is the deltoid muscle of the arm.
11. Cleanse the administration site with an antibacterial swab.
12. Insert the needle into the tissue at a 90-degree angle (Figure 7–6).
13. Aspirate the syringe to make sure the needle is not in a blood vessel. If blood enters the syringe, withdraw the needle and prepare another site for another attempt, *using a new needle.*
14. Inject the drug slowly.
15. Remove and properly dispose of the needle.
16. Gently massage the injection site. (This aids in drug absorption as well as patient comfort.)
17. Cover the site with an adhesive bandage strip.
18. Confirm and document administration of the drug.
19. Closely monitor the patient and report any changes.

Intravenous Bolus Injection

Once an intravenous infusion (intravenous lifeline) has been established, this enables the administration of a bolus injection through the intravenous line. This procedure is called an **intravenous bolus injection**. In the following description of the procedure, the bolus is packaged in a single-dose, prefilled syringe. In most emergency situations, this is the case. Sometimes, however, the necessary drug is available only in an ampule or vial, from which you must draw the proper dose.

1. Perform a thorough patient assessment and history, confirming: that the drug is needed, and that the patient does not have any allergies that contraindicate the use of the drug.
2. Receive, write down, and confirm the order.

3. Prepare the appropriate equipment:
   • Correct drug (prefilled syringe with needle)
   • Antibacterial swab and alcohol prep
4. Explain the procedure to the patient.
5. Examine the drug, reconfirming that:
   • It is the correct drug
   • It has not expired
   • It is not discolored
   • There are no visible particles in the solution
6. Calculate the required dosage.
7. Assemble the prefilled syringe and expel any excess air.
8. Verify the patency of the intravenous line.
9. Clean the medication port on the intravenous administration set using an antibacterial swab.
10. Recheck the drug.
11. Insert the needle into the medication port (Figure 7–7).
12. Pinch the tubing off above the medication port.
13. Administer the drug at the appropriate rate. (Rates differ among different types of drugs.)
14. Remove the needle and clean the administration port with an antibacterial swab; properly dispose of the needle and syringe.
15. Release the pinched intravenous line.
16. Flush the intravenous line by opening the line wide open for 30 seconds to 1 minute.
17. Confirm and document administration of the drug.
18. Closely monitor the patient and report any changes.

Intravenous Infusion (Piggyback)

1. Perform a thorough patient assessment and history, confirming that the drug is needed, and that the patient does not have any allergies that contraindicate the use of the drug.
2. Receive, write down, and confirm the order.
3. Prepare the appropriate equipment:
   • Correct drug (prefilled syringe with needle)
   • Antibacterial swab and alcohol prep
   • Label for the intravenous bag

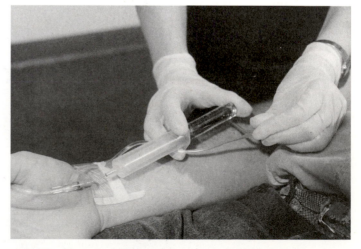

Figure 7–7 Intravenous bolus injection.
(© Delmar/Cengage Learning)

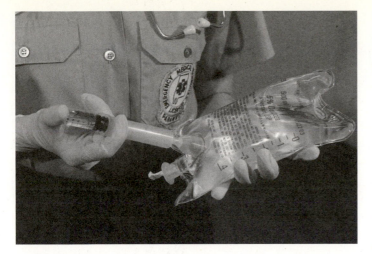

Figure 7–8 Adding medication to an intravenous bag. (© Delmar/Cengage Learning)

4. Explain the procedure to the patient.
5. Examine the drug, reconfirming that:
   - It is the correct drug
   - It has not expired
   - It is not discolored
   - There are no visible particles in the solution
6. Recheck the drug.
7. Assemble the prefilled syringe.
8. Clean the medication port on the intravenous bag with an antibacterial swab.
9. Insert the needle into the medication port of the bag and add the drug (Figure 7–8).
10. Remove the needle and cleanse the administration port with an antibacterial swab; properly dispose of the syringe and needle.
11. Thoroughly mix the drug in the intravenous bag.
12. Attach an intravenous line to the bag, "prime" the line, and attach a 1-inch by 18-gauge needle to the line.
13. Clean the medication port of the already-established intravenous line with an antibacterial swab, insert the needle, and secure with tape (Figure 7–9).

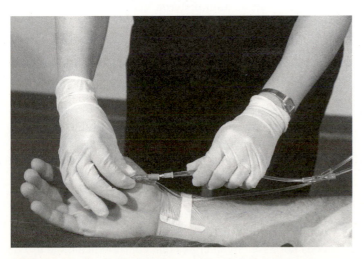

Figure 7–9 Intravenous piggyback infusion. (© Delmar/Cengage Learning)

14. Shut down the previously established intravenous line and begin flow of the piggyback drug line; set the flow to the necessary rate.
15. Label the piggyback intravenous bag with:
    - The patient's name
    - The date and time that the piggyback infusion was established
    - The name and amount of the drug added to the piggyback intravenous bag
    - The infusion flow rate
    - The name of the person who established the piggyback infusion
16. Confirm and document the establishment of the piggyback infusion.
17. Monitor the patient and report any changes.

Transtracheal Administration

1. Receive, write down, and confirm the order.
2. Examine the drug, reconfirming that:
   - It is the correct drug
   - It has not expired
   - It is not discolored
   - There are no visible particles in the solution
3. Assemble the prefilled syringe.
4. Remove the bag-valve-mask device and inject the correct amount of the drug into the endotracheal tube. Properly dispose of the needle and syringe. If the drug order is for a small dose, and you must withdraw the drug from an ampule or vial, dilute the drug with 5 to 10 mL of sterile normal saline solution or sterile water.
5. Replace the bag-valve-mask device and hyperventilate to force the drug down the tube. (Note that some endotracheal tubes have medication ports built into them.)
6. Resume normal ventilations.
7. Confirm and document the administration of the drug.
8. Monitor the patient and report any changes.

Intraosseous Infusion

Intraosseous infusion allows rapid vascular access via the bone marrow. It is used mostly to administer fluids and drugs to children 5 years of age and younger who are suffering from circulatory failure or cardiac arrest. All drugs and crystalloid solutions that can be administered intravenously can also be given by the intraosseous route.

1. Receive, write down, and confirm the order.
2. Prepare the appropriate equipment:
   - Intravenous solution, intravenous tubing, and a stopcock
   - Spinal or bone-marrow needle with a stylet (15- to 18-gauge)
   - Syringe filled with normal saline
   - Antibacterial swab and alcohol preps
3. Examine the solution, reconfirming:
   - It is the correct solution
   - It has not expired

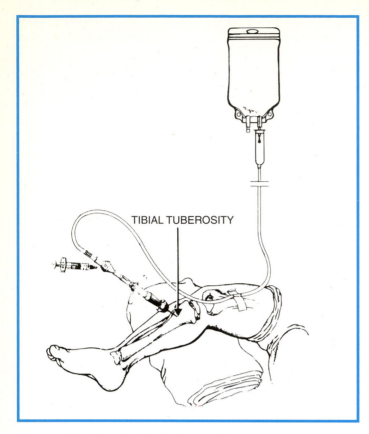

Figure 7–10 Preferred site for intraosseous drug administration (proximal tibia). (© Delmar/Cengage Learning)

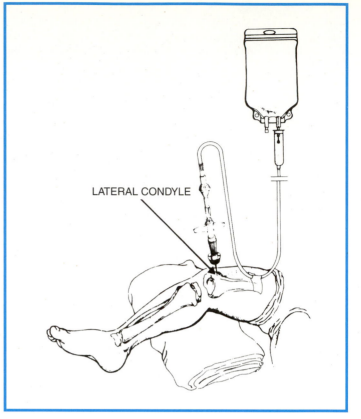

Figure 7–11 Intraosseous drug administration (distal femur). (© Delmar/Cengage Learning)

- It is not discolored
- There are no visible particles in the solution
4. Attach a line to the bag, prime the line, and attach the needle.
5. Identify bony landmarks. For example:
   - The proximal tibia: The needle will enter 1 to 3 centimeters below the tibial tuberosity just beneath the knee (Figure 7–10). The proximal tibia is the preferred site for three reasons: (1) The prominence of the bone makes it easy to find the right injection site. (2) There is little soft tissue over the bone. (3) The flat surface of the bone makes for easier needle insertion.
   - The distal femur: The needle will enter 3 centimeters above the lateral condyle just above the knee (Figure 7–11).
   - The distal tibia: The needle will enter in the flat surface of the tibia 1 to 3 centimeters above the medial malleolus at the ankle (Figure 7–12).
6. Clean the site with an antibacterial swab.
7. Insert the needle with stylet in place at a 90-degree angle to the bone or at a slight angle *away* from the joint. This is to avoid inserting the needle into the growth plate.
8. Remove the stylet.
9. Attempt to aspirate bone marrow. If no marrow enters the needle, inject a small amount of saline solution into the site. If there is resistance to the injection, or if saline

solution infiltrates the soft tissue around the site, the needle is not in the bone marrow.
10. Stabilize the needle (although it should stand unsupported).
11. Connect the tubing and begin the infusion.
12. Confirm and document the establishment of the intraosseous infusion.
13. Monitor the patient and report any changes.

Once the intraosseous infusion has been established, drugs can be administered via intravenous bolus or piggyback.

Intravenous Access via the External Jugular Vein

The external jugular vein in the neck connects into the central circulation via the subclavian vein. Fluids and drugs reach the central circulation of the body rapidly when administered via the external jugular vein. Intravenous access via the external jugular vein should only be done on the unresponsive patient.

1. Perform a thorough patient assessment and history, confirming that the drug is needed, and that the patient does not have any allergies that contraindicate the use of the drug.
2. Receive, write down, and confirm the order.

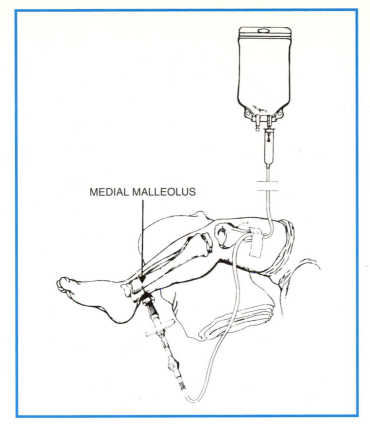

MEDIAL MALLEOLUS

Figure 7-12 Intraosseous drug administration (distal tibia). (© Delmar/Cengage Learning)

3. Prepare the appropriate equipment:
   - Appropriate intravenous fluid and administration set
   - Appropriate indwelling catheter
   - Antibacterial swab and ointment and alcohol preps
   - Sterile gauze pads
   - 1/2- to 1-inch tape
   - Sharps container
4. Position the patient supine, with the head turned away from the side to be cannulated.
5. After locating the vein, prepare the site.
6. Apply gentle traction on the vein just below the clavicle.
7. Approach the site midway between the angle of the jaw and the clavicle, aiming toward the shoulder, and puncture at a 30-degree angle.
8. Upon entry into the vein, note a flashback of blood, and advance the needle and catheter approximately 2 mm to stabilize the needle in the vein.
9. Remove the needle and properly dispose in the sharps container.
10. Connect the intravenous tubing and slowly open to allow fluid to flow. Confirm that the fluid is flowing freely without evidence of infiltration.
11. Apply antibacterial ointment and cover with sterile gauze pad or adhesive bandage.
12. Use tape to secure the intravenous tubing and catheter in place.

13. Adjust flow rate.
14. Confirm and document the successful completion of the infusion.
15. Monitor the patient and report any changes.

Patient-Administered Nitrous Oxide–Oxygen Mixture

Inhalation of a 50% mixture of nitrous oxide and oxygen produces central nervous system depression, as well as rapid pain relief.

1. Perform a thorough patient assessment and history, confirming: that the drug is needed, and that the patient does not have any allergies or medical conditions that contraindicate the use of the drug.
2. Prepare the appropriate equipment:
   - Nitrous oxide tank
   - Oxygen tank
   - Demand-valve with attached face mask
3. Open the valves on both tanks.
4. Explain the procedure to the patient, and advise the patient of the possible side effects that may be experienced.
5. Place the patient in a sitting position and instruct the patient on the use of the device.
6. Explain that if the patient begins to feel uncomfortable, to remove the mask and breath normally.
7. Monitor the patient and report any changes.

Epinephrine Autoinjector

Many people who experience allergic reactions carry epinephrine autoinjectors. The adult dose delivered from one of these autoinjectors is 0.3 mg of epinephrine. The pediatric autoinjector dose is 0.15 mg of epinephrine. There may be instances when the EMS professional will be required to use the autoinjector to administer the epinephrine.

1. Perform a thorough patient assessment and history, confirming that the drug is needed, and that the patient does not have any allergies that contraindicate the use of the drug.
2. Receive, write down, and confirm the order.
3. Explain the procedure to the patient.
4. Examine the autoinjector for name, dose, and expiration date.
5. Remove the safety cap from the autoinjector and place on the patient's outer thigh.
6. Press until you hear the autoinjector function. Hold in place for approximately 5 seconds.
7. Gently massage the injection site for approximately 15 seconds.
8. Monitor the patient and report any changes.

Umbilical Vein Catheterization

In cases when the neonate patient (less than 1 week of age) is in need of an intravenous line and/or medications and peripheral access is impossible, the umbilical vein route can be used.

1. Perform a thorough patient assessment and history, confirming that the infusion is needed.
2. Receive, write down, and confirm the order.
3. Prepare the appropriate equipment:
   - Intravenous fluid and administration set
   - Indwelling catheter
   - Antibacterial swab and ointment and alcohol preps
   - Sterile gauze pads
   - 1/2- to 1-inch tape
   - Sharps container
4. Explain to the patient's caregiver(s) the procedure and the possible complications that might result.
5. If necessary, restrain the child.
6. Clean and drape the umbilicus and umbilical area.
7. Loosely tie umbilical tape around base of the umbilicus.
8. There are two umbilical arteries and one umbilical vein. Locate the umbilical vein. It has a thin wall and larger lumen compared with the thick walls and small lumen of the umbilical arteries. Trim the umbilical vein approximately 1 cm to provide a fresh opening.
9. Insert the tip of a sterile hemostat into the lumen of the umbilical vein, and gently open the hemostat to dilate the vein.
10. Advance a heparintized-saline flushed umbilical catheter into the umbilical vein approximately 2 to 4 inches, noting blood return. The catheter is now in the inferior vena cava of the child.
11. Attach a three-way stopcock to the catheter and flush with 1 mL of heparin solution.
12. Secure the catheter with umbilical tape.
13. Attach the intravenous line to the stopcock to allow for the administration of fluids and drugs.
14. Monitor the child and report any changes.

Drug Administration to the Pediatric Patient

Drug administration to the pediatric population requires special consideration. A standard drug dosage is nearly nonexistent in children. One reason for this is that drug metabolism in the liver of neonates is slow because of immaturity. When children reach the age of 1, most pharmacokinetic patterns are similar to those of the adult, except for those of the liver. At age 1, liver metabolizing enzymes are increased, causing children to metabolize drugs at a faster rate than adults. Children generally reach adult metabolizing parameters at puberty. Therefore, drugs primarily eliminated by metabolism through the liver (hepatic) may require dosage adjustments or may require an increase in the dosing frequency.

Renal excretion is decreased for children under 1 year of age. Adult parameters for glomerular filtration are reached between 3 and 6 months. Tubular filtration does not mature for children until approximately 1 year of age. The renal excretion rate during childhood may increase and exceed that of the adult. This may cause drug under-dosing problems.

Drugs are generally ordered according to either body weight or the body surface area of children. However, calculations based on the child's body weight are generally inaccurate. Therefore, ordering drugs based on body surface area (BSA) should be used. The BSA nomogram utilizes conversions from weight and height to determine drug dosages for children. Using the weight and height relationship, the BSA nomogram can provide a more precise guide to the maturity of the child's organs and metabolic rate of functioning for pharmacokinetics. Drug dosing should be focused to the individual child according to the amount of drug per square meter of body surface area. The BSA rule for pediatric dosages is:

Approximate pediatric dose = Child's BSA in square meters × Adult dose/1.73

For example, using the BSA nomogram, a child with a weight of 10 kg and a height of 34 inches is considered to have a BSA (m^2) of 0.5. The dosage calculation is:

Child's approximate dose = 0.5 × Adult dose/1.73

Drug Administration to the Geriatric Patient

As people become older, they undergo a variety of physiologic changes that may increase their sensitivity to drugs. The loss of body weight, for example, may require initiation of therapy of a lower adult dose. Some older patients are obese, some weigh no more than a large child, and some weigh more and some weigh less. Yet, some of these patients are prescribed the standard adult doses. Other physiologic changes that may occur with age include:

- Blood-brain barrier: easily penetrated by fat-soluble drugs. This may cause confusion.
- Baroreceptor response: reduced response exaggerates the hypotensive effects of antihypertensives.
- Liver: reduced size can result in toxicity of some drugs.
- Kidneys: decreased blood flow can cause normal dosages to actually become toxic.
- Poor peripheral venous tone: exaggerates the hypotensive effects of antihypertensive drugs.
- Stomach: slower stomach emptying and an increase in gastric pH can cause stomach irritation with some drugs.

Estimates have suggested that up to 80% of adverse drug reactions in the geriatric population are dose related. The physiologic changes related to aging may result in a decrease in drug metabolism, poor distribution in the body, and poor renal excretion.

Contaminated Sharps and Equipment Disposal

Body fluids can contain infectious material that not only endangers EMS personnel, but family, friends, and bystanders. Because the patient may be infected with a pathogen without showing any signs or symptoms, EMS professionals must treat every patient as though he or she is infected.

Starting intravenous fluids and administering drugs involves coming in contact with needles and body fluids. One of the most common problems in health care is inadvertent needle sticks. Needle sticks can easily transmit diseases between the patient and EMS personnel. It is extremely important that needles and other sharps are properly handled before and after each patient use. There are some common-sense precautions that must be taken while using sharps.

- *Slow down:* more lives are saved because of accuracy, not speed. That is also true when it comes to handling sharps and avoiding accidents. When using sharps, take the time to perform the task correctly and safely. You must also be aware of the sudden bumps, turns, and so forth that you encounter in the back of an ambulance or in a helicopter. These environments can create hazards that can contribute to accidents using sharps. Remember, we have a tendency to make more mistakes when in a hurry.
- *Immediately dispose of used sharps:* never throw used sharps on the floor, on the "buddy" bench, or anywhere other than in an approved sharps container.
- *Avoid recapping needles:* this is especially true in a moving vehicle. If a needle must be recapped, never use two hands. Use only one hand on a stable surface.

CONCLUSION

EMS personnel must be knowledgeable and competent in every drug administration procedure called upon to perform. Again, a strong knowledge base of medical protocols and the routes of each medication is essential. When an emergency arises, time is precious. In an emergency, the EMS professional is required to quickly identify the drug(s) to be given, the necessary dosage, and the most appropriate route. It is important to build a knowledge base that allows comfort with the protocols and drugs administered routinely within the EMS system. Practice and prepare extensively to be able to administer drugs in a safe, rapid, and systematic manner.

STUDY QUESTIONS

1. You have responded to a patient in cardiac arrest. Why is an intramuscular injection not recommended for this situation?

2. The rate of action of a drug is determined by the drug concentration and the route by which the drug is administered. Of the four routes of drug administration listed below, which lists routes in order from fastest to slowest rate of drug absorption?
   a. Intramuscular, oral, subcutaneous, intravenous
   b. Intravenous, endotracheal, oral, intramuscular
   c. Oral, subcutaneous, intramuscular, intravenous
   d. Intraosseous, intramuscular, subcutaneous, oral

3. Which of the following steps is not appropriate when administering a drug by intravenous bolus injection?
   a. Verify the patency of the intravenous line before administering the drug
   b. Pinch the intravenous tubing off above the medication injection port
   c. Flush the intravenous line after drug administration
   d. Recap the needle and save the unused drug

4. Explain why the BSA nomogram is preferred over using a child's body weight formula for calculating drug dosage.

5. List the seven rights of drug administration, and explain the importance of each.

6. As an EMS professional treating the geriatric population, discuss the alterations in health status of concern with drug therapies.

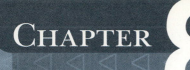

◁ ◁ ◁ ◁ ◁ ◁ ◁ ◁ ◁ ◁ ◁ ◁ ◁ ◁ ◁ ◁ ◁ ◁ ◁

CHAPTER 8

THERAPEUTIC DRUG CLASSIFICATIONS

Therapeutic Drug Classifications

OBJECTIVES

On completion of this chapter and the study questions, you should be able to:
- Describe and list the mechanisms of action for each drug classification in the chapter.
- Describe and list the indications for each drug classification in the chapter.
- Describe and list the contraindications for each drug classification in the chapter.
- Describe and list the precautions for each drug classification in the chapter.
- Describe and list the side effects for each drug classification in the chapter.
- Define amebicides and trichomonacides.
- Define antihypertensive.
- Define and discuss the importance of vitamins.

KEY TERMS

Alkylating drugs
Alpha$_1$-adrenergic blocking drugs
Amebicides
Aminoglycosides
Amphetamines and derivatives
Angiotensin-converting enzyme (ACE) inhibitors
Antianemic drugs
Antianginal drugs—nitrates/nitrites
Antiarrhythmic drugs
Anticoagulants
Anticonvulsants
Antidiabetic drugs: hypoglycemic drugs (oral)
Antidiabetic drugs: insulins
Antihistamines (H$_1$ blockers)
Antihyperlipidemic drugs—HMG—CoA reductase inhibitors
Antihypertensive drugs

Antibiotics
Antimalarial drugs
Antineoplastic (chemotherapeutic) drugs
Antipsychotic drugs, phenothiazines
Antithyroid drugs
Antiviral drugs
Barbiturates
Beta-adrenergic blocking drugs
Calcium channel blocking drugs
Calcium salts
Cardiac glycosides
Cephalosporins
Cholinergic blocking drugs
Corticosteroids
Diuretics, loop
Diuretics, thiazides
Estrogens
Histamine H$_2$ antagonists

Laxatives
Narcotic analgesics
Narcotic antagonists
Neuromuscular blocking drugs
Nonsteroidal anti-inflammatory drugs
Penicillins
Skeletal muscle relaxants, centrally acting
Sympathomimetic adrenergic drugs
Tetracyclines
Theophylline derivatives
Thyroid drugs
Tranquilizers/antimanic drugs/hypnotics
Trichomonacides
Tricyclic antidepressant drugs
Vitamins

INTRODUCTION

The classification of a drug is the pharmacologic class to which the drug has been assigned. This information is useful in learning to categorize drugs. For example, the drug albuterol is classified as a sympathomimetic. Sympathomimetics stimulate beta$_2$-receptors of the bronchi, leading to bronchodilation. Therefore, whenever a drug (albuterol, epinephrine, terbutaline) is classified as a sympathomimetic, the reader should know how the drug works, or its mechanism of action. Understanding the drug classification should make it easier to rationalize and understand when to use a drug, its contraindications, and precautions.

The drug classifications contained in this chapter are broad-based and cover many subclassifications that are covered under the individual drugs. For example, the drug epinephrine is a sympathomimetic. However, it can also be classified as a direct-acting adrenergic drug, as well as a bronchodilator. These subclassifications are covered when epinephrine is presented (not in this chapter), thereby eliminating unnecessary duplication.

Therapeutic Drug Classifications

Alkylating Drugs

Mechanism of Action

Alkylating drugs donate an alkyl radical (carbonium ion) in place of a hydrogen atom to biologically important macromolecules resulting in inactivation of the molecule, and halting cell division. This affects replication of cancerous and other cells, especially in rapidly proliferating tissues, such as the bone marrow and intestinal epithelium.

Indications for Use

Alkylating drugs are used in treating certain types of malignancies.

EMS Considerations

See also Antineoplastic drugs.

Alpha$_1$-Adrenergic Blocking Drugs

Mechanism of Action

Alpha$_1$-adrenergic blocking drugs block postsynaptic alpha$_1$-adrenergic receptors. This results in dilation of both arterioles and veins that lead to a decrease in B/P (especially diastolic B/P).

Indications

Alpha$_1$-adrenergic blocking drugs can be used alone or in combination with diuretics or beta-adrenergic blocking drugs to treat hypertension.

Contraindications

Alpha$_1$-adrenergic blocking drugs should not be used in patients who are hypersensitive to these types of drugs.

Precautions

Use alpha$_1$-adrenergic blocking drugs with caution in patients with impaired hepatic function.

Adverse Reactions and Side Effects

CNS: Dizziness, depression, anxiety, drowsiness, nervousness.
Respiratory: Dyspnea, bronchitis, bronchospasm, epistaxis, increased cough.
CV: Palpitations, postural hypotension, hypotension, tachycardia, chest pain, arrhythmia.
GI: Dry mouth, diarrhea, constipation, abdominal pain, nausea and vomiting.
Ophthalmic: Blurred vision, abnormal vision, conjunctivitis.

Overdose Management

Keep patient supine. Treat shock with volume expanders or vasopressors.

EMS Considerations

1. Monitor ECG and vital signs frequently.
2. Assess for heart and lung disease. Some drugs may cause vasospasm with Prinzmetal or vasospastic angina.
3. Monitor older patients closely because they may develop orthostatic hypotension.

Amebicides and Trichomonacides

General Statement

An **amebicide** is a drug that kills amoebae. A **trichomonacide** is anything that kills trichomonads.

Amoebae often migrate from the GI tract to other parts of the body. Frequently affected are the lungs, liver, or spleen. The amoebae colonize forming abscesses that can rupture causing infection. Unfortunately, no one drug can cure amebic infestations.

Infestation with Trichomonas vaginalis causes vaginitis. This is treated with various locally applied antitrichomonal drugs, as well as effective amebicides. Also, oral administration of metronidazole to both sexual partners may be given to prevent reinfection.

Patients can also become infected by the protozoan *Giardia lamblia*, which is transmitted in the feces. Symptoms include diarrhea, abdominal pain, and weight loss.

EMS Considerations

None.

Aminoglycosides

Mechanism of Action

Aminoglycosides are a class of antibiotics that includes gentamicin and tobramycin. These broad-spectrum antibiotics are believed to inhibit protein synthesis by binding irreversibly to ribosomes, leading to the production of nonfunctional proteins.

Indications

Aminoglycosides are powerful antibiotics *not* to be used for minor infections. These drugs are to be used to treat gram-negative bacteria causing bone and joint infections, septicemia, skin and soft tissue infections, respiratory tract infections, intra-abdominal infections, postoperative infections, and UTIs. Aminoglycosides are also used to treat gram-positive bacteria infections when other less-toxic drugs are ineffective or contraindicated.

Contraindications

Aminoglycosides should not be used in patients hypersensitive to these drugs, or in patients who require long-term therapy.

Precautions

Aminoglycosides should be used with caution on patients with impaired renal function or hearing impairment, or infants and older patients, because they are more sensitive to toxic effects.

Adverse Reactions and Side Effects

CNS: Headache, tremor, depression, lethargy, dizziness, vertigo.
Respiratory: Laryngeal edema, respiratory depression (infants).
Ototoxicity: Tinnitus, hearing impairment.
GI: Diarrhea, increased salivation, nausea and vomiting.

EMS Considerations

1. Assess for allergic reactions.
2. Monitor vital signs.
3. Increase fluids to prevent renal tubule irritation.
4. Observe for neuromuscular blockade with muscle weakness leading to apnea, when given with a muscle relaxant.

Amphetamines and Derivatives

Mechanism of Action

Amphetamines act as central nervous system stimulants, causing an increase in motor activity, mental alertness, and causing slight euphoric effects.

Indications

Amphetamines are used in patients to treat narcolepsy and certain types of mental depression.

Contraindications

Amphetamines should not be used in patients with hyperthyroidism, diabetes mellitus, hypertension, narrow-angle glaucoma, angina pectoris, and CV disease.

Precautions

Use amphetamines with caution in elderly patients, and in patients with psychopathic personality traits.

Adverse Reactions and Side Effects

CNS: Nervousness, dizziness, depression, headache, and insomnia.
Respiratory: Dyspnea, pulmonary hypertension.
CV: Arrhythmias, palpitations, hyper- or hypotension.
GI: Nausea and vomiting, diarrhea, dry mouth, metallic taste.
Dermatologic: Symptoms of allergy.

EMS Considerations

Monitor ECG and vital signs. Assess for arrhythmias, tachycardia, or hypertension. Cardiovascular changes with psychotic syndrome may indicate toxicity.

Angiotensin-Converting Enzyme (ACE) Inhibitors

Mechanism of Action

ACE inhibitors are drugs that convert antiotensin I to angiotensin II. The process occurs in the lungs, resulting in a decrease in blood pressure.

Indications

ACE inhibitors are used alone or in combination with other antihypertensives for the treatment of hypertension. Some ACE inhibitors can be used for the treatment of CHF or to treat left ventricular dysfunction.

Contraindications

ACE inhibitors should not be used in patients with a history of angioedema caused by previous treatment with an ACE inhibitor.

Precautions

Use ACE inhibitors with caution in patients during their second and third trimesters of pregnancy, as these drugs may cause injury or death to the fetus. Geriatric patients may develop more profound side effects to ACE inhibitors.

Adverse Reactions and Side Effects

CNS: Headache, dizziness, fatigue, nervousness, sleep disturbances.
Respiratory: Dyspnea, chronic cough.
CV: Hypotension, palpitations, angina pectoris, MI, orthostatic hypotension.
GI: Diarrhea, dry mouth, abdominal pain, nausea and vomiting.

Overdose Management

To restore blood pressure, administer volume expander (NS or LR) and supportive measures for treatment of shock.

EMS Considerations

Monitor vital signs. Check B/P in both arms (lying, sitting, standing). Report any evidence of angioedema (facial swelling, swelling of the extremities, tongue, mucous membranes, and airway). Monitor for airway obstruction and if present, treat with SC epinephrine (1:1000 solution).

Antianemic Drugs

Mechanism of Action

Anemia is a deficiency in the number of red blood cells (RBCs) or in the hemoglobin level in the RBCs. The normal daily iron intake for males is 12–20 mg and for females is 8–15 mg. There are two types of anemia; (1) iron-deficiency, which is the excess loss or destruction of blood cells, and (2) megaloblastic anemia, which is a deficient production of blood cells.

Indications

Antianemic drugs are used prophylatically or for the treatment of iron deficiency and iron-deficiency anemias.

Contraindications

Antianemic drugs should not be used in patients with peptic ulcers, ulcerative colitis, cirrhosis of the liver, or in patients with normal iron balance.

Precautions

Use antianemic drugs with caution, because of the possibility of allergic reactions.

EMS Considerations

Eggs, milk, coffee, and tea consumed with a meal or 1 hour after a meal may inhibit absorption of dietary iron. Ingestion of calcium and iron supplements with food can decrease iron absorption. Do not crush or chew sustained-release antianemic drugs.

Antianginal Drugs—Nitrates/Nitrites

Mechanism of Action

Both nitrates and nitrites relax vascular smooth muscle. This causes a decrease in venous return to the heart by blood pooling, causing a decrease in preload. The oxygen requirements of the heart are reduced and there is more efficient redistribution of blood flow through collateral blood vessels. Both diastolic and systolic blood pressures are decreased.

Indications

Antianginal drugs—Nitrates/Nitrites are used to treat, and used prophylactically for, acute angina pain. Nitrates are first-line treatment for unstable angina.

Contraindications

Should not be used in patients sensitive to nitrites because this may result in severe hypotension. Also should not be used in patients with severe anemia, recent heart trauma, postural hypotension, closed-angle glaucoma, impaired hepatic function, hypertrophic cardiomyopathy, hypotension, or in patients who have had a recent MI.

Precautions

Use these drugs with caution in patients with glaucoma, and in patients during lactation.

Adverse Reactions and Side Effects

Respiratory: Bronchitis, pneumonia.
CNS: Headaches, dizziness, restlessness, weakness, vertigo, anxiety, confusion, apprehension.
CV: Postural hypotension, angina, tachycardia, palpitations, paradoxic bradycardia, PVCs, arrhythmias.
GI: Diarrhea, dry mouth, abdominal pain, nausea and vomiting.
Miscellaneous: Perspiration, muscle twitching, blurred vision.

EMS Considerations

Monitor vital signs, especially for hypotension. Assess for sensitivity to nitrites that include nausea and vomiting, pallor, restlessness, and CV collapse.

Antiarrhythmic Drugs
General Statement

Antiarrhythmic drugs are classified into the following four groups:

- Group I: These drugs decrease the rate of entry of sodium during cardiac membrane depolarization, and decrease the rate of rise of phase "O" of the cardiac membrane action potential. Group I antiarrhythmics are further listed in subgroups according to their effects on action potential duration.
  - Group IA: Depress phase "O" and prolong the duration of the action potential. Examples: procainamide and quinidine.
  - Group IB: Slightly depress phase "O" and shorten the action potential. Examples: lidocaine and phenytoin.
  - Group IC: Slight effect on repolarization but marked depression of phase "O" of the action potential. Significant slowing of conduction. Examples: flecainide and propafenone.
- Group II: Competitively block beta-adrenergic receptors and depress phase "4" depolarization. Examples: acebutolol and propranolol.
- Group III: Prolong the duration of the relative refractory period without changing the phase of depolarization of the resting membrane potential. Examples: amiodarone and sotalol.
- Group IV: Slow conduction velocity and increase the refractoriness of the AV node. Example: verapamil.

Precautions

Antiarrhythmic drugs can cause toxic side effects that can be confused with the original purpose for administering the drug in the first place. For example, these drugs can actually cause new or worsening arrhythmias.

EMS Considerations

Assess heart sounds and vital signs. Obtain and document ECG, assessing the patient for extent of palpitations, chest pain, "missed beats," or fainting episodes. Monitor B/P and pulse. Avoid heart rates < 50/bpm or > 120/bpm.

Anticoagulants
Mechanism of Action

Anticoagulant drugs are divided into three classes: (1) *anticoagulants*, that are drugs that prevent or slow coagulation; (2) *thrombolytics*, which increase the rate that blood clots are dissolved; and (3) *hemostatics*, drugs that prevent or stop internal bleeding.

Indications

Anticoagulants are used to treat venous thrombosis, pulmonary embolism, acute coronary occlusions with MIs, and strokes that are caused by emboli or cerebral thrombi.

Anticoagulants are also used prophylactically for rheumatic heart disease, atrial fibrillation, and for the prevention of transient attacks of cerebral ischemia.

Contraindications

Anticoagulants should not be used in patients with hemorrhagic tendencies, impaired renal function, or severe hypertension.

Precautions

Anticoagulants should be used with caution in pregnant women because they may cause hypoprothrombinemia (deficiency of blood clotting factor II in the blood) in the infant. Geriatric patients may be more susceptible to the effects of anticoagulants.

Adverse Reactions and Side Effects

See individual drugs.

EMS Considerations

Question patients about bleeding from their gums, urine, stools, vomit, and bruises. Apply pressure to all venipuncture and injection sites to prevent bleeding and hematoma formation. With SC administration, do not aspirate or massage; give the injection in lower abdomen and rotate sites.

Anticonvulsants
Mechanism of Action

An anticonvulsant drug prevents or relieves convulsions. These drugs cannot cure convulsive disorders, but do control seizures without impairing the normal functions of the CNS.

EMS Considerations

Assess the patient for orientation to time, place, affect, reflexes, and vital signs. Observe signs and symptoms of impending seizures. With IV administration, monitor for respiratory depression and cardiovascular collapse. Note any evidence of CNS side effects, such as blurred vision, slurred speech, or confusion. Observe the patient for muscle twitching, loss of muscle tone, episodes of bizarre behavior, and/or subsequent amnesia.

Antidepressants, Tricyclic
Mechanism of Action

Tricyclic antidepressants cause adaptive changes in the serotonin and norepinephrine receptor systems, resulting in changes in the sensitivies of both presynaptic and postsynaptic receptor sites. These drugs exhibit anticholinergic, sedative, antihistaminic, and hypotensive effects.

Indications

Tricyclic antidepressant drugs are used to treat endogenous and reactive depression. See also individual drugs.

Contraindications

Tricyclic antidepressants should not be used in patients with severely impaired liver function, during the acute recovery from an MI, and during concomitant use with MAO inhibitors.

Precautions

Use tricyclic antidepressants with caution in patients with CV disease, glaucoma, and in geriatric patients. These drugs are not recommended in patients under the age of 12.

Adverse Reactions and Side Effects

CNS: Confusion, anxiety, restlessness, hallucinations, nightmares, headache, dizziness.
CV: Tachycardia, hypo- or hypertension, arrhythmias, heart block, palpitations, MI.
GI: Gastric distress, unpleasant taste, cramps, increased salivation, dry mouth.

EMS Considerations

None.

Antidiabetic Drugs: Hypoglycemic Drugs (Oral)
Mechanism of Action

Hypoglycemic drugs are any drugs that lower or maintain blood sugar levels (insulin is taken parenterally to control blood sugar). Hypoglycemic drugs are generally used in addition to diet and exercise, to control blood glucose levels in type II diabetes mellitus. Oral hypoglycemic drugs act by one or more of the following mechanisms: (1) stimulate insulin release from pancreatic beta-cells, (2) the peripheral tissues become more sensitive to insulin because of an increase in the number of insulin receptors or an increased ability of circulating insulin to combine with receptors, (3) increase glucagon release and hepatic glucose production.

Indications

Antidiabetic drugs are used in (1) non-insulin-dependent type II diabetes mellitus that does not respond to diet management alone, and (2) concurrent use of insulin and an oral hypoglycemic for type II diabetics who are difficult to control with diet alone.

Contraindications

Antidiabetic drugs should not be used in patients with the following: fever, infections, pregnancy, insulin-dependent diabetes, juvenile diabetes, brittle diabetes, or in patients with impaired endocrine, renal, or liver function.

Precautions

Geriatric patients may be more sensitive to oral hypoglycemics and hypoglycemia may be more difficult to recognize in the elderly.

Adverse Reactions and Side Effects

Hypoglycemia is the most common side effect.

CNS: Fatigue, dizziness, fever, headache, weakness, vertigo.
GI: Nausea, heartburn, full feeling.
Dermatologic: Skin rash, urticaria, eczema, photophobia.

Overdose Management (Hypoglycemia)

Mild: PO glucose, and monitor the patient.
Severe: $D_{50}W$ by IV bolus and followed by infusion of D_5W or $D_{10}W$ to maintain blood glucose level above 100 mg/dL.

EMS Considerations

To decrease the incidence of gastric upset, PO drugs should be taken with food.

Antidiabetic Drugs: Insulins
Mechanism of Action

Insulin facilitates the transport of glucose into cardiac and skeletal muscle and adipose tissue. It also increases synthesis of glycogen in the liver. Insulin is a protein and is destroyed in the GI tract. Therefore, insulin must be administered SC so that it is absorbed into the bloodstream and distributed throughout the extracellular fluid. There are three classifications of insulin: (1) rapid-acting, insulin injection (Regular Insulin, Crystalline Zinc Insulin, Unmodified Insulin), (2) intermediate-acting insulin, Isophane insulin suspension (NPH), Insulin zinc suspension (Lente), and (3) long-acting insulin, Insulin zinc suspension extended (Ultra-lente).

Indications

Replacement therapy for type-I diabetes. Patients with diabetic ketoacidosis or diabetic coma, use regular insulin. Insulin is also indicated for patients with type II diabetes when other measures have failed. *Note*: Human insulin is used almost exclusively.

Contraindications

Hypersensitivity to insulin.

Precautions

Pregnant diabetic patients may have a decrease in insulin requirements during the first half of their pregnancy.

Adverse Reactions and Side Effects

Hypoglycemia: Generally caused by insulin overdose, decreased food intake, or too much exercise in relation to the insulin dose.
Allergic: Most likely occurs following intermittent insulin therapy or IV administration of large doses to insulin-resistant patients.
Insulin resistance: Usually caused by obesity.

Blurred vision, presbyopia: Generally occurs during initial treatment or in patients who have been uncontrolled for a long period of time.

Hyperglycemic rebound: Generally occurs with chronic overdosage.

EMS Considerations

1. Regular insulin may be mixed with NPH or Lente insulins.
2. Lente or Ultra-lente insulins may be mixed with each other in any proportion.
3. Administer at 90-degree angle with a 28- or 29-gauge needle.
4. Assess for hyperglycemia: thirst, polydypsia, polyuria, drowsiness, blurred vision, loss of appetite, fruity odor on breath, and flushed dry skin.
5. Assess for hypoglycemia: drowsiness, chills, confusion, anxiety, cold sweats, excessive hunger, nausea, headache, irritability, shakiness, and tachycardia.

Antihistamines (H$_1$ Blockers)
Mechanism of Action

An **antihistamine (H$_1$ Blockers)** is a drug that blocks the action of histamines on H$_1$ receptors. Antihistamines are classified as *first-generation* and *second-generation*. First-generation antihistamines bind to central and peripheral H$_1$ receptors and second-generation antihistamines are selective for peripheral H$_1$ receptors. Second-generation antihistamines tend to be less sedating, but still have beneficial effects in treating allergies.

Indications

Antihistamines are used in patients to treat allergies, hives, and other local and systemic hypersensitivity reactions. Some first-generation antihistamines can also be used to treat insomnia, motion sickness, or vertigo.

Contraindications

Hypersensitivity to the drug, narrow-angle glaucoma, and use with MAO inhibitors.

Precautions

Use antihistamines with caution in patients with convulsive disorders, and in patients with respiratory disease. Geriatric patients may experience dizziness, excessive sedation, syncope, and hypotension.

Overdose Management

Hypotension can be treated with a vasopressor such as norepinephrine, or dopamine. *Do not use epinephrine.* For convulsions, use a short-acting depressant such as diazepam. Ice packs and a cool sponge-bath are effective in reducing fever in children.

Adverse Reactions and Side Effects

CNS: Drowsiness, dizziness, lack of coordination, fatigue, confusion, headache, nervousness.

Respiratory: Thickening of bronchial secretions, wheezing, respiratory depression, chest tightness.

CV: Postural hypotension, palpitations, bradycardia, tachycardia, ECG changes (flattening of "T" wave, prolongation of "Q-T" interval).

GI: Epigastric distress, diarrhea, nausea and vomiting.

EMS Considerations

Document vital signs, CV status, and lung sounds. Note characteristics of secretions.

Antihyperlipidemic Drugs—HMG—CoA Reductase Inhibitors
Mechanism of Action

Antihyperlipidemic drugs—HMG—CoA reductase inhibitors increase HDL cholesterol, and decrease LDL cholesterol and plasma triglycerides. The maximum response to these drugs is generally seen in 4–6 weeks.

Indications

These drugs are used as an adjunct to diet in patients to decrease elevated total LDL cholesterol when other nondrug approaches have not been adequate.

Contraindications

Antihyperlipidemic drugs should not be used in pregnant patients, children, and patients with active liver disease.

Precautions

Use with caution in patients who have ingested large amounts of alcohol, or who have a history of liver disease.

Adverse Reactions and Side Effects

CNS: Headache, dizziness, tremor, vertigo, anxiety, depression.
Respiratory: Cough.
GI: Diarrhea, abdominal cramps, heartburn, nausea and vomiting.

EMS Considerations

None.

Antihypertensive Drugs
General Statement

Blood pressure for adults over 18 years of age is classified as follows: Optimal = <120/<80 mm Hg, Normal = <130/<85 mm Hg, High Normal = 130−139/85−89 mm Hg, Stage 1 Hypertension = 140−159/90−99 mm Hg, Stage 2 Hypertension = 160−179/100−109 mm Hg, and Stage 3 Hypertension = 180 or greater/110 or greater mm Hg. The goal of antihypertensive treatment is a B/P of <140/90 mm Hg. There are two exceptions; (1) Hypertensive diabetics = <135/85 mm Hg, and (2) Patients with renal insufficiency = <130/85 mm Hg.

EMS Considerations

None.

Antibiotics

Mechanism of Action

There are two classes of antibiotics: (1) *Bacteriostatic* drugs arrest the multiplication and further development of infectious agents, or (2) *Bactericidal* drugs kill and eradicate all living microorganisms.

Indications

The correct drug depends on the type of illness, sensitivity of the infecting agent, and the patient's previous experience with a drug.

Contraindications

Hypersensitivity to the drug.

Adverse Reactions and Side Effects

Anti-infective drugs generally have few toxic effects. However, casual use of a drug may cause resistant strains which are insensitive to a particular anti-infective drug.

EMS Considerations

Monitor patient's vital signs and assess for hives, rashes, or difficulty breathing, which may indicate hypersensitivity.

Antimalarial Drugs

Mechanism of Action

Antimalarial drugs work by (1) causing inhibition of the parasite to grow, (2) causing membrane damage to the parasite, (3) interference with hemoglobin digestion by the parasite, and (4) interference with synthesis of nucleoprotein by the parasite.

Indications

Antimalarial drugs are used for the treatment or prophylaxis of acute attacks of malaria.

Contraindications

Hypersensitivity.

Precautions

Antimalarial drugs should be used with caution in patients with hepatic, severe GI, neurologic, and blood disorders.

Adverse Reactions and Side Effects

CNS: Headache, fatigue, nervousness, anxiety, irritability, confusion.
CV: Hypotension, ECG changes (inversion of T wave, widening of "QRS" complex).
GI: Diarrhea, cramps, epigastric distress, nausea and vomiting.

EMS Considerations

None.

Antineoplastic (Chemotherapeutic) Drugs

Mechanism of Action

Choice of which antineoplastic (chemotherapeutic) drug to use is dependent on the cell type of the tumor, and the site of tumor growth. All antineoplastic drugs are cell poisons, affecting both neoplastic and normal cells. However, neoplastic cells are more active and multiply more rapidly than normal cells and, therefore, are more affected by the antineoplastic drugs.

Indications

Antineoplastic drugs are used for the prevention of growth and proliferation of malignant cells.

Contraindications

Hypersensitivity to the drug. Should not use antineoplastic drugs on patients during the first trimester of pregnancy.

Precautions

Use antineoplastic drugs with caution in patients with preexisting bone marrow depression, kidney or liver dysfunction, and in patients with previous recent chemotherapy usage.

Adverse Reactions and Side Effects

Bone marrow depression is the major danger of antineoplastic therapy.

CNS: Depression, confusion, dizziness, headache, fatigue, fever, weakness.
GI: Nausea and vomiting, diarrhea, abdominal cramps.

EMS Considerations

None.

Antipsychotic Drugs, Phenothiazines

Mechanism of Action

Antipsychotic drugs phenothiazines, do not cure mental illness, but relieve the patient of symptoms such as despondency, and activate the immobile and withdrawn patient, making him/her more accessible to psychotherapy. Phenothiazine drugs block postsynaptic dopamine receptors, which lead to a reduction of psychotic symptoms.

Contraindications

Antipsychotic drugs should not be used in patients with severe CNS depression, in patients with a history of seizures, and in patients taking anticonvulsant drugs. These drugs are also contraindicated in patients with CV disorders, renal disease, and in patients with glaucoma. Antipsychotic drugs should not be given to children with chickenpox, CNS infections, or in children with measles.

Precautions

Antipsychotic drugs should be used with caution in patients with asthma, emphysema, or acute respiratory tract infections. Use with caution in geriatric patients because they have a tendency to accumulate high plasma levels of the drug because of a leaner body mass, and lower total body water.

Adverse Reactions and Side Effects

CNS: Depression, drowsiness, dizziness, fatigue.
CV: Orthostatic hypotension, hyper- or hypotension, tachycardia, fainting.
GI: Dry mouth, diarrhea, constipation.

EMS Considerations

To lessen injection (IM) dilute solutions in saline. Monitor vital signs, assess B/P in both arms in a reclining position, standing, and sitting positions, 2 minutes apart. If administered IV, monitor flow rate and B/P closely.

Antithyroid Drugs
Mechanism of Action

Antithyroid drugs inhibit the production of thyroid hormones by the thyroid gland.

Indications

Antithyroid drugs are used as an adjunct in patients to treat thyroid storm. They are also used to reduce mortality caused by alcoholic liver disease.

Contraindications

Do not use antithyroid drugs in patients who are lactating, because the drugs could cause hypothyroidism in the infant.

Precautions

Use antithyroid drugs with caution in patients with cardiovascular disease.

Adverse Reactions and Side Effects

CNS: Headache, drowsiness, vertigo, depression.
GI: Epigastric pain, taste loss, nausea and vomiting.

EMS Considerations

None.

Antiviral Drugs
Mechanism of Action

Viruses must enter living cells to reproduce and grow. There are enzymes and mechanisms that are unique to viruses and a number of drugs have been developed that inhibit viral activity. For example, drugs have been developed that prevent penetration of the virus into cells. Other drugs have been developed that inhibit enzymes needed for DNA synthesis.

EMS Considerations

None.

Barbiturates
Mechanism of Action

Barbiturates produce all levels of CNS depression. Some barbiturates are effective anticonvulsants. The depressant and anticonvulsant effects are related to the barbiturates' ability to increase or mimic the inhibitory activity of the neurotransmitter GABA on nerve synapses.

Indications

Barbiturates are used for sedation, hypnotic, anticonvulsant and for the control of acute convulsive conditions.

Contraindications

Barbiturates should not be used in patients who are hypersensitive to the drugs, patients with severe trauma, pulmonary disease (dyspnea, obstruction), edema, uncontrolled diabetes, or in patients who present with an excitatory response when given the drug.

Precautions

Use barbiturates with caution in patients with CNS depression, CV, hepatic or renal damage, and in patients with a history of alcoholism who have shown tendencies toward suicide. Geriatric patients have a tendency to have an increased sensitivity toward barbiturates.

Adverse Reactions and Side Effects

CNS: Drowsiness, agitation, confusion, CNS depression, nervousness, dizziness, headache, hallucinations, vertigo, excitement, appearance of being under the influence of alcohol.
Respiratory: Dyspnea, coughing, larngospasm, bronchospasm, apnea.
CV: Bradycardia, hypotension, syncope, circulatory collapse.
GI: Nausea and vomiting.

EMS Considerations

When barbiturates are administered, monitor the patient closely for correct flow rate. Rapid injection may cause respiratory depression, dyspnea, and shock.

Beta-Adrenergic Blocking Drugs
Mechanism of Action

Beta-adrenergic blocking drugs combine reversibly with beta-adrenergic receptors to block the response to sympathetic nerve impulses, circulating catecholamines, or adrenergic drugs. Beta-adrenergic receptors are classified as either beta$_1$ or beta$_2$. Beta$_1$-receptors are predominantly in the cardiac muscle, affecting HR, contractility, AV conduction and CO.

Beta$_2$-receptors are predominantly in the bronchi and vascular musculature, affecting airway and vasculature resistance.

Indications

An example of a beta-adrenergic blocking drug is atenolol that predominantly blocks beta$_1$ activity. However, see individual drugs for specific indications.

Contraindications

Beta-adrenergic blocking drugs should not be used in patients with sinus bradycardia, high-degree AV blocks, cardiogenic shock, and CHF unless it is secondary to tachyarrhythmias that can be treated with beta-blocking drugs. Beta-adrenergic blocking drugs are also contraindicated in patients with chronic bronchitis, bronchial asthma, emphysema, or severe COPD.

Precautions

Beta-adrenergic blockers should be used with caution in patients with diabetes, cerebrovascular insufficiency, and impaired hepatic and renal function.

Adverse Reactions and Side Effects

CV: Bradycardia, hypotension, CHF, angina, edema, arrhythmias, flushing, SOB, palpitations.
Respiratory: Dyspnea, cough, wheezing, bronchospasms, bronchial obstruction, laryngospasm.
CNS: Dizziness, fatigue, depression, hallucinations, headache, nervousness.
GI: Diarrhea, dry mouth, cramps, bloating, nausea and vomiting.

EMS Considerations

Monitor HR and B/P. Observe for increasing dyspnea, coughing, or any difficulty in breathing, or any symptoms of CHF. With a diabetic patient, monitor for symptoms of hypoglycemia (tachycardia, hypotension).

Calcium Channel Blocking Drugs

Mechanism of Action

Calcium channel blocking drugs inhibit the influx of calcium through the cell membrane, which results in a depression of automaticity and conduction velocity in both smooth and cardiac muscle.

Indications

An example of a calcium channel blocker, is nifedipine, which is used to treat patients with chronic stable angina without vasospasm. See individual drugs for uses of calcium channel blockers.

Contraindications

Calcium channel blockers should not be used in patients with sick sinus syndrome or high-degree AV block (except with a functioning pacemaker).

Precautions

Use calcium channel blockers with caution in patients with hypertension, because they have a higher risk of heart attack.

EMS Considerations

None.

Calcium Salts

Mechanism of Action

Calcium salts are used to supplement patients who are in need of additional calcium. Calcium is necessary for maintaining the normal function of nerves, muscles, and the permeability of cell membranes and capillaries.

Indications

Calcium salts are used to treat depletion of electrolytes, hypocalcemia, and poisoning from magnesium and other substances.

Contraindications

Calcium salts should not be used in patients with renal or cardiac disease.

Precautions

Calcium should be used with caution in patients with cor pulmonale, respiratory acidosis, and in patients with renal disease or failure.

Adverse Reactions and Side Effects

CNS: Confusion, delirium, stupor, lethargy.
CV: Hypotension, syncope, cardiac arrhythmias, cardiac arrest.
GI: Abdominal pain, dry mouth, nausea and vomiting.

EMS Considerations

Administer slowly, monitoring for bradycardia, hypotension, and cardiac arrhythmias. Do not mix calcium salts with any other drug in the IV line.

Cardiac Glycosides

Mechanism of Action

Cardiac glycosides increase the force and velocity of myocardial contraction (positive inotropic effect). This occurs by increasing the refractory period of the AV node and increasing total peripheral resistance.

Indications

Cardiac glycosides are used in patients with CHF, to control rapid ventricular rates caused by atrial flutter, or atrial fibrillation, and in patients with PSVT.

Contraindications

Cardiac glycosides should not be used in patients with digitalis toxicity, and in patients in both ventricular fibrillation and tachycardia.

Precautions

Use cardiac glycosides with caution in patients with ischemic disease, and heart and lung disease, including emphysema and partial heart block. These drugs should be used with caution in patients with carditis associated with rheumatic fever or viral myocarditis.

Adverse Reactions and Side Effects

CV: Changes in rate, rhythm, irritability of the heart, bigeminy, couplets, ectopic beats, ventricular fibrillation.
CNS: Headaches, fatigue, stupor.
GI: Anorexia, excessive salivation, abdominal pain, diarrhea, nausea and vomiting.

EMS Considerations

None.

Cephalosporins
Mechanism of Action

Cephalosporins are broad-spectrum antibiotics. They interfere with a final step in the formation of the bacterial cell wall resulting in unstable cell membranes that undergo lysis. Cephalosporins also cause an inhibition of cell growth and division.

Contraindications

Cephalosporins should not be used in patients who are hypersensitive to cephalosporins or related antibiotics.

Precautions

Use cephalosporins with caution in patients with impaired renal or hepatic function.

Adverse Reactions and Side Effects

CNS: Headache, fatigue, vertigo, dizziness, confusion.
CV: Hypotension.
GI: Diarrhea, abdominal cramps, heartburn, nausea and vomiting.

EMS Considerations

Parenteral solutions administered too rapidly may cause pain and irritation. The IV drugs should be infused over 30 minutes unless otherwise indicated.

Cholinergic Blocking Drugs
Mechanism of Action

Cholinergic blocking drugs prevent acetylcholine from combining with receptors on the postganglionic parasympathetic nerve terminal. This blocking causes reduction of smooth muscle spasms, blockade of vagal impulses to the heart, decreased secretions, production of mydriasis, and various CNS effects.

Indications

An example of a cholinergic blocker is atropine that is used to treat symptomatic sinus bradycardia. See individual drugs for their effects.

Contraindications

Cholinergic blocking drugs should not be used in patients with glaucoma, tachycardia, myocardial ischemia, and unstable cardiovascular states.

Precautions

Cholinergic blockers should be used with caution in patients with CHF, cardiac arrhythmias, hypertension, and chronic lung disease.

Adverse Reactions and Side Effects

CNS: Dizziness, drowsiness, nervousness, headache, restlessness.
CV: Palpitations.
GI: Dry mouth, heartburn, nausea and vomiting.

EMS Consideration

Monitor vital signs and ECG. Assess for hemodynamic changes and intraventricular heart blocks. Note any complaint of palpitations.

Corticosteroids
Mechanism of Action

Corticosteroids are any of several steroid hormones secreted by the adrenal gland. These hormones influence many metabolic pathway processes and all organ systems and are essential for life. For example, these processes include carbohydrate metabolism, protein metabolism, fat metabolism, and water and electrolyte balance.

Indications

Corticosteroids are used in patients for anti-inflammatory or immunosuppressant therapy.

Contraindications

Corticosteroids should not be used in patients with CHF or other cardiac disease, hypertension, wide-angle glaucoma, or patients with infection, because these drugs can mask infection.

Precautions

Use corticosteroids with caution in patients with diabetes mellitus, convulsive disorders, and in patients with renal or hepatic insufficiency.

Adverse Reactions and Side Effects

CNS: Headache, vertigo, restlessness, seizures.
CV: Hypertension, CHF, ECG changes, cardiac arrhythmias.
GI: Diarrhea, gastric irritation, nausea and vomiting.

EMS Considerations

None.

Diuretics, Loop
Mechanism of Action

Loop Diuretics inhibit reabsorption of sodium and chloride in the proximal and distal tubules and the loop of Henle.

Indications

An example of a loop diuretic is furosemide that is used to treat edema associated with CHF. See individual drugs for their indications.

Contraindications

Loop diuretics should not be used in patients who may be hypersensitive to the drugs, or in patients with severe electrolyte depletion.

Precautions

The administration may produce dehydration and/or hypotension. Monitor patients closely.

EMS Considerations

Monitor patients closely for signs of electrolyte imbalance:

- Hyponatremia
- Hypernatremia
- Water intoxication
- Metabolic acidosis
- Metabolic alkalosis
- Hypokalemia
- Hyperkalemia

Diuretics, Thiazides
Mechanism of Action

Thiazide diuretics cause diuresis by decreasing the rate that sodium and chloride are reabsorbed by the distal renal tubules of the kidney.

Indications

Thiazide diuretics are used in patients to treat edema, CHF, and hypertension.

Contraindications

Thiazide diuretics should not be used in patients with impaired renal function or advanced hepatic cirrhosis.

Precautions

Use thiazide diuretics with caution in patients with advanced heart failure, renal disease, or in hepatic cirrhosis, because they are likely to develop hypokalemia.

Adverse Reactions and Side Effects

CNS: Dizziness, lightheadedness, headache, vertigo, restlessness.
CV: Orthostatic hypotension, MIs in geriatric patients with advanced arteriosclerosis.
GI: Epigastric distress, diarrhea, nausea and vomiting.

EMS Considerations

Determine the extent of any edema by assessing skin turgor, mucous membranes, extremities, and lung fields.

Estrogens
Mechanism of Action

Estrogens combine with receptors in the cytoplasm of cells, resulting in an increase in protein synthesis. Estrogens aid in bone maintenance, increase elastic elements in the skin, cause sodium and fluid retention, and tend to keep plasma cholesterol at a lower level.

Indications

Estrogens are used for hormone replacement in postmenopausal women.

Contraindications

Estrogens should not be used in patients with breast, genital, or any other estrogen-dependent cancers.

Precautions

Estrogens should be used with caution in patients with asthma, epilepsy, migraine, cardiac failure, or in patients with renal insufficiency.

Adverse Reactions and Side Effects

CNS: Mental depression, dizziness, change in libido, headache, fatigue, nervousness, CVA, subarachnoid hemorrhage.
CV: MI, pulmonary embolism.
GI: Abdominal cramps, bloating, nausea and vomiting.

EMS Considerations

None.

Histamine H$_2$ Antagonists
Mechanism of Action

Histamine H$_2$ antagonists are competitive blockers of histamine, inhibiting all phases of gastric acid secretion.

Indications

Reduces both daytime and nighttime gastric acid secretions. However, see individual drugs for uses.

Contraindications

Histamine H_2 antagonists should not be used in patients who are hypersensitive to these types of drugs.

Precautions

Use histamine H_2 antagonists with caution in patients with impaired hepatic and renal function.

Adverse Reactions and Side Effects

CNS: Headache, fatigue, dizziness, confusion, insomnia.
CV: Arrhythmias when given rapid IV (rare).
GI: Diarrhea, abdominal discomfort, nausea and vomiting.

EMS Considerations

None.

Laxatives
Mechanisms of Action

Laxatives act by either stimulating the smooth muscles of the bowel or by changing the consistency of the stools.

Indications

Laxatives are used for the short-term treatment of constipation.

Contraindications

Laxatives should not be used in patients with undiagnosed abdominal pain. Laxatives may cause rupture of the abdomen or intestinal hemorrhage in patients with appendicitis, or intestinal obstruction.

Adverse Reactions and Side Effects

CNS: Dizziness, fainting, weakness.
CV: Palpitations, electrolyte imbalance.
GI: Perianal irritation, nausea and vomiting.

EMS Considerations

None.

Narcotic Analgesics
Mechanism of Action

Narcotic analgesics attach to specific receptors located in the CNS resulting in diminished transmission of pain impulses as well as depressing respiration.

Indications

Narcotic analgesics are used to treat pain from various causes such as MI, burns, postpartum, and so forth.

Contraindications

Narcotic analgesics should not be used in patients with asthma, emphysema, convulsive states, diabetic acidosis, and obesity.

Precautions

Use narcotic analgesics with caution in patients with head injury, pulmonary heart disease, and patients with depleted blood volume.

Adverse Reactions and Side Effects

CNS: Dizziness, lightheadedness, headache, fainting.
Respiratory: Depression, arrest.
CV: Flushing, changes in HR and B/P.
GI: Nausea, vomiting, anorexia.

EMS Considerations

Obtain baseline vital signs. Closely monitor vital signs. Do not administer these drugs when respiratory rate is <12/min or the systolic B/P is <90 mm Hg unless ventilatory support is ready. Tell the patient that a warm feeling and flushing is normal when therapeutic doses are given. Patients may perspire profusely.

Narcotic Antagonists
Mechanism of Action

Narcotic antagonists block the action of narcotic analgesics by displacing them from their receptor sites, or by preventing narcotics from attaching to the opiate receptors.

EMS Considerations

Determine the cause of respiratory depression. Observe the patient for appearance of withdrawal symptoms, and/or airway obstruction.

Neuromuscular Blocking Drugs
Mechanism of Action

Neuromuscular blocking drugs compete with acetylcholine for receptor sites in the muscle cells, causing paralysis. Paralysis occurs in the following order: eyelids, difficulty in swallowing/talking, weakening of the extremities and neck, followed by relaxation of the trunk and spine.

Indications

Neuromuscular blocking drugs are used for the management of airway control. See individual drugs.

Contraindications

Hypersensitivity to any of these drugs.

Precautions

Neuromuscular blocking drugs should be used with caution in patients with renal, hepatic, endocrine, or pulmonary impairment.

Adverse Reactions and Side Effects

Respiratory: Respiratory paralysis.
CV: Cardiac arrhythmias, bradycardia, hypotension, cardiac arrest.
GI: Excessive salivation.

EMS Considerations

Monitor vital signs frequently and respiratory status continuously.

Nonsteroidal Anti-Inflammatory Drugs

Mechanism of Action

Nonsteroidal anti-inflammatory drugs work by decreasing prostaglandin synthesis. Their anti-inflammatory effect is similar to aspirin.

Indications

Nonsteroidal anti-inflammatory drugs are used to treat inflammatory disease, including rheumatoid arthritis, gout, and other musculoskeletal diseases.

Contraindications

Nonsteroidal anti-inflammatory drugs should not be used in patients who are hypersensitive to aspirin. They are also contraindicated in persons under the age of 14.

Precautions

Use with caution in patients with a history of GI disease, reduced renal function, and in geriatric patients.

Adverse Reactions and Side Effects

CNS: Dizziness, vertigo, headache, nervousness, lightheadedness.
Respiratory: Bronchospasm, laryngeal edema, dyspnea, SOB.
CV: CHF, hypotension, hypertension, arrhythmias, palpitations, tachycardia, chest pain.
GI: Intestinal ulceration, heartburn, dry mouth, nausea and vomiting.

EMS Considerations

Note hypersensitive reactions to aspirin. Nonsteroidal anti-inflammatory drugs exacerbate asthma.

Penicillins

Mechanism of Action

Penicillins kill bacteria by binding to their cytoplasmic membranes, inhibiting cell wall synthesis. Penicillins work best on young organisms, and have little effect on mature, resting cells.

Indications

Penicillins are used to combat many types of gram-positive, gram-negative, and anaerobic organisms.

Contraindications

Penicillins should not be used in persons hypersensitive to these drugs.

Precautions

Penicillins should be used with caution in patients with a history of asthma, or hay fever.

Adverse Reactions and Side Effects

CNS: Dizziness, fatigue, hyperactivity.
GI: Diarrhea, abdominal cramps, increased thirst.

EMS Considerations

IM or IV administration of penicillins may cause a great deal of local irritation: therefore, inject slowly.

Skeletal Muscle Relaxants, Centrally Acting

Mechanism of Action

Centrally acting skeletal muscle relaxants decrease muscle tone and involuntary movement by depressing spinal polysynaptic reflexes.

Indications

Centrally acting skeletal muscle relaxants are used to treat musculoskeletal and neurologic disorders associated with muscle spasms, muscle spasms caused by trauma, and inflammation.

Precautions

Use centrally acting skeletal muscle relaxants with caution in patients with decreased liver or renal function.

Adverse Reactions and Side Effects

CNS: Drowsiness, headaches, fatigue, irritability, nervousness.
GI: Diarrhea, epigastric pain, nausea and vomiting.

EMS Considerations

None.

Sympathomimetic (adrenergic) Drugs

Mechanism of Action

Sympathomimetic (adrenergic) drugs act by mimicking the action of norepinephrine or epinephrine by combining with alpha and/or beta receptors, or, by causing the release of the natural neurohormones from their storage sites at the nerve terminals.

Indications

See the individual drugs.

Contraindications

Sympathomimetics should not be used in patients with tachycardia caused by arrhythmias, or in patients with tachycardia or heart block caused by digitalis toxicity.

Precautions

Use sympathomimetics with caution in patients with CAD, arrhythmias, hypertension, or a history of CVA.

Adverse Reactions and Side Effects

Respiratory: Dyspnea, dry throat, cough.
CV: Tachycardia, palpitations, arrhythmias, angina, hypertension.
CNS: Anxiety, drowsiness, dizziness, headache.
GI: Heartburn, drowsiness, nausea and vomiting.

EMS Considerations

Obtain baseline general physical condition, including vital signs and ECG. Document lung assessment of cough and sputum production.

Tetracyclines
Mechanism of Action

Tetracyclines inhibit protein synthesis by binding to the ribosomal 50s subunit.

Indications

Tetracyclines are used to treat patients with infections caused by sexually transmitted diseases such as produced by rickettsia, chlamydia, and mycoplasma. These drugs can also be used as an alternative to penicillin for uncomplicated gonorrhea.

Contraindications

Do not use tetracyclines to treat persons hypersensitive to these drugs.

Precautions

Use tetracyclines with caution in patients with impaired kidney function.

Adverse Reactions and Side Effects

CNS: Dizziness, lightheadedness.
GI: Diarrhea, thirst, epigastric distress, nausea and vomiting.

EMS Considerations

Administer IM into large muscle mass to avoid extravasation into subcutaneous or fatty tissue.

Theophylline Derivatives
Mechanism of Action

Theophylline derivatives stimulate the CNS, relax bronchial smooth muscles and pulmonary blood vessels, produce diuresis, and increase the rate and force of cardiac contractions.

Indications

Theophylline derivatives are used both as prophylaxis and for the treatment of bronchial asthma, reversible bronchospasms associated with chronic bronchitis, emphysema, and COPD.

Contraindications

Theophylline derivatives should not be used in patients who are hypotensive, or patients with CAD or angina pectoris.

Precautions

Use theophylline derivatives with caution in patients with acute cardiac disease, hypertension, or severe renal or hepatic disease.

Adverse Reactions and Side Effects

CNS: Headache, dizziness, lightheadedness, vertigo.
Respiratory: Tachypnea, respiratory arrest.
CV: Hypotension, palpitations, tachycardia, life-threatening arrhythmias.
GI: Diarrhea, epigastric pain, nausea and vomiting.

EMS Considerations

Observe signs and symptoms of toxicity that include nausea, irritability, or cardiac arrhythmias.

Thyroid Drugs
Mechanism of Action

Thyroid hormones regulate growth by controlling protein synthesis and regulating energy metabolism. This increases respiratory rate, body temperature, cardiac output, heart rate, blood volume, and carbohydrate and protein metabolism.

Indications

Thyroid drugs are used to replace or supplement in hypothyroidism.

Contraindications

Thyroid drugs should not be used in patients with uncorrected adrenal insufficiency, hyperthyroidism, or AMI.

Precautions

Use thyroid drugs with caution in patients with angina pectoris, hypertension, and other cardiovascular diseases.

Adverse Reactions and Side Effects

CV: Arrhythmias, palpitations, angina, increased heart rate.
CNS: Headache, nervousness, irritability.
GI: Diarrhea, cramps, nausea and vomiting.

EMS Considerations

Report any symptoms or history of CAD. Monitor vital signs and cardiac rhythms. Report if the heart rate goes to >100 beats/min.

Tranquilizers/Antimanic Drugs/Hypnotics

Mechanism of Action

Tranquilizers/antimanic drugs/hypnotics are thought to affect the limbic system and reticular formation to reduce anxiety by increasing or facilitating the inhibitory neurotransmittor activity of GABA.

Indications

These types of drugs are used as antianxiety agents, hypnotics, anticonvulsants, and muscle relaxants.

Contraindications

Do not use these classifications of drugs in patients who are hypersensitive to them, or in patients with narrow-angle glaucoma, or in patients being treated for psychiatric disorders.

Precautions

Use these drugs with caution in patients with impaired hepatic or renal function.

Adverse Reactions and Side Effects

CNS: Drowsiness, confusion, sedation, dizziness, vertigo, depression, headache.
Respiratory: Respiratory depression, sleep apnea.
CV: Hypertension, hypotension, bradycardia, tachycardia, palpitations, cardiovascular collapse.
GI: Diarrhea, increased appetite, nausea and vomiting.

EMS Considerations

Monitor B/P before and after IV administration.

Vitamins

General Statement

Vitamins are essential, noncaloric substances required for normal metabolism. They are produced by living organisms such as plants and animals, and are obtained by diet. Vitamins are necessary for promoting growth, health, and life. They are necessary for the metabolic processes responsible for transforming foods into tissue and energy. However, vitamins do not provide energy because they do not contain calories. Table 8–1 lists the common vitamin requirements for the body, Table 8–2 shows the vitamins and their uses, and Table 8–3 shows the vitamin deficiency states.

Table 8–1 Common Vitamin Requirements. (© Delmar/Cengage Learning)

Vitamin	RDA	Physiologic Effects Essential for:
A (retinol, retinaldehyde, retonic acid)	1400–6000 IU	Growth & development epithelial tissue maintenance; reproduction prevents night blindness
B complex:		
B-1 (thiamine)	0.3–1.5 mg	Energy metabolism: normal nerve function
B-2 (riboflavin)	0.4–1.8 mg	Reactions in energy cycle that produce ATP; oxidation of amino acids and hydroxy acids; oxidation of purines
B-3 Niacin (nicotinic acid, nicotinamide)	5–19 mg	Synthesis of fatty acids and cholesterol; blocks FFA; conversion of phenylalanine to tyrosine
B-6 (pyridoxine, pyridoxal, pyridoxamine)	0.3–2.5 mg	Amino acid metabolism; glycogenolyis, RBC/Hb synthesis; formation of neurotransmitters; formation of antibodies
Folacin (folic acid, pteroylglutamic acid)	50–800 µg	DNA synthesis, formation of RBCs in bone marrow with cyanocobalamine
Pantothenic acid (calcium pantothenate, dexpanthenol)	10 mg	Synthesis of sterols, steroid hormones, porphyrins; synthesis and degradation of fatty acids; oxidative metabolism of carbohydrates, gluconeogenesis
B-12 (cyanocobalamin, hydroxocobalamin, extrinsic factor)	0.3–4.0 µg	DNA synthesis in bone marrow; RBC production with folacin; nerve tissue maintenance
B-7 (Biotin)	No recommendation	Synthesis of fatty acids, generation of tricarboxylic acid cycle; formation of purines Coenzyme in CHO metabolism

(continues)

Table 8–1 (continued)

Vitamin	RDA	Physiologic Effects Essential for:
C (ascorbic acid, ascorbate)	60 mg	Formation of collagen; conversion of cholesterol to bile acids; protects Vit. A and E and polyunsaturated fats from excessive oxidation; absorption and utilization of iron; converts folacin to folinic acid; some role in clotting, adrenocortical hormones, and resistance to cancer and infections
D (calcitriol, cholecalciferol, dihydrotachysterol, ergocalciferol, viosterol)	400 IU	Intestinal absorption and metabolism of calcium and phosphorus as well as renal reabsorption; release of calcium from bone and resorption
E (tocopherol)	4–15 IU	May oppose destruction of Vit. A and fats by oxygen fragments called free radicals; antioxidant; may affect production of prostaglandins which regulate a variety of body processes
K (menadione, phytonadione)	No recommendation	Formation of prothrombin and other clotting proteins by the liver; blood coagulation

Table 8–2 Vitamins and Uses. (© Delmar/Cengage Learning)

Vitamin	Effect	Uses
A (retinoic acid)	Reduces formation of comedones; keratin production suppression	Acne, psoriasis, ichthyosis, Darier's disease xerophthalmia, intestinal infections, prevents night blindness
Niacin	Reduction of blood cholesterol and triglycerides; blocks FFA release	Hypercholesterolemia, hyperbetalipoproteinemia
D (dihydrotachysterol)	Maintains calcium and phosphorus levels in bone and blood	Hypoparathyroidism: increase intestinal absorption of calcium
C	Reduces urine pH; converts methemoglobin to hemoglobin	Idiopathic methemoglobin; recurrent UTIs in high risk clients; aids in iron absorption
E	Reduces endogenous perioxidases	Hemolytic anemia in premature infants; protects cell membranes from oxidation
K	Increases liver production of thrombin	Warfarin toxicity; essential for blood coagulation

Table 8–3 Vitamin Deficiency States. (© Delmar/Cengage Learning)

Vitamin	Deficiency	Signs & Symptoms
A	Xerophthalmia	Progressive eye changes: night blindness to xerosis of conjunctiva and cornea with scarring
	Keratomalacia	Degeneration of epithelial cells with hardening and shrinking
B-6	Beriberi	Fatigue, weight loss, weakness, irritability; headaches, insomnia, peripheral neuropathy, CHF, cardiomyopathy
Niacin	Pellagra	Depression, anorexia, beefy red glossitis, cheilosis, dermatitis
B-12	Pernicious anemia	Macrocytic, megaloblastic anemia; progressive neuropathy R/T demyelination
C	Scurvy	Joint pain, growth retardation, anemia, poor wound healing with increased susceptibility to infection; petechial hemorrhages
D	Rickets (child) Osteomalacia (adult)	Demineralization of bones and teeth with bone pain and skeletal muscle deformities
E	Hemolytic anemia in low birth weight infants	Macrocytic anemia; increased hemolysis of RBCs and increased capillary fragility
K	Hemorrhagic disease in newborns	Increase tendency to hemorrhage (Rx)

CONCLUSION

The classification of drugs is the orderly grouping of drugs that have the same or similar mechanisms of action. Attempting to memorize each individual drug as to its mechanism, indications, contraindications and precautions is a tedious method to learning drugs. However, by placing drugs in orderly groups as to how they work eliminates much of the repetition in the learning process. Therefore, it is best to place drugs in their groups or classifications to give a more systematic approach to learning.

▷ STUDY QUESTIONS

1. Your patient is a 60-year-old female experiencing an asthma attack. Which class of drug would you expect to administer to her?
   a. Alpha$_1$-adrenergic blocking drug
   b. Antihistamine (H$_1$ blocker)
   c. Corticosteroid
   d. Sympathomimetic

2. While conducting your medication assessment, your 55-year-old male patient states that he is taking a pill for high cholesterol. Drugs that lower cholesterol are classified as:
   a. Sulfonamides
   b. ACE inhibitors
   c. Antihyperlipidemic drugs
   d. Anticoagulants

3. A(n) _____ can be used to treat high blood pressure.
   a. Antiarrhythmic
   b. Neuromuscular blocker
   c. Theophylline derivative
   d. Thyroid drug

4. Briefly explain the importance of vitamins in our diet.
   _____
   _____
   _____
   _____
   _____
   _____
   _____

5. A patient suffering from a urinary tract infection would most likely be taking:
   a. Sulfonamides
   b. Tetracyclines
   c. Anti-inflammatories
   d. A general anti-infective

6. A common classification of drugs used to treat anxiety is:
   a. Neuromuscular blocking drug
   b. Tricyclic antidepressant
   c. Antipsychotic drug
   d. Aminophylline

7. A common respiratory side effect from taking antihistamines (H$_1$ blockers) is:
   a. Dizziness
   b. Postural hypotension
   c. Acute labyrinthitis
   d. Thickening of bronchial secretions

8. A common cardiovascular side effect of a sympathomimetic drug is:
   a. Hypotension
   b. Bradycardia
   c. Tachycardia
   d. Flushing

9. Drugs that displace previously given narcotics from their receptor sites are called:
   a. Narcotic antagonists
   b. Narcotic analgesics
   c. Neuromuscular blockers
   d. Parasympathetic blockers

10. A common contraindication for administering a beta-adrenergic blocking drug is:
    a. Sinus bradycardia
    b. Sinus tachycardia
    c. Hypertension
    d. Ventricular arrhythmias

CHAPTER 9

DRUGS USED TO TREAT PULMONARY EMERGENCIES

Therapeutic Classifications of Drugs Used for Respiratory Emergencies

Adrenergics
Ephedrine sulfate
Epinephrine
Metaproterenol sulfate
Racemic epinephrine
Salmeterol xinafoate

Antiasthmatics
Cromolyn sodium
Zafirlukast
Zileuton

Anticholinergics
Atropine
Ipratropium bromide

Antihistamines
Diphenhydramine
  hydrochloride
Promethazine hydrochloride

Bronchodilators
Albuterol
Albuterol/ipratropium
Aminophylline
Bitolterol mesylate
Levalbuterol
Terbutaline sulfate

Corticosteroids
Fluticasone propionate
Hydrocortisone
Triamcinolone

Diuretic
Furosemide

Electrolyte
Magnesium sulfate

Glucocorticoids
Beclomethasone dipropronate

Dexamethasone
Methyprednisolone

Inotropic
Milrinone

Neuromuscular Blocking Drugs
Pancuronium bromide
Rocuronium bromide
Succinylcholine chloride
Vecuronium bromide

**Nondepolarizing Skeletal
  Muscle Relaxants**
Atracurium
Tubocurarine chloride

Medicinal Gas
Oxygen

OBJECTIVES

On completion of this chapter and the study questions, you should be able to:

• Describe the use of pulse oximetry in the out-of-hospital setting.

- Describe the use of capnography (end-tidal carbon dioxide detection) in the out-of-hospital setting.
- Describe the out-of-hospital management of asthma and status asthmaticus.
- Describe the following adrenergic drugs: ephedrine, epinephrine, metaproterenol, racemic epinephrine, and salmeterol.
- Describe the following antiasthmatic drugs: cromolyn, zafirlukast, and zileuton.
- Define the following anticholinergic drugs: atropine and ipratropium.
- Define the following antihistamine drugs: diphenhydramine and promethazine.
- Describe the following bronchodilator drugs: albuterol, albuterol/ipratropium, aminophylline, bitolterol, and levalbuterol.
- Describe the following corticosteroid drugs: fluticasone, hydrocortisone, and triamcinolone.
- Describe the diuretic drug furosemide.
- Describe the following glucocorticoid drugs: beclomethasone, dexa-methasone, and methyprednisolone.
- Describe the inotropic drug milrinone.
- Describe the following neuromuscular blocking drugs: atracurium, pancuronium, rocuronium, succinylcholine, tubocurarine, and vecuronium.
- Describe oxygen (medicinal gas) and magnesium sulfate (electrolyte).
- Describe the steps in performing rapid-sequence intubation (RSI).

KEY TERMS

Adrenergic	Bronchodilator	Glucocorticoid
Antiasthmatic	Capnography	Leukotriene
Anticholinergic	Corticosteroids	Neuromuscular blocking agent
Antihistamine	End-tidal carbon dioxide	Pulse oximetry
Asthma	($ETCO_2$) detector	Status asthmaticus

CASE STUDY

You are called to a local playground for a child having trouble breathing. When you arrive you find a 13-year-old male who is complaining of chest tightness and having trouble breathing. You find out that your patient had been playing "touch football" with his friends. He admits to you that he has asthma, and should not have been playing football.

Your initial assessment reveals your patient has wheezing with labored breathing, is pale, and has a rapid heart rate.

1. According to local protocol, your first-line drug for asthma is albuterol at an initial dose of:
   a. MDI, 2 inhalations (180 mcg).
   b. MDI, 1 inhalation (90 mcg).
   c. 50 mg slow IV.
   d. 0.01 mcg/kg, SQ.

2. A respiratory side effect of albuterol you should be assessing for is:
   a. Hypertension.
   b. Epistaxis.
   c. Fatigue.
   d. Epigastric pain.

INTRODUCTION

Responding to a pulmonary (respiratory) emergency is a common occurrence for EMS professionals. A familiar scenario consists of a patient in a sitting position, leaning forward, and fighting to breathe, using accessory muscles. Wheezing is usually present, but may become fainter as the patient's condition becomes more severe. The problem—an acute asthma attack.

Fighting for breath can be a terrifying and potentially fatal experience. The EMS professional must be able to act quickly and accurately when treating pulmonary emergencies. In many such emergencies, a calm EMS professional and 100% humidified oxygen are all that is required to provide the patient with relief. However, if needed, several drugs are effective in relieving pulmonary distress.

Except for oxygen, most of the drugs presented in this chapter therapeutically work as bronchodilators. A bronchodilator acts by relaxing the smooth muscles of the bronchial airways and pulmonary blood vessels, making it easier for the patient to breathe.

Most bronchodilators are classified pharmacologically as adrenergic drugs. Adrenergic drugs primarily act on beta$_2$-receptors, relaxing bronchial smooth muscles. When beta$_2$-receptors are stimulated, however, beta$_1$-receptors are also stimulated, to a lesser extent. Beta$_1$-stimulation causes the heart to increase in both rate and contractile force.

Pulse oximetry has become the standard of care in out-of-hospital emergency medicine. The pulse oximeter is another tool we can use to help objectively determine the oxygenation status of our patients. It should be immediately applied to the patient to help establish baseline vital signs. The normal SpO$_2$ should be between 95-100%. If the SpO$_2$ reading is below 95%, but above 90% (91-94%), the patient is experiencing mild hypoxia and should be administered humidified oxygen. The patient is experiencing moderate hypoxia when the SpO$_2$ reading is below 91%, but above 85% (86-90%). In this case the patient needs to be continually assessed, and administered 100% humidified oxygen. A SpO$_2$ reading below 86% is an indication that the patient is experiencing severe hypoxia, and should be given 100% humidified oxygen, and possibly advanced airway assistance.

Capnography, the continuous monitoring of carbon dioxide levels in expired air of mechanically ventilated patients, has also become the standard of care in out-of-hospital emergency medicine. A common device used for this purpose is the end-tidal carbon dioxide (ETCO$_2$) detector. When the ETCO$_2$ detector indicates a lack of carbon dioxide in expired air, the endotracheal (ET) tube is most likely in the esophagus, and the patient should be reintubated. The reverse is also true; when the ETCO$_2$ detector indicates the presence of carbon dioxide in the expired air, the ET tube is most likely placed properly.

It is important not to rely on any one device when assessing your patient. Both the pulse oximeter and the ETCO$_2$ detector are to be used only as adjuncts when performing pulmonary assessments and ET tube placement.

Asthma

Asthma is a disease caused by a narrowing and inflammation of the tracheobronchial tree by various stimuli. When this occurs, patients generally present with wheezing, shortness of breath, and coughing. Most patients have mild/moderate asthma. However, some patients have continuous asthma attacks called **status asthmaticus**, which may be fatal.

The recurrence and severity of asthma attacks is influenced by *triggers,* or the causes of the asthma attack. Some examples of asthma triggers include such influences as allergens, dust, various medicines, dyes, odors, exercise, or exposure to occupational hazards.

Generally, asthma occurs most often in children or young adults. However, asthma can occur at any age. Asthma occurs more often in boys than girls before puberty; however, in adults, asthma is equally distributed between the sexes.

The successful treatment of an asthma attack is focused on correcting hypoxia, reversing bronchospasm, and treating inflammatory changes. Oxygen is an important part of asthma treatment in most attacks. Beyond oxygen, mild asthma attacks are managed well with beta-agonists such as albuterol. Patients experiencing moderate asthma attacks often may require multiple medications, including long-acting beta-agonists, **corticosteroids**, and **leukotriene** antagonists.

Severe asthma attacks may require high doses of beta-agonists and steroids. Airway patency via endotracheal (ET) intubation and mechanical ventilation may also be required for severe asthma attacks.

Individual Drugs

ALBUTEROL

(al-BYOU-ter-ohl)
Pregnancy Class: C
Proventil, Ventolin, Volmax (Rx)
Classifications: Albuterol is a direct-acting adrenergic drug, bronchodilator (beta agonist)

Mechanism of Action

Albuterol causes bronchodilation by stimulating $beta_2$-receptors of the bronchi. Also has minimal $beta_1$-stimulation.

Indications

Albuterol is used to treat bronchial asthma, bronchospasm caused by bronchitis, and reversible chronic obstructive pulmonary disease (COPD).

Contraindications

Albuterol should not be used in patients who are lactating.

Precautions

Because of its mild $beta_1$ (cardiac) effects, albuterol should be used with caution in patients with heart disease, hypertension, and patients with diabetes.

How Supplied

Metered dose inhaler: 0.09 mg/inh.

Route and Dosage

Adult: Metered dose inhaler—patients over 12 years of age: 2 inhalations (180 mcg) every 4–6 hours. (Ventolin may be used in patients over 4 years of age).
Nebulizer: 2.5 to 5 mg every 20 minutes. Do not exceed three doses.
Pediatric: Metered dose inhaler: 1 inhalation (90 mcg) every 4 hours.
Nebulizer: 0.15 mg/kg every 20 minutes. Do not exceed three doses.

Adverse Reactions and Side Effects

CNS: Headache, fatigue, lightheadedness, irritability, aggressive behavior.
Respiratory: Epistaxis, hoarseness, nasal congestion, an increase in sputum.
CV: Hypertension, tachycardia, arrhythmias, chest pain.
GI: Dry mouth, epigastric pain.

EMS Considerations

1. Some patients may only require 1 inhalation; monitor closely.
2. Instruct the patient to inhale through the nose and exhale through pursed lips. This prolongs expiration and keeps the airway open longer.

Drug Interactions

None.

ALBUTEROL/IPRATROPIUM

(al-BYOU-ter-ohl/i-pra-TROE-pee-um)
Pregnancy Class: C
Combivent, DuoNeb,(Rx)
Classification: combination bronchodilator

Mechanism of Action

Stimulates $beta_2$ receptors and antagonizes the acetylcholine receptor causing bronchodilation.

Indications

If a first-line bronchodilator is ineffective, used to treat COPD or acute asthma during transport.

Contraindications

Do not give albuterol/ipratropium to patients with a known allergy to peanuts or soybeans.

Precautions

Use with caution in patients with asthma, cardiovascular disease, or in patients with closed-angle glaucoma.

How Supplied

14.7 g canister, which supplies 200 doses.

Route and Dosage

Adult: 2 inhalations (240 mcg albuterol and 42 mcg ipratropium) every 6 hours by metered dose inhaler.

Adverse Reactions and Side Effects

Resp.: bronchospasm, cough
CV: arrhythmias
CNS: headache
GI: nausea

AMINOPHYLLINE

(am-in-OFF-ih-lin)
Pregnancy Class: C
Aminophyllin, Truphyllin (Rx)
Classification: Bronchodilator

Mechanism of Action

Aminophylline relaxes bronchial smooth muscles. It also stimulates the heart and the respiratory center in the brain. Aminophylline contains approximately 80% theophylline.

Indications

Aminophylline is used to treat respiratory problems caused by asthma, COPD, pulmonary edema, and CHF.

Contraindications

Do not give aminophylline to patients who are hypersensitive to the drug, or to patients who are experiencing uncontrolled cardiac arrhythmias because aminophylline can exacerbate the arrhythmias.

Precautions

Aminophylline should be used with caution in patients with edema.

How Supplied

5 mg/mL injection.

Route and Dosage

Adult: 5 mg/kg IV infusion over 20 minutes.

Pediatric: Consult your protocols and/or medical control.
NOTE: Ideally, in patients who are currently receiving a theophylline/ aminophylline preparation, the loading dose should be deferred until the serum theophylline concentration is determined. However, when there is sufficient respiratory distress in these patients to warrant a small risk, half the usual loading dose (2.5 mg/kg) may be administered if no laboratory confirmation of serum theophylline levels is available.
To prepare infusion: Add 250–500 mg of aminophylline to 50–100 mL of IV solution.

Adverse Reactions and Side Effects

CNS: Nervousness, anxiety, headache, seizures.
CV: Arrhythmias, tachycardia, palpitations.
GI: Nausea, vomiting.

EMS Considerations

1. Rapid administration of aminophylline (>25 mg/min) can cause severe hypotension or ventricular fibrillation. If available, use an infusion pump or a device to regulate infusion rate.
2. Monitor vital signs closely; aminophylline may cause transitory lowering of B/P.

Drug Interactions

None.

ATRACURIUM BESYLATE

(ah-trah-KYOUR-ee-um)
Pregnancy Class: C
Tracrium (Rx)
Classification: Nondepolarizing skeletal muscle relaxant

Mechanism of Action

Atracurium prevents the action of acetylcholine by competing for cholinergic receptors.

Indications

Atracurium is used as a skeletal muscle relaxant during endotracheal (ET) intubation.

Contraindications

Atracurium should not be used in patients with electrolyte disorders or in patients with bronchial asthma.

Precautions

Use atracurium with caution in patients during labor and delivery, and in patients who are experiencing histamine release.

Route and Dosage

Adults and children over 2 years of age: 0.4–0.5 mg/kg by IV bolus.

How Supplied

10 mg/mL.

Adverse Reactions and Side Effects

Respiratory: Dyspnea, laryngospasm.
CV: Tachycardia, flushing.

EMS Considerations

Atropine may be used if bradycardia develops. Do not mix atracurium with alkaline solutions, including lactated ringers (LR).

Drug Interactions

None.

ATROPINE SULFATE

(AH-troh-peen)
Pregnancy Class: C
Classification: Anticholinergic drug

Mechanism of Action

Atropine an **anticholinergic drug**, competes with the neurotransmitter acetylcholine for receptor sites, blocking the stimulation of parasympathetic nerve fibers.

Indications

Atropine can be used for the treatment of exercise-induced bronchospasm.

Contraindications

Atropine should not be used in patients suffering from acute bronchospasm, as a more rapid response is required.

Precautions

Atropine should be used with caution in patients with hypertension and cardiovascular disease, because of the increased workload placed on the heart.

Route and Dosage

Administered using a small-volume nebulizer by adding 0.5–1.0 mg of atropine to 2–3 mL of normal saline.

How Supplied

Atropine is supplied in ampules or vials that contain 1.0 mg in 1mL of solution.

Adverse Reactions and Side Effects

CNS: Anxiety, dizziness, headache, nervousness.
CV: Palpitations.
GI: Nausea and vomiting, dry mouth.

EMS Considerations

The patient's lung sounds should be assessed and peak flow rate measured before and after administration.

Drug Interactions

None.

BECLOMETHASONE DIPROPIONATE

(be-kloh-METH-ah-zohn)
Pregnancy Class: C
Beclovent (Rx)
Classification: Glucocorticoid

Mechanism of Action

Beclomethasone has properties that help regulate the metabolic pathways that involve protein, carbohydrates, and fat that help produce an anti-inflammatory effect.

Indications

Beclomethasone is used in chronic therapy for patients experiencing bronchial asthma.

Contraindications

Beclomethasone should not be used in patients with status asthmaticus or in patients who are hypersensitive to the drug.

Precautions

The safe use of beclomethasone in patients under the age of 6 has not been established.

How Supplied

Metered dose inhaler: 0.042 mg/inh, 0.084 mg/inh.

Route and Dosage

Adult: 2–4 inhalations (84–168 μg) t.i.d.–q.i.d. Maximum dose: 20 inhalations (840 μg) daily.
Pediatric (6–12 years of age): 1–2 inhalations (42–84 μg) t.i.d.–q.i.d. Maximum dose: 10 inhalations (420 μg) daily.

Adverse Reactions and Side Effects

CNS: Headache.
Respiratory: Pharyngitis, coughing, epistaxis, nasal burning.

EMS Considerations

1. If the canister is cold, the therapeutic effects may be decreased.
2. To administer:
   - Shake canister thoroughly.
   - Ask the patient to exhale as completely as possible.
   - Have the patient inhale deeply while pressing the canister down with forefinger.
   - After inhalation, ask the patient to hold his/her breath as long as possible; then exhale slowly.
   - At least 1 minute must elapse between doses.
3. If the patient is also receiving bronchodilators by inhalation (i.e., albuterol) use the bronchodilator first which will open the airway and increase the penetration of the beclomethasone.

Drug Interactions

None.

BITOLTEROL MESYLATE

(bye-TOHL-ter-ohl)
Pregnancy Class: C
Tornalate Aerosol (Rx)
Classification: Bronchodilator

Mechanism of Action

Bitolterol combines with $beta_2$-adrenergic receptors producing dilation of the bronchioles. Bitolterol has little $beta_1$-adrenergic effect.

Indications

Bitolterol is used to treat bronchitis, emphysema, and COPD. It may be used with theophylline and/or steroids.

Contraindications

Known hypersensitivity.

Precautions

Safety has not been established in children less than 12 years of age. Use with caution in the following: ischemic heart disease, hypertension, diabetes mellitus, cardiac arrhythmias caused by increased afterload, and in patients with seizure disorders.

How Supplied

Metered dose inhaler: 0.37 mg/inh.

Route and Dosage

Patients over 12 years of age: 2 inhalations at an interval of 1–3 min.

Adverse Reactions and Side Effects

CNS: Lightheadedness.
CV: Premature ventricular contractions (PVCs).

EMS Considerations

To correctly administer bitolterol, the inhaler must be upright. Have the patient exhale completely. Then instruct the patient to breathe in slowly and deeply, squeezing the canister and mouthpiece between the thumb and forefinger. The patient should then hold his/her breath for 10 seconds and then slowly exhale.

Drug Interactions

Additive effects with other beta-adrenergic bronchodilators.

CROMOLYN SODIUM

(CROM-moh-lin)
Pregnancy Class: B
Intal (Rx)
Classifications: Antiasthmatic, antiallergic drug

Mechanism of Action

Prevents the release of histamine, slow-reacting substance of anaphylaxis, and other substances causing hypersensitivity reactions.

Indications

Cromolyn is an adjunct drug used in the management of severe bronchial asthma.

Contraindications

Cromolyn should not be used in patients who are hypersensitive to the drug or in patients experiencing status asthmaticus.

Precautions

Cromolyn should be used with caution in patients who are lactating.

How Supplied

Metered dose inhaler: 0.8 mg/inh.

Route and Dosage

Adult: Prophylaxis for bronchial asthma: 20 mg q.i.d. Adjust dosage as required. Prophylaxis for bronchospasm: 20 mg single dose. Not recommended for out-of-hospital pediatric use.

Adverse Reactions and Side Effects

Respiratory: Bronchospasm, cough.
CNS: Dizziness, headache, drowsiness.
GI: Nausea.

EMS Considerations

None.

Drug Interactions

None.

DEXAMETHASONE

(dex-ah-METH-ah-zohn)
Decadron (Rx)
Classification: Glucocorticoid

Mechanism of Action

Dexamethasone is a long-acting steroid that suppresses inflammation and normal immune response.

Indications

Dexamethasone is used to treat severe allergic reactions.

Contraindications

There are no contraindications for a single out-of-hospital dose of dexamethasone.

Precautions

Use dexamethasone in pregnant patients only if the benefits outweigh risks. Also use with caution in patients with hypertension and CHF, as dexamethasone can cause fluid retention.

Route and Dosage

Adult: 4 mg administered by slow IV bolus.
Pediatric: Not recommended in the out-of-hospital setting.

How Supplied

24 mg/mL in 5- and 10-mL ampules.

Adverse Reactions and Side Effects

CNS: Headache, restlessness, depression, vertigo.
CV: Hypertension, CHF.
GI: Abdominal distention, nausea and vomiting.

EMS Considerations

Dexamethasone is sensitive to temperature extremes.

Drug Interactions

None.

DIPHENHYDRAMINE HYDROCHLORIDE

(dye-fen-HY-drah-meen)
Pregnancy Class: B
Benadryl (Rx)
Classification: Antihistamine (H$_1$-receptor antagonist)

Mechanism of Action

Diphenhydramine competes with histamine for H$_1$ receptor sites. It has significant anticholinergic properties. Diphenhydramine blocks the effects of histamine, including vasodilation, increased gastrointestinal tract secretions, increased heart rate, and hypotension.

Indications

Diphenhydramine is used in addition to epinephrine for the symptomatic relief of allergic symptoms caused by histamine release.

Contraindications

Do not administer diphenhydramine to patients experiencing acute asthma attacks, because it thickens bronchial secretions.

Precautions

Administer diphenhydramine with caution to patients with cardiovascular disease or hypertension.

Route and Dosage

Adult: 10–50 mg by slow IV bolus or deep IM injection at a rate of approximately 1 mL/min. Note that some patients may require up to 100 mg.
Pediatric: 2–5 mg/kg by slow IV bolus or deep IM injection. Note that the usual dosage is 10–30 mg.

How Supplied

10 mg/mL, 50 mg/mL ampules or vials.

Adverse Reactions and Side Effects

CNS: Drowsiness, dizziness, headache, and (possible) paradoxic excitement in children.
Respiratory: Wheezing, thickening of bronchial secretions, tightness of the chest.
CV: Palpitations, hypotension.
Eyes: Blurred vision.
GI: Dry mouth, diarrhea, nausea and vomiting.

EMS Considerations

Assess the patient's airway patency, lung sounds, respiratory function, frequently.

Drug Interactions

None.

EPHEDRINE SULFATE

(eh-FED-rin)
Pregnancy Class: C
Ephed II (Rx)
Classification: Adrenergic drug

Mechanism of Action

Ephedrine, an **antihistamine**, releases norepinephrine, having a direct effect on both alpha- and beta-receptors. This causes increased B/P by arteriolar constriction, cardiac stimulation, and bronchodilation.

Indications

Ephedrine is used to treat bronchial asthma and reversible bronchospasms associated with obstructive pulmonary disease.

Contraindications

Ephedrine should not be used in patients who have diabetes, pregnancy where blood pressure is greater than 130/80 mm Hg, and patients who are lactating.

Precautions

Ephedrine should be used with caution in patients with ischemic heart disease, because it can cause hypertension and angina.

Route and Dosage

Adult: 12.5–25 mg slow IV.
Pediatric: 3 mg/kg slow IV.

How Supplied

50 mg/mL ampules or vials.

Adverse Reactions and Side Effects

CNS: Nervousness, confusion, hallucinations.
Respiratory: Difficulty breathing.
CV: Angina.

EMS Considerations

Monitor vitals signs frequently. Also assess mental status and pulmonary function.

Drug Interactions

Dexamethasone: Ephedrine decreases effect of dexamethasone.
Diuretics: Diuretics decrease response to sympathomimetics.
Furazolidone: Increase pressor effect leading to possible hypertensive crisis and intracranial hemorrhage.
Guanethidine: Decrease effect of guanethidine by displacement from its site of action.
Halothane: Serious arrhythmias caused by sensitization of the myocardium to sympathomimetics by halothane.
MAO Inhibitors: Increase pressor effect leading to possible hypertensive crisis and intracranial hemorrhage.
Methyldopa: Effect of ephedrine decreases in methyldopa-treated clients.
Oxytocic drugs: Severe persistent hypertension.

EPINEPHRINE

(ep-ih-NEF-rin)
Pregnancy Class: C
Adrenalin, EpiPen (Rx)
Classification: Adrenergic drug

Mechanism of Action

Epinephrine is a catecholamine that stimulates both alpha-adrenergic and beta-adrenergic receptors in the sympathetic nervous system. Stimulation of $beta_1$-receptors increases the rate and force of cardiac contractions, resulting in an increase in cardiac output. Stimulation of $beta_2$-adrenergic receptors relaxes the bronchial smooth muscles, thereby increasing vital lung capacity. Epinephrine's stimulation of alpha receptors causes the arterioles of the bronchioles to constrict, which can help reduce edema. Alpha-adrenergic stimulation also produces peripheral vasoconstriction, which aids in raising arterial blood pressure.

Indications

Epinephrine is used to treat acute bronchial asthma, bronchospasms caused by emphysema, chronic bronchitis, and in patients experiencing anaphylaxis.

Contraindications

Epinephrine should not be administered to patients experiencing cardiac arrhythmias.

Precautions

Epinephrine should be used with caution in patients with cardiac disease, diabetes, or in patients with hypertension.

Route and Dosage

(Bronchodilation) Adult: 0.3–0.5 mg (0.3–0.5 mL) SC of a 1:1000 solution.
Pediatric: 0.01 mg/kg (0.01 mL/kg) SC of a 1:1000 solution.
(Mild/moderate anaphylaxis) Adult: 0.3–0.5 mg (0.3–0.5 mL) of a 1:1000 solution SC. Autoinjector, IM, 0.3 mg; repeat doses may be necessary.
(Severe anaphylaxis) Adult: 0.3–0.5 mg slow IV bolus (3–5 mL of a 1:10,000 solution). In addition to the IV bolus, an IV infusion may be necessary at 1 mg/min but not to exceed 4 mg/min.
To prepare infusion: Add 2 mg of a 1:1000 solution to 500 mL of IV solution, making a concentration of 4 mg/mL.
(Mild/moderate anaphylaxis) Pediatric: 0.01 mL/kg of a 1:1000 solution SC. Autoinjector, IM, 0.15 mg; repeat injections may be necessary.
(Severe anaphylaxis) Pediatric: 0.1 mL/kg of a 1:10,000 solution by IV bolus.

How Supplied

1 mg/mL ampule, 1 mg/10mL prefilled syringe. Also comes in multi-dose vials.

Adverse Reactions and Side Effects

CNS: Headache, nervousness, tremor.
CV: Arrhythmias, hypertension, chest pain.
GI: Nausea, vomiting.

EMS Considerations

Monitor patient closely; pay special attention to blood pressure, pulse, and ECG status. Assess lung sounds before and after administration. An IV bolus injection of a 1:1000 solution may cause sudden hypertension or cerebral edema.

Drug Interactions

Beta-adrenergic blocking agents: Initial effectiveness in treating glaucoma of this combination may decrease over time.
Chymotrypsin: Epinephrine, 1:100, will inactivate chymotrypsin in 60 minutes.

FLUTICASONE PROPIONATE

(flu-TIH-kah-sohn)
Pregnancy Class: C
Flovent (Rx)
Classification: Corticosteroid

Mechanism of Action

Fluticasone has anti-inflammatory properties that aid in the reduction of airway constriction in patients experiencing asthma.

Indications

Fluticasone is used in the prevention and maintenance in the treatment of asthma in patients over 4 years of age.

Contraindications

Fluticasone should not be used in patients who have experienced nasal surgery or nasal trauma until healing has occurred.

Precautions

Fluticasone should be used with caution in patients experiencing bacterial or viral infections, and during lactation.

Route and Dosage

Adults and children over 4 years of age: 100 μg by metered-dose inhaler.

How Supplied

0.11 mg/inh, 0.22 mg/inh, 0.44 mg/inh.

Adverse Reactions and Side Effects

CNS: Headache, dizziness.
Respiratory: Epistaxis, nasal burning, nasal dryness.
GI: Nausea and vomiting.

EMS Considerations

None.

Drug Interactions

None.

FUROSEMIDE

(fur-OH-se-mide)
Pregnancy Class: C
Lasix, (Rx)
Classification: Diuretic

Mechanism of Action

Furosimide inhibits the reabsorption of sodium and chloride in the kidneys.

Indications

Furosimide can be used to treat pulmonary edema and congestive heart failure (CHF).

Contraindications

Do not give furosimide to patients with: hypovolemia, hypotension, hypokalemia. Suspect kypokalemia if the patient is on long-term diuretic therapy of if the ECG shows prominent P waves, diminished T waves, or the presence of U waves. Known hypersensitivity to furosemide.

Precautions

Patients hypersensitive to sulfonamides or thiazide diuretics may be hypersensitive to furosemide. Administration to furosemide may result in dehydration and hypotension; geriatric patients are at increased risk.

Route and Dosage

Adult: 0.5–1.0 mg/kg by slow IV bolus over 1–2 minutes.
Pediatric: 1 mg/kg by slow IV bolus over 1–2 minutes.

Adverse Reactions and Side Effects

CV: hypotension and arrhythmias
CNS: dizziness and headache
GI: nausea, vomiting, diarrhea
Fluids and electrolytes: potassium depletion, metabolic alkalosis

How Supplied

10 mg/mL

EMS Considerations

Because of furosemide's diuretic effect, monitor the patient's blood pressure closely. Assess lung sounds before giving furosemide and monitor them closely after administration.

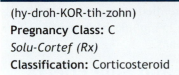

HYDROCORTISONE

(hy-droh-KOR-tih-zohn)
Pregnancy Class: C
Solu-Cortef (Rx)
Classification: Corticosteroid

Mechanism of Action

Hydrocoritsone has anti-inflammatory properties that are used in the treatment of severe anaphylaxis.

Indications

Hydrocoritsone is used in the treatment of severe, anaphylaxis, asthma, or COPD.

Contraindications

None.

Precautions

Only one dose of hydrocortisone should be administered in the out-of-hospital setting.

Route and Dosage

Adult: 15–240 mg IV. If an IV cannot be started, hydrocortisone can be administered IM at 100–500 mg.

How Supplied

50 mg/mL vials.

Adverse Reactions and Side Effects

CNS: Headache, vertigo.
CV: CHF, fluid retention, hypertension.
GI: Nausea.

EMS Considerations

Administer IV solution at a rate of 100 mg over 30 seconds. Doses greater than 500 mg should be infused over 10 minutes.

Drug Interactions

None.

IPRATROPIUM BROMIDE

(eye-prah-TROH-pee-um)
Pregnancy Class: B
Atrovent (Rx)
Classification: Anticholinergic

Mechanism of Action

Ipratropium blocks the action of acetylcholine, which inhibits parasympathetic stimulation. This action causes bronchodilation and dries bronchial secretions.

Indications

Ipratropium is used to treat patients with COPD, including chronic bronchitis and emphysema.

Contraindications

Ipratropium should not be used in patients hypersensitive to the drug or hypersensitive to atropine.

Precautions

Use ipratropium with caution in patients with narrow-angle glaucoma, and in patients who are lactating. Safety has not been determined in children.

Route and Dosage

2 inhalations (36 µg). Additional inhalations may be needed, but should not exceed 12 inhalations/day.

How Supplied

0.018 mg/inh.

Adverse Reactions and Side Effects

CNS: Headache, dizziness, nervousness, fatigue, difficulty in coordination, tremor.
CV: Tachycardia, palpitations, flushing.
Respiratory: Cough, dyspnea, worsening of COPD symptoms.
GI: Dry mouth, GI distress, nausea.

EMS Considerations

Ipratropium may be mixed with albuterol in the nebulizer if used within 1 hour. Perform detailed pulmonary assessment before and after administration.

Drug Interactions

None.

LEVALBUTEROL

(leev-al-BYOO-ter-ole)
Pregnancy Class: C
Xopenex (Rx)
Classification: Bronchodilator

Mechanism of Action

Levalbuterol binds beta$_2$ adrenergic receptors in airway smooth muscle causing bronchodilation.

Indications

Levalbuterol is given for short-term control of bronchospasm due to reversible airway disease.

Contraindications

Known hypersensitivity to levalbuterol or albuterol.

Precautions

Levalbuterol should be used with caution in patients with cardiovascular disease, hypokalemia, and in patients with a history of seizures.

Route and Dosage

Adults: 0.63 mg by nebulization three times daily.
Pediatrics: 0.16–1.25 mg by nebulization (single dose).

How Supplied

0.31 mg/3mL vials; 0.63 mg/3 mL vials; 1.25 mg/3mL vials; 1.25 mg/0.5 mL unit-dose vials.

Adverse Reactions and Side Effects

Resp.: increased cough, paradoxical bronchospasm, nasal edema
CV: tachycardia
CNS: dizziness, headache, nervousness, anxiety
GI: dyspepsia

EMS Considerations

Before giving levalbuterol, obtain baseline ECG and vital signs and monitor patient closely.

MAGNESIUM SULFATE

(mag-NEE-see-um SUL-fayt)
Pregnancy Class: A
Classification: Electrolyte

Mechanism of Action

Magnesium sulfate is an essential element for muscle contraction and nerve transmission.

Indications

Magnesium sulfate can be used as an adjunct medication to treat moderate to severe asthma in patients who respond poorly to beta-agonists.

Contraindications

Magnesium should not be used in patients with heart block or who have myocardial damage, or in patients with hypertension.

Precautions

Use magnesium sulfate with caution in patients with renal disease, because magnesium sulfate is removed from the body solely by the kidneys.

Route and Dosage

Adult: 2 grams in 100 mL of IV solution, given over 2–5 minutes.
Pediatric: 25–50 mg/kg IV over 10–20 minutes. Dilute in D_5W before administration.

How Supplied

Supplied in both vials and prefilled syringes at 40 mg/mL, 80 mg/mL, 100 mg/mL, and 125 mg/mL. Magnesium sulfate comes as 10% and 50% solutions.

Adverse Reactions and Side Effects

CNS: Drowsiness, respiratory depression.
CV: Bradycardia, hypotension, arrhythmias.
Miscellaneous: Itching, flushing, hypothermia.

EMS Considerations

Rapid IV administration may cause respiratory or cardiac arrest. An overdose of magnesium sulfate may cause respiratory depression and/or heart block. To reverse these effects, hyperventilate the patient using 100% humidified oxygen and administer an IV bolus of 10% calcium gluconate at 5–10 mEq (10–20 mL).

Drug Interactions

CNS depressants (general anesthetics, sedative-hypnotics, narcotics): Additive CNS depression.
Digitalis: Heart block when Mg intoxication is treated with calcium in digitalized clients.
Neuromuscular blocking agents: Possible additive neuromuscular blockage.

METAPROTERENOL SULFATE

(met-ah-proh-TER-ih-nohl)
Pregnancy Class: C
Alupent (Rx)
Classifications: Adrenergic, bronchodilator

Mechanism of Action

Metaproterenol is a strong $beta_2$-adrenergic agonist, having a strong effect on pulmonary receptors, relaxing bronchial smooth muscles. This results in an increase in lung capacity and a decrease in airway resistance. Its minimal $beta_1$-adrenergic effects produce CNS and cardiac stimulation.

Indications

Metaproterenol is a bronchodilator used to treat asthma, bronchitis, emphysema, and other conditions associated with reversible bronchospasms.

Contraindications

Do not use metaproterenol in patients with preexisting cardiac arrhythmias associated with tachycardia.

Precautions

Use metaproterenol with caution in patients with hypertension, coronary artery disease, CHF, or diabetes.

Route and Dosage

(Hand-held nebulizer) Adult: Usual dose is 10 inhalations (range 5–15 inhalations) of undiluted 5% solution.
(IPPB) Adult: 0.3 mL (range: 0.2–0.3 mL) of a 5% solution diluted to 2.5 mL saline.

How Supplied

Metered-dose inhaler: 0.65 mg/inh.
Solution: 0.4%, 0.6%, 5%.

Adverse Reactions and Side Effects

CNS: Nervousness, tremor, headache.
CV: Hypertension, arrhythmias, chest pain.
GI: Diarrhea, nausea, vomiting.
Miscellaneous: Backache, skin reactions.

EMS Considerations

Excessive use of inhalers can result in tolerance and paradoxic bronchospasm. Assess patient's B/P, pulse rate, respirations, and lung sounds before and after administration. Measure patient's peak flow rate before and after drug administration.

Drug Interactions

Possible potentiation of adrenergic effects if used before or after other sympathomimetic bronchodilators.

METHYLPREDNISOLONE

(meth-ill-pred-NISS-oh-lohn)
Pregnancy Class: C
Solu-Medrol (Rx)
Classification: Glucocorticoid

Mechanism of Action

Methylprednisolone decreases the body's inflammatory response as well as suppresses the body's immune system.

Indications

Methylprednisolone is used in the treatment of severe anaphylaxis, asthma, or COPD.

Contraindications

Do not administer methylprednisolone to patients who are hypersensitive to adrenocorticoid preparations.

Precautions

Use methylprednisolone with caution in patients with renal disease, diabetes, hypertension, seizures, and CHF.

Route and Dosage

Adult: 100–200 mg by IV bolus or IM if an IV cannot be established. Methylprednisolone comes in powdered form and must be reconstituted before use.
Pediatric: Methylprednisolone is not recommended for out-of-hospital use.

How Supplied

Vials containing 125 mg.

Adverse Reactions and Side Effects

CNS: Depression, euphoria, headache, restlessness.
CV: Hypertension, CHF.
GI: Nausea, vomiting.
Miscellaneous: Fluid retention, increased intraocular pressure.

EMS Considerations

Methylprednisolone used with diuretics may cause additive hypokalemia.

Drug Interactions

Erythromycin: Increases effect of methylprednisolone caused by decreased breakdown by liver.
Troleandomycin: Increases effect of methylprednisolone caused by decreased breakdown by liver.

MILRINONE

(MILL-ri-none)
Pregnancy Class: C
Primacor (Rx)
Classification: Inotropic

Mechanism of Action

Milrinone dilates the vascular smooth muscle, decreasing both preload and afterload. It also increases myocardial contractility.

Indications

Milrinone is given to treat CHF that is unresponsive to conventional therapy.

Contraindications

Milrinone should not be given to patients with severe aortic or pulmonic valvular heart disease.

Precautions

Milrinone should be used with caution in patients with a history of arrhythmias or in patients with abnormal digoxin levels.

Route and Dosage (Adults only)

IV loading dose: 50 mcg/kg followed by an *IV infusion:* 0.50 mcg/kg/minute

How Supplied

Injection: 1 mg/mL in 10, 20, and 50 mL vials
Premixed infusion: 20 mg/100 mL and 40 mg/200 mL

Adverse Reactions and Side Effects

CV: hypotension, angina, ventricular arrhythmias
CNS: headache, tremor

EMS Considerations

None

OXYGEN

(OX-ah-gin)
Classification: Medicinal gas

Mechanism of Action

Oxygen is required to enable the cells to break down glucose into a usable energy form. Oxygen is a colorless, odorless, tasteless gas, essential to respiration. At sea level, oxygen makes up approximately 10–16% of venous blood and 17–21% of arterial blood. Oxygen is carried from the lungs to the body's tissues by hemoglobin in the red blood cells. The administration of oxygen increases arterial oxygen tension (PaO_2) and hemoglobin saturation. This improves tissue oxygenation when circulation is adequately maintained.

Indications

Oxygen is used (1) to treat severe chest pain that may be caused by cardiac ischemia, (2) to treat hypoxemia from any cause, and (3) in the treatment of cardiac arrest.

Contraindications

None, for emergency use.

Precautions

If the patient has a history of COPD, begin oxygen administration at lower flow rates, increasing flow rates as necessary.

Route and Dosage

Adult (Inhalation): Several devices are used to administer oxygen, including masks, nasal cannulas, positive pressure devices, and volume-regulated ventilators. Some of the more commonly used oxygen devices and their delivery capacities include:

- *Nasal cannula:* O_2 concentrations of 24–44% at flow rates of 1–6 L/min.
- *Simple face mask:* O_2 concentrations of 40–60% at flow rates of 8–10 L/min.
- *Face mask with oxygen reservoir (non-rebreather):* O_2 concentration of 60% at a flow rate of 6 L/min. An O_2 concentration of almost 100% can be achieved with a flow rate of 10 L/min.

- *Venturi mask:* O_2 concentrations:
    - 24% at 4 L/min.
    - 28% at 4 L/min.
    - 35% at 8 L/min.
    - 40% at 8 L/min.
- *Mouth-to-mask:* With supplemental O_2 at 10 L/min., O_2 concentrations can reach 50%. Without supplemental O_2 concentration reaches only approximately 17%.

Pediatric: Same as the adult.

Adverse Reactions and Side Effects

Respiratory: In rare cases of COPD oxygen administration may reduce respiratory drive. This is not a reason to withhold oxygen, but rather monitor the patient closely.
Miscellaneous: Oxygen that is not humidified may dry out or be irritating to mucous membranes. Therefore, use humidified oxygen whenever possible.

EMS Considerations

Reassure patients who are anxious about face masks but who require high concentrations of oxygen.

Drug Interactions

None.

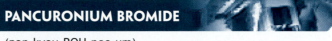

PANCURONIUM BROMIDE

(pan-kyou-ROH-nee-um)
Pregnancy Class: C
Pavulon (Rx)
Classification: Neuromuscular blocking drug

Mechanism of Action

Pancuronium competes with acetylcholine for the receptor sites in the muscle cells, causing paralysis. Muscle paralysis is sequential in the following order: heaviness of the eyelids, difficulty in swallowing and talking, diplopia, progressive weakening of the extremities and neck, relaxation of the truck and spine. The respiratory system is affected last. Pancuronium does not affect consciousness.

Indications

Pancuronium is used to produce muscle relaxation to facilitate endotracheal (ET) intubation.

Contraindications

None, when used for emergency ET intubation.

Precautions

None, when used for emergency ET intubation.

Route and Dosage

Adults and children over 1 month of age: 0.06–0.1 mg/kg IV bolus.

How Supplied

1 mg/mL, 2 mg/mL.

Adverse Reactions and Side Effects

Respiratory: Bronchospasm, apnea, respiratory insufficiency.
CV: Increased heart rate, hypotension.
Miscellaneous: Salivation, skin rash, flushing.

EMS Considerations

Monitor vital signs, and ECG. Pancuronium can cause vagal stimulation producing bradycardia, hypotension, and arrhythmias. Pancuronium does not affect consciousness. Therefore, explain all procedures and provide emotional support for the patient.

Drug Interactions

Azathioprine: Reverses effects of pancuronium.
Bacitracin: Additive muscle relaxation.
Enflurane: Increased muscle relaxation.
Isoflurane: Increased muscle relaxation.
Metocurine: Increased muscle relaxation but duration is not prolonged.
Quinine: Increases effect of pancuronium.
Sodium colistimethate: Increased muscle relaxation.
Succinylcholine: Increases intensity and duration of action of pancuronium.
Tetracyclines: Additive muscle relaxation.
Theophyllines: Decreases effects of pancuronium; also, possible cardiac arrhythmias.
Tricyclic antidepressants with halothane: Administration of pancuronium may cause severe arrhythmias.
Tubocurarine: Increased muscle relaxation but duration is not prolonged.

PROMETHAZINE HYDROCHLORIDE

(proh-METH-ah-zeen)
Pregnancy Class: C
Phenergan (Rx)
Classification: Antihistamine

Mechanism of Action

Promethazine competes with histamine at H_1 histamine receptors, preventing or reversing the effects of histamine.

Indications

Promethazine is used as an adjunct drug in the treatment of anaphylaxis.

Contraindications

Promethazine should not be used in comatose patients, in patients with CNS depression, or in patients who are lactating.

Precautions

Use promethazine with caution in geriatric patients. These patients are more likely to experience confusion, dizziness, and hypotension.

Route and Dosage

Adult: 25–50 mg IV or IM in combination with an equal dose of an analgesic and hypnotic as per protocol. Atropine may also be required as per protocol.
Pediatric, 2–12 years of age: 1.2 mg/kg in combination with an equal dose of analgesic or barbiturate as per protocol. May also be required to administer atropine as per protocol.

How Supplied

25 mg/mL, 50 mg/mL.

Adverse Reactions and Side Effects

CNS: Headache, dizziness, drowsiness, confusion, restlessness.
Respiratory: Thickening of bronchial secretions, wheezing, chest tightness.
CV: Palpitations, bradycardia, reflex tachycardia, QT prolongation, postural hypotension.
GI: Diarrhea, nausea, vomiting.

EMS Considerations

None.

Drug Interactions

None.

RACEMIC EPINEPHRINE

(ra-CEE-mic ep-ih-NEF-rin)
Pregnancy Class: C
microNEFRIN, Vaponefrin (Rx)
Classification: Adrenergic drug

Mechanism of Action

Racemic epinephrine stimulates both alpha-adrenergic and beta-adrenergic receptors. It is usually administered to pediatric patients for its $beta_2$ effects, which cause bronchial smooth muscle relaxation.

Indications

Racemic epinephrine is used to treat laryngotracheobronchitis (croup), and patients with severe dyspnea during long transport times.

Contraindications

Do not use racemic epinephrine in patients with epiglottitis.

Precautions

Excessive use of racemic epinephrine may cause bronchospasm, probably by rebound effect.

Route and Dosage

Adult: Not usually indicated for out-of-hospital use.
Pediatric: 0.25–0.5 mL/kg by inhalation. To administer, add 0.25–0.5 mL of a 2.25% epinephrine solution (1:1000 solution) to 2–3 mL of normal saline and administer via a nebulizer.

How Supplied

Racemic epinephrine is supplied in nebulizer bottles containing 7.5 mL, 15 mL, or 30 mL.

Adverse Reactions and Side Effects

CNS: Headache, anxiety, fear, nervousness.
Respiratory: Respiratory weakness.
CV: Palpitations, tachycardia, arrhythmias.
GI: Nausea, vomiting.

EMS Considerations

Assess patient vital signs frequently, because adverse reactions and side effects can develop rapidly.

Drug Interactions

None.

ROCURONIUM BROMIDE

(roh-kyou-ROH-nee-um)
Pregnancy Class: B
Zemuron (Rx)
Classification: Neuromuscular blocking drug

Mechanism of Action

Rocuronium competes with acetylcholine for receptor sites causing muscular paralysis. Must be accompanied by adequate sedation. Rocuronium does not affect consciousness or pain threshold.

Indications

Rocuronium is used as an adjunct to facilitate rapid sequence or routine intubation.

Contraindications

None during emergency intubation.

Precautions

Rocuronium should be used with caution in patients with pulmonary hypertension, valvular heart disease, or in patients with significant hepatic disease.

Route and Dosage

Adults and children: 0.6–1.2 mg/kg slow IV in appropriately premedicated patients.

How Supplied

10 mg/mL.

Adverse Reactions and Side Effects

Respiratory: Symptoms of asthma (bronchospasm, wheezing, rhonchi).
CV: Arrhythmias, abnormal ECG, tachycardia, transient hypotension and hypertension.
GI: Nausea and vomiting.

EMS Considerations

None.

Drug Interactions

None.

SALMETEROL XINAFOATE

(sal-MET-er-ole)
Pregnancy Class: C
Serevent (Rx)
Classification: Beta$_2$-adrenergic agonist

Mechanism of Action

Salmeterol is selective for beta$_2$-adrenergic receptors, located in the bronchi. This causes relaxation of the bronchial smooth muscles.

Indications

Salmeterol is used for the long-term treatment of asthma or bronchospasm associated with COPD.

Contraindications

Salmeterol should not be used in patients to treat acute symptoms of asthma, or in patients who are lactating.

Precautions

Use salmeterol with caution in patients with impaired hepatic function, cardiac arrhythmias, and hypertension.

Route and Dosage

Adult and children over 12 years of age: Two inhalations (42 mcg) approximately 12 hours apart by metered-dose inhaler.

How Supplied

21 mcg/inh.

Adverse Reactions and Side Effects

Respiratory: Paradoxic bronchospasms, bronchitis.
CV: Chest pain, palpitations, increased B/P, tachycardia.
CNS: Headache, nervousness, dizziness, fatigue.
GI: Stomach pain.
Musculoskeletal: Joint pain, back pain, muscle cramps.

EMS Considerations

Shake canister well before using at room temperature. Therapeutic effects may diminish if cold.

Drug Interactions

MAO Inhibitors: Potentiation of the effect of salmeterol.
Tricyclic antidepressants: Potentiation of the effect of salmeterol.

SUCCINYLCHOLINE CHLORIDE

(suck-sin-ill-KOH-leen)
Pregnancy Class: C
Anectine (Rx)
Classification: Depolarizing neuromuscular blocking drug

Mechanism of Action

Succinylcholine prevents muscles from contracting by prolonging time during which the receptors at the neuromuscular junction cannot respond to acetylcholine.

Indications

Succinylcholine is used as an adjunct to facilitate endotracheal (ET) intubation.

Contraindications

Succinylcholine should not be used in patients with acute narrow-angle glaucoma or penetrating eye injuries.

Precautions

Use succinylcholine with caution in patients with fractures. Patients with fractures may receive additional trauma caused by succinylcholine-induced muscle spasms.

Route and Dosage

Adult: 1.5 mg/kg IV bolus.
Pediatric: 1–2 mg/kg IV bolus.

How Supplied

20 mg/mL, 50 mg/mL, 100 mg/mL.

Adverse Reactions and Side Effects

Respiratory: Apnea, respiratory depression.
CV: Bradycardia or tachycardia, hypertension, hypotension.
Skeletal muscles: Muscle spasms, muscle pain.
GI: Salivation.

EMS Considerations

To reduce salivation, you can premedicate the patient with atropine as per protocol. For IV infusion, use 1 or 2 mg/mL solution of succinylcholine in D_5W or 0.9% NaCl. Succinylcholine is not compatible with alkaline solutions.

Drug Interactions

Aminoglycoside antibiotics: Additive skeletal muscle blockade.
Amphotericin B: Increased effect of succinylcholine caused by induced electrolyte imbalance.
Antibiotics, nonpenicillin: Additive skeletal muscle blockade.
Beta-adrenergic blocking agents: Additive skeletal muscle blockade.
Chloroquine: Additive skeletal muscle blockage.
Cimetidine: Cimetidine inhibits pseudocholinesterase.
Clindamycin: Additive skeletal muscle blockade.
Cyclophosphamide: Increased effect of succinylcholine by decreased breakdown of drug in plasma by pseudocholinesterase.
Cyclopropane: Increased risk of bradycardia, arrhythmias, sinus arrest, apnea, and malignant hyperthermia.
Diazepam: Decreased effect of succinylcholine.
Digitalis glycosides: Increased chance of cardiac arrhythmias, including ventricular fibrillation.
Echothiophate iodide: Increased effect of succinylcholine by decreased breakdown of drug in plasma by pseudocholinesterase.
Furosemide: Increased skeletal muscle blockade.
Halothane: Increased risk of bradycardia, arrhythmias, sinus arrest, apnea, and malignant hyperthermia.
Isoflurane: Additive skeletal muscle blockade.
Lidocaine: Additive skeletal muscle blockade.
Lincomycin: Additive skeletal muscle blockade.
Lithium carbonate: Increased skeletal muscle blockade.
Magnesium salts: Additive skeletal muscle blockade.
Narcotics: Increased risk of bradycardia and sinus arrest.
Nitrous oxide: Increased risk of bradycardia, arrhythmias, sinus arrest, apnea, and malignant hyperthermia.
Oxytocin: Increased effect of succinylcholine.
Phenelzine: Increased effect of succinylcholine.
Phenothiazines: Increased effect of succinylcholine.
Polymyxin: Additive skeletal muscle blockade.
Procainamide: Increased effect of succinylcholine.
Procaine: Increased effect of succinylcholine by inhibiting plasma pseudocholinesterase activity.
Promazine: Increased effect of succinylcholine.
Quinidine: Additive skeletal muscle blockade.
Quinine: Additive skeletal muscle blockade.
Tacrine: Increased effect of succinylcholine.
Thiazide diuretics: Increased effect of succinylcholine caused by induced electrolyte imbalance.
Thiotepa: Increased effect of succinylcholine by decreased breakdown of drug in plasma by pseudocholinesterase.

Trimethaphan: Increased effect of succinylcholine by inhibiting plasma pseudocholinesterase activity.

TERBUTALINE SULFATE

(ter-BYOU-tah-leen)
Pregnancy Class: B
Brethaire, Brethine (Rx)
Classification: Bronchodilator

Mechanism of Action

Terbutaline is a beta$_2$-adrenergic agonist, having strong effects on pulmonary receptors. Terbutaline relaxes bronchial smooth muscles, resulting in an increase in lung capacity and a decrease in airway resistance.

Indications

Terbutaline is used in patients with asthma, bronchitis, emphysema, and pulmonary obstructive disease.

Contraindications

Do not administer terbutaline to patients who are hypersensitive to adrenergic amine drugs.

Precautions

Use terbutaline with caution in patients with cardiac disease, diabetes, and in children less than 12 years of age.

Route and Dosage

Adults and children over 12 years of age, SC: 0.25 mg. This may be repeated in 15–30 minutes if necessary.
Adults and children over 12 years of age, inhalation: 0.2–0.5 mg (1–2 inhalations) q 4–6 hours. Inhalations should be separated by 60 sec intervals.

How Supplied

Metered-dose inhaler: 0.2 mg/inh.
Injection: 1 mg/mL.

Adverse Reactions and Side Effects

Respiratory: Wheezing.
CV: Atrial premature beats, PVCs, bradycardia, tachycardia, ST wave changes.
CNS: Stimulation.

EMS Considerations

Auscultate and document lung assessments. Observe respiratory patients for evidence of lung tolerance and bronchospasm.

Drug Interactions

None.

TRIAMCINOLONE

(try-am-SIN-oh-lohn)
Pregnancy Class: C
Azmacort (Rx)
Classification: Corticosteroid

Mechanism of Action

Triamcinolone has anti-inflammatory properties that produce bronchodilation in reversible airway obstruction.

Indications

Triamcinoline is used in patients with pulmonary emphysema accompanied by bronchospasm or bronchial edema.

Contraindications

Triamcinoline should not be used in patients with CHF, cardiac disease, or hypertension.

Precautions

Use triamcinoline with caution in patients with decreased renal function or renal disease.

Route and Dosage

Adult, metered-dose inhaler: 2 inhalations (200 mcg) or 4 inhalations (400 mcg).
Pediatric, 6–12 years of age, metered-dose inhaler: 1–2 inhalations (100–200 mcg).

How Supplied

100 mcg/inh.

Adverse Reactions and Side Effects

CNS: Dizziness, syncope.

EMS Considerations

None.

Drug Interactions

None.

TUBOCURARINE CHLORIDE

(too-boh-kyour-AR-een)
Pregnancy Class: C
Classification: Nondepolarizing neuromuscular blocking drug

Mechanism of Action

Tubocurarine competes with acetylcholine for the receptor sites of muscle cells.

Indications

Tubocurarine can be used as a muscle relaxant during endotracheal (ET) intubation.

Contraindications

Tubocruarine should not be used in patients where the release of histamine is dangerous.

Precautions

Use tubocurarine with caution during pregnancy and in children.

Route and Dosage

Adults: 6–9 mg (40–60 units) by IV bolus.
Children up to 4 weeks of age: 0.3 mg/kg IV.
Infants and children: 0.6 mg/kg IV bolus.

How Supplied

3 mg/mL.

Adverse Reactions and Side Effects

Respiratory: Allergic reactions.
CV: Circulatory collapse.

EMS Considerations

Tubocurarine is incompatible with alkaline solutions.

Drug Interactions

Acetylcholine: Acetylcholine antagonizes effect of tubocurarine.
Anticholinesterases: Anticholinesterases antagonize effect of tubocurarine.
Calcium salts: Increase effect of tubocurarine.
Diazepam: Diazepam may cause malignant hyperthermia with tubocurarine.
Potassium: Antagonizes effect of tubocurarine.
Propranolol: Increase effect of tubocurarine.
Quinine: Increased effect of tubocurarine.
Succinylcholine chloride: Increased relaxant effect of both drugs.

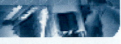

VECURONIUM BROMIDE

(veh-kyour-OH-nee-um)
Pregnancy Class: C
Norcuron (Rx)
Classification: Nondepolarizing neuromuscular blocking drug

Mechanism of Action

Vecuronium is a competitive nondepolarizing drug that competes with acetylcholine for receptor sites in the muscle cells, preventing the muscles from contracting.

Indications

Vecuronium causes skeletal muscle relaxation to facilitate endotracheal (ET) intubation.

Contraindications

Vecuronium should not be used in patients who are hypersensitive to the drug.

Precautions

Use vecuronium with caution in pediatric and elderly patients, and in patients with renal impairment.

Route and Dosage

Adult and children over 10 years of age, IV: 0.08–0.1 mg/kg.

How Supplied

Powder for injection: 10 mg, 20 mg.

Adverse Reactions and Side Effects

Respiratory: Bronchospasms, respiratory paralysis.
CV: Arrhythmias, bradycardia, hypotension, cardiac arrest.
GI: Excessive salivation.

EMS Considerations

Monitor vital signs and ECG. Vecuronium can cause vagal stimulation resulting in bradycardia, hypotension, and arrhythmias.

Drug Interactions

Bacitracin: Increased muscle relaxation following high IV or IP doses of bacitracin.
Sodium colistimethate: Increased muscle relaxation following high IV or IP doses of sodium colistimethate.
Tetracyclines: Increased muscle relaxation following high IV or IP doses of tetracyclines.
Succinylcholine: Increased effect of vecuronium.

ZAFIRLUKAST

(zah-FIR-loo-kast)
Pregnancy Class: B
Accolate (Rx)
Classification: Antiasthmatic

Mechanism of Action

Zafirlukast is a competitive antagonist of selective leukotriene receptors. These receptors are components of slow-reacting substances of anaphylaxis. Zafirlukast inhibits bronchoconstriction caused by sulfur dioxide and cold air in patients with asthma. It also reverses bronchoconstriction caused by grass, cat dander, ragweed, and mixed antigens.

Indications

Zafirlukast is used for prophylaxis and chronic treatment of asthma in adults and in children over 12 years of age.

Contraindications

Zafirlukast should not be used in patients experiencing an acute asthma attack, including status asthmaticus.

Precautions

Use zafirlukast with caution in patients over 65 years of age.

Route and Dosage

Adults and children over 12 years of age, tablets: 20 mg.

How Supplied

20 mg tablets.

Adverse Reactions and Side Effects

CNS: Headache, dizziness.
GI: Diarrhea, abdominal pain, nausea and vomiting.

EMS Considerations

None.

Drug Interactions

Aspirin: Increased plasma levels of zafirlukast.
Erythromycin: Decreased plasma levels of zafirlukast.
Terfenadine: Decreased plasma levels of zafirlukast.
Theophylline: Decreased plasma levels of zafirlukast.
Warfarin: Significant increase in PT.

ZILEUTON

(zye-LOO-ton)
Pregnancy Class: C
Zyflo (Rx)
Classification: Antiasthmatic

Mechanism of Action

Zileuton inhibits the formation of leukotrienes. Leukotrienes are substances that induce smooth muscle contraction. Zileuton reduces bronchoconstriction caused by cold air challenge in asthmatics.

Indications

Zileuton is used in the prophylaxis and chronic treatment of asthma in adults and children over 12 years of age.

Contraindications

Zileuton should not be used in patients experiencing acute asthma attacks, including status asthmaticus.

Precautions

Use zileuton with caution in patients who have a large intake of alcohol or who have a past history of liver disease.

Route and Dosage

Adults and children over 12 years of age, tablets: 600 mg.

How Supplied

Tablets: 600 mg.

Adverse Reactions and Side Effects

CNS: Headache, dizziness, insomnia, nervousness.
GI: Flatulence, constipation, nausea and vomiting.

EMS Considerations

None.

Drug Interactions

None.

Rapid-Sequence Intubation (RSI)

Situations may arise when endotracheal intubation is not immediately possible. For example, a patient may resist ventilation because of pain. A semiconscious or combative patient may also resist ventilation. In situations such as these, it may be necessary to administer a series of drugs designed to temporarily paralyze the patient so an ET tube can be inserted.

Rapid-sequence intubation is necessary to facilitate intubation in the conscious or semiconscious patient. A potent sedative is administered simultaneously with a **neuromuscular blocking agent** so the patient can tolerate intubation so the airway can be effectively controlled.

Indications for rapid-sequence intubation include acute intracranial lesions, overdose, status epilepticus, combative patients requiring immediate intubation and possible cervical spine fracture where immobilization is not possible because of delirium, and so forth. Before performing the actual intubation, the patient is given a brief neurologic assessment involving level of consciousness, motor response, verbal response, and pupillary response.

Procedure for Rapid-sequence Intubation

- Assemble equipment:
  - Bag-valve-mask connected to oxygen. The patient should be preoxygenated with 100% oxygen using a manual resuscitator.
  - Suction
  - Endotracheal tubes
  - Laryngoscope handle and blades
  - Cricothyrotomy tray
  - Medications

- Perform neurologic assessment while oxygenating patient with 100% oxygen
- Premedicate the patient as follows:
  - *Head-injured patients:* Fentanyl, 50–100 mcg IVP when the Glasgow Coma Scale is less than 13.
  - *Non-head-injured patients:* Midazolam 2–2.5 mg slow IVP (also used for head-injured patients whose Glasgow Coma Scale is 13 or greater)
  - *Pediatric/adolescent patients:* Atropine 0.01 mg/kg IVP for control of possible bradycardia, which may develop because of vagal stimulation during intubation.
  - *Head-injured patients, patients with CNS injury, hypertensive crisis, or cardiac instability:* Lidocaine 1 mg/kg IVP for ICP management.
- Administer succinylcholine, 1.5 mg/kg IVP.
- Apply cricoid pressure until intubation is successfully completed.
- If fasciculations occur, wait until they stop, and ventilate patient using a bag-valve-mask. When the patient's jaw relaxes, causing a decreased resistance to ventilations, proceed with intubation.
- If the patient cannot be intubated during the first 20 seconds, stop the procedure and ventilate using a bag-valve-mask for approximately one minute. If the patient does not adequately relax after the initial dose of succinylcholine, a second dose should be given at 1–1.5 times the initial dose.
- If repeated intubation attempt fails, ventilate the patient using a bag-valve-mask until an alternative airway can be obtained. At this point, a cricothyrotomy may be indicated.
- If bradycardia develops during the intubation procedure, the patient should be ventilated with 100% oxygen. If this is unsuccessful, administer atropine at 0.5 mg IVP.

- Once intubation is complete, inflate the ET cuff, release cricoid pressure, and confirm tube placement, and document the procedure.

Succinylcholine is the most often used short-acting neuromuscular blocking agent for rapid-sequence intubation. After it is given, the patient undergoes fasciculations and muscle cramps, which are followed by flaccid paralysis. The patient will generally experience paralysis within 30–60 seconds. Paralysis will last approximately 4–6 minutes.

Side effects, which may develop, include:

- *Respiratory:* Respiratory depression, apnea, wheezing.
- *CV:* Bradycardia, sinus arrest, hypertension or hypotension.
- *Eyes:* Intraocular pressure.
- *GI:* Nausea, vomiting.

Rapid-sequence intubation protocols may also include the following neuromuscular blocking agents:

- *Pancuronium bromide:* Onset of paralysis within approximately 3 minutes, with a therapeutic duration of approximately 40 minutes.
- *Tubocurarine chloride:* Has a rapid onset and therapeutic effects of approximately 30–90 minutes. The major concern with tubocurarine is its significant histamine release, which results in hypotension.
- *Atracurium and Vecuronium:* Both drugs are short acting, non-depolarizing muscle relaxants. They have an onset time of approximately 2–3 minutes, and a therapeutic duration of approximately 20–40 minutes.

CONCLUSION

Having to fight for each breath can be very frightening for a patient. Rapid assessment and proper recognition of presenting signs and symptoms by the EMS professional can be life saving.

The most important drug used during a respiratory emergency is oxygen. However, conditions such as reversible airway obstruction caused by asthma or COPD may require additional drug options such as bronchodilators, antiasthmatics, or anti-inflammatory drugs. It is important to know each drug classification included in your protocols and how they work so each patient can receive rapid, appropriate treatment.

▶ STUDY QUESTIONS

1. Bronchodilators are used to treat reversible airway obstruction. They work by:
   a. Decreasing edema
   b. Reducing carbon dioxide content
   c. Relaxing the bronchial smooth muscles
   d. Increasing breathing by stimulation of the CNS

2. Briefly explain the rationale for giving atropine to pediatric patients who are candidates for RSI.
   _____
   _____
   _____
   _____
   _____
   _____

3. To administer albuterol to a 13-year-old patient, the dosage needed is:
   a. One-half the adult dose
   b. One inhalation (90 mcg). Repeat as necessary.
   c. Two inhalations (180 mcg)
   d. Three inhalations (270 mcg)

4. Aminophylline is contraindicated in patients:
   a. Who suffer from uncontrolled cardiac arrhythmias
   b. With hypertension
   c. With CHF
   d. Over 60

5. The adult dosage for epinephrine to treat bronchial asthma is:
   a. 0.3–0.5 mg by IV bolus of a 1:10,000 solution
   b. 0.3–0.5 mg SC of a 1:1000 solution
   c. 3–5 mg SC of a 1:1000 solution
   d. 0.01 mg/kg SC of a 1:1000 solution

6. Briefly explain the mechanism of action for a drug classified as an anticholinergic.
   _____
   _____
   _____
   _____
   _____
   _____

7. Why is it important to use oxygen that is humidified?
   _____
   _____
   _____
   _____
   _____
   _____
   _____

8. Briefly explain the mechanism of action for a drug classified as a neuromuscular blocker.

_____

_____

_____

_____

_____

_____

9. Terbutaline is used to treat asthma and COPD by relaxing bronchial smooth muscles. The initial adult dose when given SC is:
   a. 0.25 mg
   b. 25 mg
   c. 0.5 mg
   d. 50 mg

10. The terbutaline dosage for an 8-year-old patient is:
    a. 0.25 mg
    b. 0.5 mg
    c. 1.0 mg
    d. Not recommended

▶ EXTENDED CASE STUDY

You are dispatched to a home for a "man fallen." When you arrive you find a conscious 58-year-old man who had fallen in the kitchen "hours ago." On initial assessment you find he is oriented, but pale, signs of peripheral cyanosis, rapid/deep respirations without noticeable distress, and a rapid pulse rate.

The information gained from your initial assessment may be misleading and may also give you a false sense of security. The patient is alert and oriented, but yet his vital signs suggest he may quickly become a high-priority patient. For example, indicators of the following:

- Pallor = associated with poor perfusion.
- Canosis = hypoxemia –a broad variety of conditions including asthma, pneumonia, COPD, CHF, trauma, etc.
- Rapid respirations = respiratory or cardiac problems.
- Rapid heart rate = many conditions including shock, respiratory or cardiac compromise, etc.

Due to your initial findings, this patient should be considered a high priority. The patient must be evaluated for potential respiratory and cardiac problems. For example, examine the patient for chest symmetry, breath sounds, pulses, SpO_2, and ECG evaluation. The patient should be placed on humidified oxygen to treat his hypoxia and for possible shock.

While placing the patient on oxygen and an ECG monitor, the following is determined by your partner:

- Patient has a 40-year habit of smoking 2 packs of cigarettes per day; he states that his doctor has told him that he has "mild COPD."
- Diminished breath sounds with rhonchi bilaterally.
- Vital signs =
  - Resp: 40/min; productive cough
  - HR: 130 beats/min and regular
  - B/P: 90/58 mm Hg
  - SpO_2: 78%
  - Temp: 102.1 F

You must now try to determine a probable chief complaint to effectively continue treatment and communicate your findings and treatment to the receiving facility.

This patient's history of smoking and COPD, make him at risk for pneumonia. This is supported by his presentation with fever and productive cough. Therefore, immediate treatment should include transport (as per local protocol), high flow oxygen to address his hypoxia and developing shock, and an IV to run at least 10 mL/kg to address developing shock. While enroute to the receiving facility, reassess your patient every 3–5 minutes and have advanced life support equipment ready to intervene, if needed.

CHAPTER 10

DRUGS USED TO TREAT CARDIOVASCULAR EMERGENCIES

Therapeutic Classifications of Drugs Used for Cardiovascular Emergencies

Analgesics
Butorphanol
Hydromorphone
Meperidine
Morphine
Nalbuphine
Nitrous oxide-oxygen mixture
Pentazocine

Angiotensin-Converting Enzyme (ACE) Inhibitors
Captopril
Enalapril
Lisinopril
Ramipril

Antianginals
Amyl nitrite inhalant
Diltiazem
Labetolol
Metoprolol
Nifedipine
Nitroglycerin
Propranolol

Verapamil

Antiarrhythmics
Adenosine
Amiodarone
Atenolol
Atropine
Digoxin
Diltiazem
Esmolol
Ibutilide
Isoproterenol
Labetolol
Lidocaine
Magnesium sulfate
Metoprolol
Nifedipine
Nitroprusside
Procainamide
Propranolol
Verapamil

Anticoagulant
Heparin

Anticonvulsant
Phenytoin

Antihypertensives
Atenolol
Bumetanide
Diazoxide
Diltiazem
Enalaprilat
Furosemide
Hydralazine
Labetolol
Metoprolol
Nifedipine
Nitroprusside
Propranolol
Verapamil

Antiplatelet
Acetylsalicyclic acid

Antitussive
Hydromorphone

Bronchodilators
Epinephrine

Isoproterenol
Cardiac Stimulators
Epinephrine
Isoproterenol
Coronary Vasodilator
Nitroglycerin
Diuretics
Bumetanide
Furosemide
Electrolyte
Magnesium sulfate
Electrolyte Modifiers
Calcium chloride
Calcium gluceptate
Calcium gluconate
Hydrogen Ion Buffer

Sodium bicarbonate
Inotropics
Amrinone
Digoxin
Dobutamine
Dopamine
Medicinal Gases
Nitrous oxide-oxygen mixture
Oxygen
Peripheral Vasoconstrictors
Dopamine
Epinephrine
Norepinephrine
Vasopressin
Thrombolytic Enzymes
Alteplase

Anisoylated plasminogen
Streptokinase activator
Reteplase
Streptokinase
Vasodilators
Amrinone
Amyl nitrite inhalant
Diazoxide
Enalaprilat
Nitroprusside
Vasopressors
Dopamine
Epinephrine
Norepinephrine

OBJECTIVES

On completion of this chapter and the study questions, you should be able to:

- Describe in detail the following analgesic drugs: butorphanol, hydromorphone, meperidine, morphine, nalbuphine, nitrous oxide-oxygen mixture, and pentazocine.
- Describe in detail the following ACE inhibitors: captopril, enalapril, lisinopril, and ramipril.
- Describe in detail the following antianginal drugs: amyl nitrite inhalant, diltiazem, labetolol, metoprolol, nifedipine, nitroglycerin, propranolol, and verapamil.
- Describe in detail the following antiarrhythmic drugs: adenosine, amiodarone, atenolol, atropine, digoxin, diltiazem, esmolol, ibutilide, isoproterenol, labetolol, lidocaine, magnesium sulfate, metoprolol, nifedipine, nitroprusside, procainamide, propranolol, and verapamil.
- Describe in detail the anticoagulant: heparin.
- Describe in detail the anticonvulsant: phenytoin.
- Describe in detail the following antihypertensive drugs: atenolol, bumetanide, diazoxide, diltiazem, enalaprilat, furosemide, hydralazine, labetolol, metoprolol, nifedipine, nitroprusside, propranolol, and verapamil.
- Describe in detail the antiplatelet drug: acetylsalicyclic acid.
- Describe in detail the antitussive: hydromorphone.
- Describe in detail the bronchodilators: epinephrine and isoproterenol.
- Describe in detail the following cardiac stimulators: epinephrine and isoproterenol.
- Describe in detail the coronary vasodilator: nitroglycerine.
- Describe in detail the following diuretics: bumetanide and furosemide.
- Describe in detail the electrolyte magnesium sulfate.
- Describe in detail the following electrolyte modifiers: calcium chloride, calcium gluceptate, and calcium gluconate.
- Describe in detail the hydrogen ion buffer: sodium bicarbonate.
- Describe in detail the following inotropic drugs: amrinone, digoxin, dobutamine, and dopamine.

- Describe in detail the following medicinal gases: nitrous oxide-oxygen mixture and oxygen.
- Describe in detail the peripheral vasoconstrictors: dopamine, epinephrine, norepinephrine, and vasopressin.
- Describe in detail the following thrombolytic drugs: alteplase, anisoylated plasminogen streptokinase activator, reteplase, and streptokinase.
- Describe in detail the following vasodilators: amrinone, amyl nitrate inhalant, diazoxide, enalaprilat, and nitroprusside.
- Describe in detail the following vasopressor drugs: dopamine, epinephrine, and norepinephrine.

KEY TERMS

ACE Inhibitors
Adams-Stokes syndrome
Analgesic
Antianginal
Antiarrhythmic
Anticoagulant

Antihypertensive
Antiplatelet
Beta-blockers
Cardiogenic shock
Congestive heart failure
Diuretic
Hydrogen ion buffer

Hypertensive crisis
Inotropic Agents
Nitrates
Sick sinus syndrome
Wolff-Parkinson-White syndrome

CASE STUDIES

1. Your patient is a 52-year-old man who says, "My heart feels like it is racing." The ECG monitor shows ventricular tachycardia (Figure 10-1). At the present time, the patient is hemodynamically stable. In this situation, which of the following drugs should be administered?
   a. Amiodarone
   b. Verapamil
   c. Lidocaine
   d. Atropine

2. You respond to a 46-year-old man who complains of severe substernal chest pain that radiates to his left shoulder, arm, and hand. He is short of breath and very apprehensive. The ECG monitor shows a sinus tachycardia at a regular rate of 120 beats/min (Figure 10-2). After assessing vital signs, you note that they are within normal limits. Initial treatment should include oxygen, reassurance, and:
   a. Nitroglycerin
   b. Amiodarone
   c. Adenosine
   d. Morphine

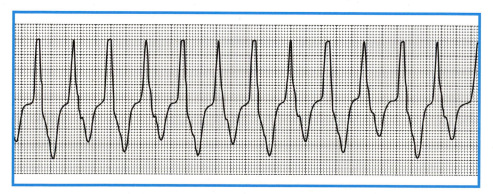

Figure 10-1 Ventricular tachycardia. (© Delmar/Cengage Learning)

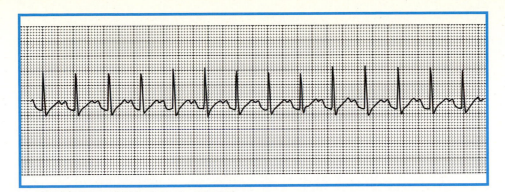

Figure 10-2 Sinus tachycardia. Rate: 120 beats/min. (© Delmar/Cengage Learning)

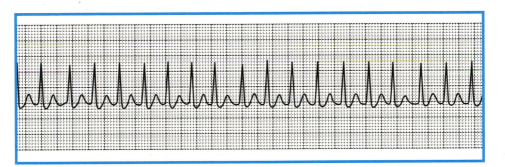

Figure 10-3 Paroxysmal supeaventricular tacycardia. Rate: 100 beats/min. (© Delmar/Cengage Learning)

3. EMS is called to a 67-year-old woman who says that her heart feels like it is "fluttering." The ECG monitor indicates the patient is experiencing paroxysmal supraventricular tachycardia at a regular rate of 180 beats/min (Figure 10-3). Vital signs are currently within normal limits and she is tolerating the rhythm fairly well. Which is the drug of choice to treat stable paroxysmal supraventricular tachycardia?
   a. Isoproterenol
   b. Procainamide
   c. Adenosine
   d. Verapamil

Ventricular Ectopy

Response: EMS responds to a complaint of chest pain and shortness of breath. When EMS arrives, a 53-year-old man is found lying on the living room sofa complaining of substernal chest pain that radiates to his left shoulder and jaw. The patient says that he was watching television when the pain began, about an hour ago. He had passed the pain off as indigestion until it began radiating into his shoulder and jaw. He weighs 250 pounds, has no previous cardiac history, and is not taking any medications. The initial examination reveals the following:

Level of consciousness: Alert and oriented, but apprehensive.
Respirations: 30/min.
Breath sounds: Clear bilaterally.
Blood pressure: 160/96.
Skin condition: Cool, clammy.

ECG Interpretation: After connecting the patient to the ECG monitor, the monitor shows a rhythm like the one shown in Figure 10-4. The rhythm is interpreted as a sinus rhythm with multifocal premature ventricular contractions (PVCs). Multifocal PVCs should be treated immediately. These PVCs are considered malignant, because the ectopic activity causing them originates from more than one area of the ventricles. The fact that the PVCs are multifocal, coupled with the patient's presenting signs and symptoms, indicate that the chances are high that the multifocal PVCs will deteriorate to ventricular fibrillation, placing the patient in cardiopulmonary arrest. Other malignant PVCs may include:

Unifocal PVCs that occur more than six times/min.
Closely coupled PVCs.
PVCs that occur in short bursts of three or more in succession (salvos).
PVCs that occur on the preceding T wave (R-on-T phenomenon).

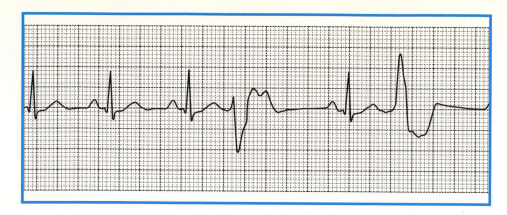

Figure 10-4 Sinus rhythm with multifocal premature ventricular contractions (PVCs).
(© Delmar/Cengage Learning)

Management: After initial evaluation, the first step is reassurance. Reassurance may relieve some of the patient's apprehension, which in turn, may help reduce the frequency of the PVCs. The initial drugs to be considered when treating this patient include oxygen, aspirin, nitroglycerin, and possibly morphine. Next, place the patient on 4-6 L of humidified oxygen (100%). The oxygen flow can be increased if necessary. Oxygen by itself may aid in controlling PVCs. As the patient is short of breath, it may be appropriate to place him in a comfortable position such as sitting or semisitting.

Aspirin is given as soon as possible to patients who are experiencing chest pain. It works by decreasing platelet aggregation, thereby decreasing the incidence of an MI. The initial dose of aspirin should be 160-325 mg.

The next drug to be considered is nitroglycerin. Nitroglycerin increases cardiac blood flow by dilating coronary arteries and improving collateral flow to ischemic regions of the heart. The dosage of nitroglycerin is 0.3-0.4 mg sublingual tablet or sublingual spray every 5 minutes for 15 minutes (3 total doses).

If the nitroglycerin is ineffective, the next drug to be considered is morphine. Morphine alters the perception of pain and produces generalized CNS depression. It is commonly used for patients who may be experiencing an MI. The dosage for morphine is 4-10 mg IV.

It is vital to make the best possible use of treatment time. Establish the IV lifeline and start initial drug therapy at the scene. Then, however, the patient should be moved to the ambulance for transport to the appropriate emergency facility. All other treatment and monitoring should be done enroute. Appendix C includes tables that contain the Emergency Cardiac Care Guidelines based on the American Heart Association's 2008 Handbook of *Emergency Cardiovascular Care for Health-Care Providers*.

INTRODUCTION

The leading cause of death in the United States is cardiovascular disease. Often, the initial presentation of cardiovascular disease occurs as an emergency in the out-of-hospital setting. EMS providers play an integral role in the treatment of cardiovascular emergencies. The drug therapy for cardiovascular emergencies is the most extensive of any disease state in which EMS personnel provide drug treatment.

This chapter focuses on drugs used in out-of-hospital cardiovascular emergencies. Several categories of drugs are discussed in this chapter. Many of the drugs provide multiple therapeutic actions and are included in several therapeutic categories. Within specific categories the drugs work via various mechanisms of action and each is presented in detail within the chapter. Antiarrhythmic drugs are administered to terminate cardiac *arrhythmias*. These drugs are classified according to their mechanism of action and their effects on the *action potential* of cardiac cells. Inotropic agents are utilized to increase the force of contractions and improve *cardiac output* in the setting of cardiogenic shock. Antihypertensives act through various mechanisms to reduce blood pressure, while *vasopressors* cause vasoconstriction to increase blood pressure. Included in this chapter are antianginal agents which are administered to decrease the workload on the heart, reduce the oxygen demands of the heart, and increase coronary blood flow to the heart. Diuretics act to reduce *pulmonary edema* and blood pressure. This chapter also discusses the use of *thrombolytic agents* that are used to dissolve *thrombi* and, therefore, restore blood flow through obstructed vessels or within the heart.

The appropriate and timely administration of the drugs presented in this chapter has resulted in a significant decrease in morbidity and mortality associated with cardiovascular emergencies. It is vital that EMS providers be vigilant in maintaining their knowledge of these drugs.

Individual Drugs

ACETYLSALICYLIC ACID

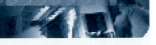

(ah-SEE-till-sal-ih-SILL-ick AH-sid)

Pregnancy Class: C (D during the first trimester)

Acuprin, Ascriptin, ASA, Aspergum, Aspirtab, Bayer Aspirin, Bufferin, Ecotrin, Empirin, Halfprin, St. Joseph Adult Chewable Aspirin

Classification: Antiplatelet, antipyretic, non-opioid analgesic, nonsteroidal anti-inflammatory agent

Mechanism of Action

Antiplatelet activity is produced by decreasing the synthesis of substances that mediate platelet aggregation and cause arteries to constrict.

Indications

To decrease the risk of death and reinfarction from nonfatal myocardial infarction. Prophylaxis of myocardial infarction in patients with symptoms of ischemic chest pain.

Contraindications

Hypersensitivity to salicylates. Bleeding disorders or thrombocytopenia. Avoid during pregnancy, especially during the third trimester, because of the potential for adverse effects on the fetus and the mother.

Precautions

Use cautiously in patients with a history of gastrointestinal bleeding or ulcer disease. Use of aspirin in patients with a history of asthma may provoke an acute attack. Avoid use in children or teenagers because of the potential for Reye's syndrome.

Route and Dosage

160–325 mg PO as soon as possible for patient presenting with acute coronary syndrome. May be given rectally (300 mg). Thereafter, 80–325 mg PO every day.

How Supplied

Tablets: 81 mg, 162.5 mg, 325 mg.
Chewable tablets: 81 mg.
Chewing gum: 227 mg.
Enteric-coated (delayed-release) tablets: 80 mg, 165 mg, 325 mg.
Suppositories: 60 mg, 120 mg, 125 mg, 130 mg, 195 mg, 200 mg, 300 mg, 325 mg.

Adverse Reactions and Side Effects

GI: GI bleeding, epigastric distress, nausea.
Hematologic: Anemia, increased bleeding time.
HEENT: Tinnitus at toxic concentrations.
Allergic: Anaphylaxis, bronchospasm, asthma-like symptoms.

EMS Considerations

Aspirin should be administered as soon as possible if myocardial infarction is suspected.

Drug Interactions

The risk of bleeding may be increased with warfarin, heparin, heparin-like agents, and thrombolytic agents.

ADENOSINE

(ah-DEN-oh-seen)
Pregnancy Class: C
Adenocard (Rx)
Classification: Antiarrhythmic

Mechanism of Action

Slows conduction through the AV node of the heart. Adenosine may also interrupt reentry pathways through the AV node.

Indications

To convert paroxysmal supraventricular tachycardia, including **Wolff-Parkinson-White syndrome** (Figure 10–5A and Figure 10–5B), to a normal sinus rhythm. Vagal maneuvers should be attempted prior to administering adenosine.

Contraindications

Hypersensitivity to adenosine. Second- or third-degree AV heart block or **sick sinus syndrome**.

Precautions

Brief periods of heart block may occur following administration of adenosine. Approximately 50–60% of patients develop some type of cardiac arrhythmia after the administration of adenosine. However, these arrhythmias generally last only a few seconds. Arrhythmias most likely to develop

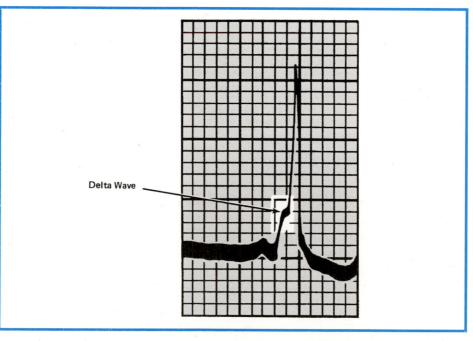

Delta Wave

Figure 10–5A Wolff-Parkinson-White syndrome is associated with a high incidence of paroxysmal tachycardia. A major defining characteristic is the initial slurring of the R wave (delta wave). Other characteristics include heart rate of about 100 beats/min, with regular rhythm; a shortened PR interval (0.06 sec); and a widened QRS complex (0.14 sec). (© Delmar/Cengage Learning)

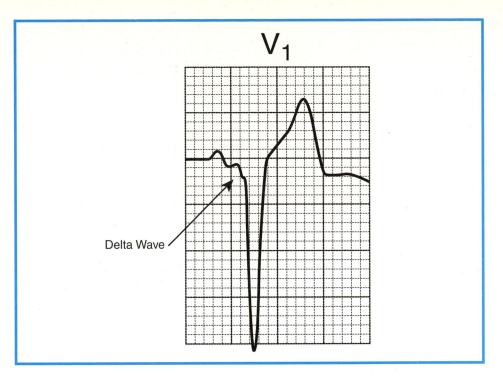

V_1

Delta Wave

Figure 10–5B The slurring of the QRS complex (delta wave). (© Delmar/Cengage Learning)

include premature ventricular contractions, premature atrial contractions, sinus bradycardia, and sinus tachycardia.

Route and Dosage

Adults and pediatrics > 50 kg: Initial dose of 6 mg rapid IV bolus, followed by a rapid IV flush of normal saline. If the initial dose is unsuccessful after 1–2 minutes, give 12 mg rapid IV bolus followed by a rapid IV flush of normal saline. Another 12 mg dose may be repeated if necessary.
Pediatric: <50 kg: initial dose 0.05–0.1 mg/kg as a rapid IV bolus. If necessary, dose may be increased by 0.05–0.1 mg/kg until SR or a maximum dose of 0.3 mg/kg is given.

How Supplied

6 mg/2 mL vial.

Adverse Reactions and Side Effects

CNS: Headache.
Respiratory: Dyspnea, may cause bronchoconstriction in asthma patients.
CV: Arrhythmias, palpitations, hypotension, chest pain, facial flushing.
GI: Nausea, metallic taste.

EMS Considerations

Assess patient vital signs frequently. Patients who develop high-grade AV heart block should not be given additional doses of adenosine.

Drug Interactions

Methylxanthines, such as theophylline or aminophylline, prevent adenosine from binding to receptor sites. Asthma or COPD patients may be taking these drugs and may require larger doses of adenosine. Dipyridamole (*Persantine Rx*) can potentiate the effects of adenosine and patients may require smaller doses of adenosine.

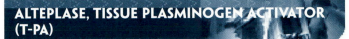

ALTEPLASE, TISSUE PLASMINOGEN ACTIVATOR (T-PA)

(AL-teh-playz)
Pregnancy Class: C
Activase (Rx)
Classification: Thrombolytic

Mechanism of Action

Binds to fibrin in a thrombus, causing a conversion of plasminogen to plasmin. This conversion results in local fibrinolysis and a decrease in circulating fibrinogen. The thrombus is dissolved which may limit the size of infarction during a myocardial infarction.

Indications

Treatment of myocardial infarction within 4–6 hours of the onset of chest pain.

Contraindications

Active internal bleeding. History of cerebral vascular accident. Intracranial or spinal trauma or surgery within the past 2 months. Severe, uncontrolled hypertension. Bleeding disorders.

Precautions

Alteplase should be administered cautiously to patients with cerebrovascular disease, hypertension, severe liver or kidney disease, or age greater than 75 years.

Route and Dosage

Adult (greater than 65 kg or 143 lb): A total of 100 mg IV over 3 hours as follows: 60 mg over the first hour. Administer the first 6–10 mg of the 60 mg by IV bolus over 1–2 minutes and the rest by IV infusion. 20 mg by IV infusion over the second hour. 20 mg by IV infusion over the third hour.

Adult (less than 65 kg or 143 lb): A total of 1.25 mg/kg IV over 3 hours as follows: 0.75 mg/kg over the first hour. Administer the first 0.075–0.125 mg/kg of the 0.75 mg/kg by IV bolus over the first 1–2 minutes. 0.25 mg/kg by IV infusion over the second hour. 0.25 mg/kg by IV infusion over the third hour.

Pediatric: Not recommended for out-of-hospital use.

To prepare alteplase: Reconstitute with sterile water for injection without preservatives immediately prior to use. Once reconstituted, the preparation contains 1 mg/mL. The reconstituted solution may be further diluted in an equal volume of normal saline or D_5W to yield a concentration of 0.5 mg/mL. Dilution should be performed by gently swirling the solution.

How Supplied

Powder for injection: 50 mg, 100 mg.

Adverse Reactions and Side Effects

CNS: Intracranial bleeding, headache.
CV: Reperfusion arrhythmias, hypotension.
GI: GI bleeding, retroperitoneal bleeding, nausea, vomiting.
HEENT: Epistaxis, gingival bleeding.

EMS Considerations

Assess vital signs every 15 minutes. ECG should be continuously monitored. Assess patient frequently for signs of bleeding.

Drug Interactions

Concurrent use with aspirin, warfarin, heparin, or heparin-like drugs may increase the risk of bleeding.

AMIODARONE

(am-ee-OH-dah-rohn)
Pregnancy Class: D
Cordarone, Pacerone (Rx)
Classification: Antiarrhythmic (Class III)

Mechanism of Action

Prolongs the action potential and refractory period of the myocardial cell resulting in slowing of the sinus rate, and increased PR and QT intervals. Additionally, amiodarone inhibits alpha- and beta-adrenergic stimulation resulting in relaxation of vascular smooth muscle, reduction of peripheral vascular resistance, and a slight increase in cardiac index.

Indications

First-line agent for the treatment of shock—refractory ventricular fibrillation and pulseless ventricular tachycardia. Treatment of polymorphic ventricular tachycardia and wide-complex tachycardia of uncertain etiology. Hemodynamically stable ventricular tachycardia refractory to cardioversion. Prophylaxis of frequently recurring ventricular fibrillation and hemodynamically unstable ventricular tachycardia. To control the rate in the treatment of refractory, sustained, or paroxysmal atrial fibrillation, paroxysmal supraventricular tachycardia, and symptomatic atrial flutter.

Contraindications

Severe sinus node dysfunction, second- and third-degree AV block, cardiogenic shock, and pregnancy and lactation. Amiodarone should not be administered to patients with bradycardia because of increased incidence of syncope.

Precautions

Safety and efficacy of amiodarone in children have not been established. Elderly patients may experience an increased incidence of adverse effects. Amiodarone should be used cautiously in patients with **congestive heart failure** because of negative inotropic effects. Use with caution in patients with a history of liver or renal dysfunction, or thyroid disease. Amiodarone should be used with caution in patients with pulmonary disease because of the potential for serious pulmonary effects, such as fibrosis.

Route and Dosage

Adults (cardiac arrest): 300 mg IV push. The initial dose may be administered undiluted or diluted with 20mL D_5W. May repeat at 150 mg in 3–5 minutes. The 150 mg dose should be prepared by adding 1 ampule or 3 mL of amiodarone to 100 mL D_5W to produce a concentration of 1.5 mg/mL. Maximum cumulative dose is 2.2 gm/24 hours.

Adults (stable wide-complex tachycardia/supraventricular tachycardia): rapid infusion: 150 mg IV over 10 minutes. May repeat 150 mg IV every 10 minutes as needed. Then 360 mg IV over 6 hours (1 mg/min).

Maintenance infusion: 540 mg IV over the remaining 18 hours (0.5 mg/min). After the first 24 hours, continue the infusion at a rate of 0.5 mg/min. The maintenance infusion should be prepared by adding 900 mg or 18 mL of amiodarone to 500 mL D_5W to produce a concentration of 1.8 mg/mL. The maintenance infusion should be prepared in a glass bottle. Amiodarone is also compatible with NS.

How Supplied

Injection: 50 mg/mL in 3-mL ampules.

Adverse Reactions and Side Effects

CNS: Dizziness, fatigue, malaise, tremor, lack of coordination, ataxia.

Respiratory: Pulmonary fibrosis or infiltrates, pneumonitis, adult respiratory distress syndrome, pulmonary edema, cough, progressive dyspnea.

CV: Congestive heart failure, worsening of arrhythmias, bradycardia, hypotension, prolonged QT interval.

GI: Hepatitis, cirrhosis, anorexia, nausea, vomiting.

Dermatologic: Photosensitivity, blue discoloration of skin, rash, ecchymosis, flushing.

HEENT: Corneal microdeposits, visual disturbances (blurred vision, halos), eye discomfort.

Other: Hypo- or hyperthyroidism, angioedema, Stevens-Johnson syndrome.

EMS Considerations

During administration of amiodarone the ECG should be monitored for increased PR and QRS intervals, increased arrhythmias, and bradycardia. Respiratory status and blood pressure should be monitored closely.

Drug Interactions

Amiodarone may cause digoxin toxicity. When used concurrently, the dose of digoxin should be decreased by 50%. Amiodarone may prolong the QT interval; other drugs that prolong the QT interval should be avoided. Concentrations of antiarrhythmics, such as procainamide and lidocaine, are increased by the administration of amiodarone. Doses of these drugs should be decreased by 30–50% if amiodarone to be administered concurrently.

Concurrent use of *beta-adrenergic blockers* or *calcium channel blockers* with amiodarone may increase the risk of bradyarrhythmias, sinus arrest, and AV block.

ANISOYLATE PLASMINOGEN STREPTOKINASE ACTIVATOR, ANISTREPLASE

(an-ih-STREP-layz)
Pregnancy Class: C
Eminase (Rx)
Classification: Thrombolytic enzyme

Mechanism of Action

Anistreplase combines with plasminogen to form a complex which converts plasminogen to plasmin. Plasmin then degrades fibrin present in clots to cause lysis of the thrombus.

Indications

Acute management of myocardial infarction to preserve ventricular function, limit infarct size, and reduce mortality.

Contraindications

Active internal bleeding, history of intracranial or intraspinal surgery or trauma within 2 months, history of cerebrovascular accident, recent trauma, intracranial neoplasm, arteriovenous malformation, or aneurysm. Known bleeding disorder, severe uncontrolled hypertension, or allergy to streptokinase.

Precautions

Safety and efficacy have not been established in pregnancy, lactation, or children. Use anistreplase cautiously in the following conditions because of risks associated with therapy: within 10 days of major surgery, cerebrovascular disease, within 10 days of GI or GU bleeding, within 10 days of trauma, SBP greater than 180 mm Hg or DBP greater than 110 mm Hg, patients older than 75 years of age, patients receiving anticoagulants, any condition in which bleeding would constitute a significant hazard or would be difficult to manage because of its location.

Route and Dosage

Adult: 30 units IV over 2–5 minutes as soon as possible after onset of symptoms.

To reconstitute powder: Slowly add 5 mL of sterile water for injection. Gently roll the vial after directing the stream of water against the side of the vial in order to prevent foaming. Do not shake the vial. Discard if not administered within 30 minutes.

How Supplied

Powder for injection: 30 Units.

Adverse Reactions and Side Effects

CNS: Intracranial hemorrhage, headache.
Respiratory: Bronchospasm, hemoptysis.
CV: Reperfusion arrhythmias, hypotension.
GI: GI bleeding, retroperitoneal bleeding.
GU: Hematuria.
Dermatologic: Ecchymoses.
Hematologic: Bleeding, anemia, thrombocytopenia.
Local: Hemorrhage at injection site.
HEENT: Gingival bleeding, epistaxis, eye hemorrhage.
Other: Anaphylaxis, fever, chills.

EMS Considerations

Obtain extensive patient history in order to facilitate rapid administration of anistreplase. Continuously monitor for evidence of bleeding, hypotension, and arrhythmias.

Drug Interactions

Aspirin, non-steroidal inflammatory drugs, warfarin, heparin, and heparin-like drugs may increase the risk of bleeding.

ATENOLOL

(a-TEN-oh-lole)
Pregnancy Class: D
Tenormin (Rx)
Classifications: antianginal, antihypertensive, beta-blocker

Mechanism of Action

Blocks the stimulation of $beta_1$-adrenergic (myocardial) receptors.

Indications

Management of hypertension, angina pectoris and used to help prevent an MI.

Contraindications

Bradycardia, heart blocks, and pulmonary edema.

Precautions: Dosage reductions may be required in patients with renal impairment, patients with asthma, and in the geriatric patient.

Route and Dosage

Adult (PO): 25–50 mg, once/day.
Adult (IV): 5 mg over 5 minutes. May repeat in 5 minutes.
Pediatric: Not recommended.

How Supplied

Tablets: 25 mg, 50 mg, 100 mg.
Injection: 0.5 mg.ml.

Adverse Reactions and Side Effects

CNS: weakness, fatigue, dizziness.
Resp.: wheezing, bronchospasm.
CV: bradycardia, hypotension, CHF.

EMS Considerations

1. Monitor BP and HR. Do not administer if HR <50 and/or SBP <90.
2. Monitor respirations; may cause dyspnea and bronchospasm.
3. With the diabetic patient, watch for symptoms of hypoglycemia (hypotension or tachycardia).

Drug Interactions

Additive hypotensive effects with other antihypertensives. May counteract other anticholinergic drugs.

ATROPINE

(AH-troh-peen)
Pregnancy Class: C
Atro-Pen (Rx)
Classification: Antiarrhythmic, cholinergic blocking agent

Mechanism of Action

Atropine blocks the action of acetylcholine on receptors on the AV and SA nodes in the heart. Stimulation of parasympathetic nerve fibers is blocked resulting in enhancement of sinus node automaticity, atrioventricular conduction, increased heart rate, and increased cardiac output.

Indications

First drug of choice for symptomatic sinus bradycardia. Symptoms may include: chest pain, shortness of breath, decreased level of consciousness, hypotension, congestive heart failure, and premature ventricular contractions in the setting of myocardial infarction.

Other indications include: Second drug after epinephrine or vasopressin for asystole or bradycardic pulseless electrical activity (PEA). May be useful for AV nodal block or ventricular asystole.

Contraindications

Hypersensitivity to atropine, acute MI, Type II, and third-degree AV block.

Precautions

Use atropine with caution in the setting of myocardial ischemia or myocardial infarction. Increases in heart rate may worsen ischemia or increase the size of the infarction. Doses <0.5 mg may result in paradoxical slowing of the heart.

Route and Dosage

Adult (symptomatic sinus bradycardia): 0.5–1 mg IV bolus. Repeat as needed every 3–5 minutes, to a total dose of 0.04 mg/kg (3 mg).
Adult (AV block at the nodal level): 0.5–1 mg IV bolus. Repeat every 3–5 minutes, to a total dose of 0.04 mg/kg (3 mg).
Adult (Asystole or Pulseless Electrical Activity-PEA): 1 mg IV/IO bolus. Repeat every 3–5 minutes, to a total of 0.04 mg/kg. A total dose of 0.04 mg/kg (3 mg) of atropine causes full vagal blockage in adults.
Pediatric: 0.02 mg/kg IV bolus. Repeat every 5 minutes as needed to a maximum total dose of 1 mg in a child and 2 mg in an adolescent. Minimum single dose of atropine is 0.1 mg. Maximum single dose in the child is 0.5 mg, and maximum single dose in the adolescent is 1 mg.

Note: Atropine can be administered through a catheter that has been passed down and beyond the tip of an established ET tube. The dosage is 2–2.5 times the IV bolus dosage, and should be diluted in 10 mL of normal saline or sterile water for the adult patient and diluted in 1–2 mL of normal saline or half-normal saline in the pediatric patient.

How Supplied

Injection: 0.05 mg/mL, 0.1 mg/mL, 0.3 mg/mL, 0.4 mg/mL, 0.5 mg/mL, 0.8 mg/mL, 1 mg/mL.

Adverse Reactions and Side Effects

CNS: Drowsiness, confusion.
CV: Tachycardia.
HEENT: Blurred vision, dilated pupils, dry eyes, dry mouth.

EMS Considerations

Doses less than the minimum may actually slow the heart rate. Excessive doses may cause ventricular tachycardia or ventricular fibrillation. Atropine given to patients with nonsymptomatic bradycardia may produce adverse effects. Atropine may be harmful if used to treat AV block at the His-Purkinje level (second-degree type II AV block and third-degree block with wide-QRS complexes).

Drug Interactions

Additive effects may occur if atropine is given with other anticholinergics.

BUMETANIDE

(byou-MET-ah-nyd)
Pregnancy Class: C
Bumex (Rx)
Classifications: Loop diuretic, antihypertensive

Mechanism of Action

Bumetanide inhibits the reabsorption of sodium and chloride in the kidneys. It increases the excretion of water, sodium, chloride, magnesium, hydrogen, calcium, and potassium. Bumetanide causes renal and peripheral vasodilation and may cause a temporary decrease in peripheral vascular resistance. Bumetanide causes diuresis and lowers blood pressure.

Indications

Treatment of edema secondary to congestive heart failure. Hypertension: bumetanide can be used alone or in combination with other antihypertensive drugs.

Contraindications

Do not administer to patients with a known hypersensitivity to bumetanide. Do not use in patients who are anuric.

Precautions

Use bumetanide with caution in patients whose electrolytes are depleted or in patients who have diabetes mellitus. Safety and efficacy in children under the age of 18 years have not been established.

Route and Dosage

Adult: 0.5–2 mg IV bolus over 2 minutes or IM. Repeat at 2–3 hour intervals if needed. The total dosage of bumetanide should not exceed 10 mg/d.
Pediatric: Not recommended for out-of-hospital use.

How Supplied

Injection: 0.25 mg/mL.

Adverse Reactions and Side Effects

CNS: Headache, dizziness.
Cardiovascular: Hypotension, possible ECG changes.
Fluid and electrolytes: Metabolic alkalosis, hypovolemia, dehydration, hypokalemia, hyponatremia.
Gastrointestinal: Nausea, vomiting.

EMS Considerations

Excessive amounts of bumetanide can ultimately lead to circulatory collapse. Closely monitor the patient, frequently assessing vital signs and lung sounds looking for edema or signs of developing dehydration.

Drug Interactions

Bumetanide administered with other antihypertensives or diuretics may cause additive hypotension and fluid depletion.

BUTORPHANOL

(byou-TOR-fah-nohl)
Pregnancy Class: C
Stadol NS (Rx)
Classifications: Narcotic agonist-antagonist, opioid partial agonist, analgesic

Mechanism of Action

Butorphanol is thought to bind to the opiate receptors in the CNS, acting as an agonist to some receptors and as an antagonist to others. Butorphanol alters the awareness of and response to pain; it also causes generalized CNS depression.

Indications

Butorphanol is used to treat moderate to severe pain of any cause.

Contraindications

Do not use butorphanol in patients who:
Are known to be hypersensitive to the drug.
Are dependent on opiates, may precipitate withdrawal.
Have suffered head injury.
Complain of abdominal pain.

Precautions

Use butorphanol cautiously in patients whose respiration is impaired. The dosage of butorphanol may have to be reduced in elderly patients because they may be more sensitive to the drug. Give butorphanol with caution to patients with a history of convulsive disorders, because it may cause seizure activity. Safety has not been established in pregnancy, lactation, or children less than 18 years of age.

Route and Dosage

Adult (IV/IO Bolus): 0.5–2 mg every 3 hours as needed. Administer at a rate of 2 mg or less over 3–5 minutes IV.
Adult (IM): 1–4 mg every 3 hours as needed.
Adult (Nasal): 1 mg (1 spray in 1 nostril). Dose may be repeated 60–90 minutes later. This sequence may be repeated in 3–4 hours.
Elderly (IV, IM): 1 mg every 4–6 hours as needed. Administer over 3–5 minutes.
Elderly (Nasal): 1 mg (1 spray in 1 nostril). Dose may be repeated 90–120 minutes later. This sequence may be repeated in 3–4 hours.
Pediatric: Not recommended for out-of-hospital use.

How Supplied

Injection: 1 mg/mL, 2 mg/mL.
Intranasal solution: 10 mg/mL, in 2.5-mL metered-dose spray pump.

Adverse Reactions and Side Effects

CNS: Headache, confusion, hallucinations.
CV: Hypotension or hypertension, palpitations.
Respiratory: Respiratory depression.
GI: Nausea, vomiting, dry mouth.

EMS Considerations

Assess patient vital signs and neurologic status very closely. Administer butorphanol cautiously; it has 5 times the potency of morphine.

Drug Interactions

Additive CNS depression may occur if butorphanol is used with alcohol, antihistamines, antidepressants, or sedative/hypnotic drugs. Use with other narcotics may diminish the analgesic effects. Butorphanol may cause acute withdrawal syndrome to patients dependent on opiate drugs.

CALCIUM GLUCONATE

(KAL-see-um GLUE-koh-nayt)
Pregnancy Class: C
Kalcinate (Rx)
Classifications: Calcium supplement, electrolyte modifier

Mechanism of Action

Calcium salts are electrolytes; they are essential for the transmission of nerve impulses that initiate the contraction of cardiac muscle.

Indications

Calcium salts are used in the emergency treatment of hyperkalemia, hypocalcemia, and as an antidote for calcium channel blocker overdose.

Contraindications

Calcium salts should not be used during resuscitative efforts unless hyperkalemia, hypocalcemia, or calcium channel blocker toxicity has been proved.

Precautions

Calcium salts should be used with caution in patients receiving digoxin because of the potential for increased cardiac irritability. Calcium salts may produce arterial vasospasm in the heart and brain; therefore, use with caution in patients with cardiac, pulmonary, and cerebrovascular disease. Do not mix with sodium bicarbonate because a precipitate will form.

Route and Dosage

Adult : 500–1000 mg IV/IO given slowly 1 mL/minute with a maximum dose of 3 g. *Pediatric:* 60–100 mg/kg IV/IO given slowly over 5–10 minutes with a maximum dose of 3 g.

How Supplied

Calcium gluconate injection: 100 mg/mL (10% solution).

Adverse Reactions and Side Effects

CNS: Syncope.
CV: Cardiac arrest, arrhythmia, bradycardia.
GI: Nausea, vomiting.
Local: Tissue necrosis at the injection site.

EMS Considerations

Giving calcium gluconate too rapidly to a patient with a pulse may cause bradycardia. Monitor ECG continuously.

Drug Interactions

Do not administer calcium gluconate with sodium bicarbonate, because if the two substances are mixed a precipitate develops. Use with caution and in smaller doses for patients taking digoxin, because calcium gluconate in the presence of digoxin increase cardiac irritability.

CAPTOPRIL

(KAP-toe-pril)
Pregnancy Class: C (first trimester); D (second and third trimesters)
Capoten (Rx)
Classifications: ACE inhibitor, Antihypertensive

Mechanism of Action

Inhibitor of angiotensin synthesis

Indications

To be used alone or with other antihypertensives, especially thiazide diuretics. Used in combination with diuretics and digitalis in the treatment of CHF not responding to conventional therapy. Also used to treat post-MI patients.

Contraindications

Not to be used in patients with a history of angioedema related to previous use of ACE inhibitors.

Precautions

Used with caution in patients with impaired renal function and during lactation.

Route and Dosage

Dosage is in tablet form and individualized. However, *initial* dosages include:
Malignant hypertension (Adult and Pediatric): 25 mg;
Heart Failure (Adult): 25 mg;
Left ventricular dysfunction after MI (Adult): 6.25 mg
Severe childhood hypertension: 0.3mg/kg

How Supplied

Tablets: 12.5 mg, 25 mg, 50 mg, and 100 mg.

Adverse Reactions and Side Effects

CNS: headache, dizziness, fatigue, confusion
Respiratory: cough, dyspnea, bronchospasm
CV: hypotension, angina, palpitations, tachycardia, MI
GI: nausea, vomiting, diarrhea, abdominal pain

EMS Considerations

None.

CLOPIDOGREL

(kloh-PID-oh-grel)
Pregnancy Class: B
Plavix (Rx)
Classification: Antiplatelet agent

Mechanism of Action

Inhibits platelet aggregation by inhibiting the binding of ATP to platelet receptors.

Indications

May reduce atherosclerotic events in patients at risk of MI, acute coronary syndrome, stroke, or peripheral vascular disease.

Contraindications

Hypersensitivity to clopidogrel, or in patients with peptic ulcer, intracranial bleeding, and in lactating patients.

Precautions

Use clopidogrel with caution in patients with a history of GI

Route and Dosage

Adult (Recent MI, Stroke, or Peripheral Vascular Disease): 75 mg PO daily.
Adult (Acute Coronary Syndrome): 300 mg initially, then 75 mg once daily.

How Supplied

Tablets, 75 mg, 300 mg.

Adverse Reactions and Side Effects

CNS: dizziness, headache, depression.
Respiratory: cough, dyspnea.
CV: chest pain, hypertension, edema.
GI: abdominal pain, diarrhea, dyspepsia, gastritis, GI bleeding.

Drug Interactions

Concurrent use of aspirin, NSAIDs, heparin or other thrombolytic drugs may increase the risk of bleeding.

DIAZOXIDE

(dye-az-OX-eyed)
Pregnancy Class: C
Hyperstat IV, Proglycem (Rx)
Classification: Peripheral vasodilator, antihypertensive

Mechanism of Action

Diazoxide relaxes the vascular smooth muscles in the peripheral arterioles. It causes vasodilation and decreases peripheral vascular resistance. Diazoxide lowers both systolic and diastolic blood pressure.

Indications

Diazoxide is used for the emergency treatment of hypertensive crisis.

Contraindications

Do not administer diazoxide to patients with known hypersensitivity to diazoxide or to thiazide diuretics.

Precautions

Use diazoxide with caution in patients with symptomatic cardiac disease. Use with caution with diabetic patients, because diazoxide can cause an increase in blood sugar (hyperglycemia).

Route and Dosage

Adult: 1–3 mg/kg, up to 150 mg in a single dose, by rapid IV bolus. Repeat in 5–15 min if needed.
Pediatric: Same as adult.

How Supplied

Injection: 15 mg/mL.

Adverse Reactions and Side Effects

CNS: Dizziness, headache, lightheadedness.
CV: Tachycardia, hypotension, arrhythmia, chest pain, edema, congestive heart failure.
Fluid and electrolytes: Sodium and water retention.
Endocrine: Hyperglycemia.

EMS Considerations

Assess patient every 5 minutes adverse reactions and side effects can develop rapidly. Patient should remain supine for approximately 30 minutes after administration. Monitor diabetic patients for signs and symptoms of hyperglycemia.

Drug Interactions

Use with other antihypertensive or nitrate drugs may cause an additive hypotensive effect. Diazoxide may decrease the effectiveness of phenytoin. Simultaneous use with diuretics may increase hyperglycemic and hypotensive effects.

DIGOXIN

(dih-JOX-in)
Pregnancy Class: C
Lanoxicaps, Lanoxin (Rx)
Classification: Therapeutic: Antiarrhythmic, inotropic

Mechanism of Action

Digoxin increases both the force and velocity of ventricular contractions while simultaneously slowing conduction through the sinoatrial and the atrioventricular node. Digoxin significantly increases both stroke volume and cardiac output.

Indications

1. Digoxin is used to control the heart's ventricular rate in the management of:
   - Atrial fibrillation.
   - Atrial flutter.
   - Paroxysmal supraventricular tachycardia (PSVT).
2. Digoxin is used to treat congestive heart failure (CHF).

Contraindications

Do not administer digoxin to patients: who are hypersensitive to digitalis preparations; with uncontrolled ventricular arrhythmias; with atrioventricular heart block.

Precautions

Use digoxin with caution with patients with recent heart muscle damage; lung disease; hypoxia; hypothyroidism. All such patients may experience increased sensitivity to the drug. Hypokalemia predisposes the patient to digoxin toxicity.

Route and Dosage

Adult: 10–15 mcg/kg by slow IV bolus. Because of its toxicity, many local protocols do not allow the out-of-hospital administration of digoxin. Administer digoxin in divided doses, beginning at 50% of the *loading dose*, with additional fractional doses of 25% of the loading dose. Administering digoxin in divided doses may avoid the development of toxicity. IV injection should be administered over a minimum of 5 minutes. May be administered either undiluted or diluted with sterile water, normal saline, or D_5W.
Pediatric: Not recommended for out-of-hospital use.

How Supplied

Injection: 0.25 mg/mL.

Adverse Reactions and Side Effects

CNS: Fatigue, headache, blurred vision, yellow vision.
CV: Bradycardia and almost any cardiac arrhythmia.
GI: Nausea, vomiting, anorexia.
HEENT: Blurred vision, yellow vision, halos.

EMS Considerations

In cases of digoxin toxicity, electrical cardioversion may cause a fatal ventricular cardiac arrhythmia. Therefore, do not attempt cardioversion unless the patient develops a life-threatening arrhythmia. If attempted, electrical cardioversion should begin at the lowest possible energy level. Digoxin may cause both severe toxicity and drug interactions in the critically ill patient. Therefore, digoxin may have a limited role in the out-of-hospital management of congestive heart failure.

Drug Interactions

Use of digoxin with beta-adrenergic blocking drugs may cause additive bradycardia. Diuretics, corticosteroids that cause potassium depletion; quinidine, and verapamil may increase the risk of toxicity.

DILTIAZEM

(dill-TIE-ah-zem)
Pregnancy Class: C
Cardizem Injectable, Cardizem Lyo-Ject (Rx)
Classifications: Antianginal, antiarrhythmic (Class IV), antihypertensive

Mechanism of Action

Inhibits the transport of calcium into myocardial and vascular smooth muscle cells. SA and AV node conduction is decreased, the AV node refractory period is prolonged, cardiac contractility and peripheral vascular resistance is decreased. These actions result in decreased blood pressure, decreased frequency and severity of anginal attacks, and suppression of arrhythmias.

Indications

Management of hypertension and angina pectoris. In addition, diltiazem is administered to control the ventricular rate in atrial fibrillation and flutter. Diltiazem may terminate these re-entrant arrhythmias. Diltiazem is used as a second-line agent after adenosine to treat refractory stable paroxysmal supraventricular tachycardia.

Contraindications

Hypersensitivity to diltiazem, hypotension, second- or third-degree AV block or sick sinus syndrome unless artificial pacemaker is in place, recent or acute myocardial infarction, pulmonary edema, Wolff-Parkinson-White syndrome with rapid atrial fibrillation or flutter, wide-complex QRS tachycardias of uncertain origin.

Precautions

Safety in pregnancy, lactation, or children has not been established. The risk of hypotension is greater in elderly patients; IV dosage and rate reductions are recommended. Diltiazem should be used with caution in patients with liver or renal dysfunction, or congestive heart failure.

Route and Dosage

Adults: 0.25 mg/kg IV/IO bolus administered over 2 minutes. May be repeated in 15 minutes if needed at a dose of 0.35 mg/kg. The initial doses may be followed with a continuous infusion at 10 mg/hr. Titrate from 5–15 mg/hr to achieve desired heart rate. The infusion may be continued for up to 24 hours. The IV bolus may be administered without further dilution. The infusion may be prepared by diluting 200 mg, 200 mg, or 100 mg of diltiazem with normal saline or D_5W to a total volume of 500, 250, or 100 mL to produce a final concentration of 0.4, 0.8, or 1 mg/mL, respectively. The contents of the monovial are reconstituted with a small amount of normal saline or D_5W expressed into the vial from a bag attached to the monovial transfer set. Once the drug is dissolved, it is transferred back to the bag for administration.
Pediatric: Not recommended for out-of-hospital use.

How Supplied

Injection: 5 mg/mL (5-,10-, and 25 mL vials).
Monovial: 100 mg freeze-dried powder.
Powder for injection: 10 mg, 25 mg.
Lyo-Ject: Consists of a dual-chamber, prefilled, calibrated syringe containing 25 mg diltiazem in one chamber and 5 mL of diluent in the other chamber.

Adverse Reactions and Side Effects

CNS: Dizziness, weakness, anxiety, headache.
Respiratory: cough, dyspnea.
CV: Arrhythmias, congestive heart failure, peripheral edema, bradycardia, hypotension, AV heart block.
GI: Nausea, vomiting.
Dermatologic: Rash, urticaria, photosensitivity, Stevens-Johnson syndrome.

EMS Considerations

Continuously monitor ECG and blood pressure during the administration of diltiazem.

Drug Interactions

Concurrent use with beta-adrenergic blockers, digoxin, or phenytoin may result in bradycardia, conduction defects, or congestive heart failure. Additive hypotension may occur with coadministration of other antihypertensives or acute alcohol ingestion. Diltiazem may cause increased blood levels of digoxin, increasing the risk of toxicity.

DOBUTAMINE

(doh-BYOU-tah-meen)
Pregnancy Class: B
Dobutrex (Rx)
Classification: Inotropic, adrenergic agent

Mechanism of Action

Stimulates beta$_1$-adrenergic receptors in the heart to increase contractility, cardiac output, and stroke volume with little effect on heart rate or blood vessels.

Indications

Dobutamine is used to treat:

1. Pulmonary congestion and low cardiac output. Increases cardiac output without significantly increasing heart rate.
2. Hypotension when vasodilator drugs cannot be used.

Contraindications

Hypersensitivity to dobutamine or bisulfites.

Precautions

Atrial fibrillation should be treated with digoxin prior to receiving dobutamine. Hypovolemia or bradycardia should be corrected before administering dobutamine. Dobutamine has been used safely in children; however, the risk of tachycardia is increased.

Route and Dosage

Adult: 2–20 mcg/kg/min by IV infusion titrated to effect. There are two ways to prepare the IV infusion:

1. Add 250 mg of dobutamine to 500 mL of D$_5$W or NS to make a concentration of 500 mcg/mL.
2. Add 500 mg of dobutamine to 250 mL of D$_5$W or NS to make a concentration of 2 mg/mL (2000 mg/mL).

Pediatric: 2–20 mcg/kg/min IV infusion titrated to effect.
Infusion preparation: Multiply the patient's body weight (in kg) by 6. This equals the amount of milligrams added to D$_5$W, D$_5$1/2NS, NS, or LR. Running the infusion at 1 mL/h will deliver 1mcg/kg/min.

How Supplied

Injection: 12.5 mg/mL in 20-, 40-, and 100-mL vials.
Premixed infusion: 250 mg/250 mL, 500 mg/500 mL, 500 mg/250 mL, 1000 mg/250 mL.

Adverse Reactions and Side Effects

CNS: Headache.
CV: Tachycardia, hypertension, chest pain, arrhythmias, premature ventricle contractions (PVCs).

Respiratory: Shortness of breath.
GI: Nausea, vomiting.

EMS Considerations

Monitor the patient closely. An increase in systolic blood pressure of 10–20 mm Hg and an increase in heart rate of 5–15 beats/min is considered normal. If the patient is hypovolemic, treat hypovolemia with IV volume expanders before giving dobutamine.

Drug Interactions

Use with nitroprusside may have a synergistic effect on increasing cardiac output. Beta-adrenergic blocking agents may cause dobutamine to be ineffective. The hypertensive potential of dobutamine may be enhanced by oxytocics or tricyclic antidepressants.

DOPAMINE

(DOH-pah-meen)
Pregnancy Class: C
Intropin (Rx)
Classifications: Inotropic agent, vasopressor, adrenergic.

Mechanism of Action

Dopamine stimulates both alpha- and beta-adrenergic receptors and dopaminergic receptors in a dose-dependent fashion. Table 10–1 lists the various dose levels of dopamine, the receptors stimulated, and the actions produced on the body. Dopamine increases blood pressure and cardiac output and improves blood flow through the kidneys.

Indications

Dopamine is used to treat hemodynamically significant hypotension (SBP <70 to 100 mm Hg) in the absence of hypovolemia. Second-line agent for symptomatic bradycardia. Dopamine is administered to increase urine output in the treatment of shock unresponsive to fluid replacement. Dopamine may be co-administered with vasopressors in dopaminergic doses to maintain renal perfusion.

Contraindications

Tachyarrhythmias, pheochromocytoma (a benign *catecholamine*-producing tumor), hypersensitivity to dopamine or bisulfites.

Precautions

Hypovolemia should be treated with fluids prior to administering dopamine. Dopamine may worsen ischemia and should be used with caution in myocardial infarction. The vasoconstrictive effects of dopamine may worsen occlusive vascular diseases. Safety has not been established in pregnancy, lactation, or children.

Table 10–1 Dosage-related responses to Dopamine

Dose	Major Receptors Stimulated	Response
1–2 mcg/kg/min	Dopaminergic	Vasodilation of renal, mesenteric, and cerebral arteries. No effect on heart or blood pressure
2–10 mcg/kg/min	Beta₁-adrenergic Alpha-adrenergic	Increased cardiac output (beta) Vasoconstriction (alpha)
10–20 mcg/kg/min	Alpha-adrenergic	Renal, mesenteric, and peripheral arterial and venous vasoconstriction, producing marked increase in systemic vascular resistance and preload
>20 mcg/kg/min	Alpha-adrenergic	Similar to the response to norepinephrine, i.e., vasoconstriction; positive inotropism

Route and Dosage

Adult: 2.5–20 mcg/kg/min IV infusion. Rate dependent on desired effect (see Table 10–1). Depending on the infusion rate, the infusion should be prepared as follows:

200 mg diluted in 250 mL of D₅W or NS = 800 mcg/mL.
400 mg diluted in 250 mL of D₅W or NS = 1600 mcg/mL.
800 mg diluted in 250 mL of D₅W or NS = 3200 mcg/mL.
800 mg diluted in 500 mL of D₅W or NS = 1600 mcg/mL.

Pediatric: 2–20 mcg/kg/min IV infusion. To administer the pediatric dosage, use the following shortcut: Multiply the patient's body weight (in kg) by 6. That product equals the number of mg of dopamine to dilute in 100 mL of D₅W; the resulting solution, administered at the rate of 1 mL/h, will yield the required dosage (1mcg/kg/min).

How Supplied

Injection for dilution: 40 mg/mL, 80 mg/mL, 160 mg/mL.
Premixed injection: 200 mg/250 mL, 400 mg/250 mL, 800 mg/250 mL 800 mg/500 mL.

Adverse Reactions and Side Effects

CNS: Headache.
CV: Arrhythmias, hypotension, palpitations, chest pain.
Respiratory: Dyspnea.
Eyes: Dilated pupils.
GI: Nausea, vomiting.
Local: Tissue necrosis at IV site.

EMS Considerations

Correct hypovolemia with IV volume expanders before giving dopamine. If dopamine is to be discontinued, do so gradually, because sudden cessation can result in acute hypotension. Patients with compromised cardiac function should receive more highly concentrated solution to prevent fluid overload. Monitor vital signs and ECG continuously.

Drug Interactions

Do not mix dopamine with alkaline drugs, because alkaline solutions may deactivate dopamine. Using dopamine with phenytoin may produce hypotension and bradycardia. Dopamine has an advantage over isoproterenol in that dopamine does not increase myocardial oxygen demand as much as isoproterenol.

EPINEPHRINE

(ep-ih-NEF-rin)
Pregnancy Class: C
Adrenalin, EpiPen (Rx)
Classification: Bronchodilator, cardiac stimulator, vasopressor

Mechanism of Action

Epinephrine is a catecholamine that stimulates alpha- and beta-adrenergic receptors in the sympathetic nervous system. Beta₁-stimulation: Increase in heart rate, increase in cardiac contractility, increase in cardiac output, increase in cardiac automaticity. Beta₂-stimulation: Relaxation of bronchial smooth muscle resulting in bronchodilation. Alpha₁-stimulation: Peripheral vasoconstriction, increase in systemic vascular resistance, increase in arterial blood pressure.

Indications

Epinephrine is a first-line drug used for all forms of cardiopulmonary arrest, including:

- Ventricular fibrillation
- Ventricular tachycardia without a pulse (to be treated as ventricular fibrillation)
- Pulseless electrical activity (PEA)
- Asystole

Epinephrine can also be used as a vasopressor when treating symptomatic severe hypotensive sinus bradycardia.

Contraindications

None, during cardiopulmonary arrest. Otherwise, do not administer epinephrine to patients hypersensitive to sympathomimetic amines.

Precautions

Epinephrine may cause myocardial ischemia and increased *myocardial oxygen demand*—administer with caution in patients with cardiac disease, elderly patients, or hyperthyroidism. Epinephrine should be administered with caution in diabetics because of the potential for hyperglycemia. Epinephrine should be administered cautiously to patients with hypertension—may lead to **hypertensive crisis**. High doses of epinephrine are no longer recommended as these have not been found to improve survival or neurologic outcome.

Route and Dosage

Adult (cardiac arrest): 1 mg (10 mL of a 1: 10,000 solution) IV/IO bolus every 3–5 minutes during the arrest. Follow each dose with 20 mL flush of IV solution. Higher doses (up to 0.2 mg/kg) may be used if the 1 mg dose fails. During cardiac arrest, epinephrine may be administered as a continuous IV infusion. To prepare, add 1 mg (1 mL of a 1:1000 solution) to 500 mL of NS or D_5W. Initial infusion rate of 1 mcg/minute titrated to effect; generally 2–10 mcg/minute.

Adult (hypotension, symptomatic sinus bradycardia): 2–10 mcg/min IV infusion, titrate to effect. To prepare, add 1 mg (1 mL of a 1:1000 solution) to 500 mL NS or D_5W. Infuse at 1–5 mL/min.

Pediatric (pulseless arrest): 0.01 mg/kg (0.1 mL/kg of a 1:10,000 solution) IV bolus or intraosseous (IO) for the initial dose. If the initial dose is via the ET tube, the dose is 0.1 mg/kg (0.1 mL/kg of a 1:1000 solution). Repeat every 3–5 minutes until IV/IO access achieved then begin with initial IV/IO dose. Subsequent doses (IV, IO) should be given at 0.1 mg/kg up to 0.2 mg/kg (0.2 mL/kg of a 1:1000 solution) every 3–5 minutes.

Pediatric (symptomatic bradycardia): 0.01 mg/kg (0.1 mL/kg of a 1:10,000 solution) administered IV bolus or IO or 0.1 mg/kg (0.1 mL/kg of a 1:1000 solution) diluted in 1–2 mL of normal or half normal saline via ET tube. A continuous IV/IO infusion may be initiated at 0.1 mcg/kg/min, titrated to effect, up to 1 mcg/kg/min. The infusion is prepared as follows: 0.6 times the body weight (in kg) equals the amount of mg of epinephrine added to 100 mL of D_5W, D_5/0.45% NaCl, normal saline, or LR. Infusing at 1 mL/hr delivers 0.1 mg/kg/min.

Note: Epinephrine can be administered through a catheter that has been passed down and beyond the tip of an established ET tube. The dosage for adults is 2–2.5 times that of the recommended IV bolus dosage and should be diluted in 10 mL of normal saline or sterile water. The dosage for pediatric patients can be increased up to 10 times the IV bolus or IO dosage and should be diluted in 1–2 mL of normal or half-normal saline.

How Supplied

1 mg/mL, 5 mg/mL.

Adverse Reactions and Side Effects

None, during cardiopulmonary resuscitation.
Otherwise:
CNS: Nervousness, restlessness, headache, tremor.
CV: Arrhythmia, angina, hypertension, tachycardia.
GI: Nausea, vomiting.
Endo: Hyperglycemia.

EMS Considerations

Epinephrine's therapeutic effects usually begin about 90 seconds after administration. However, because these effects are short-lived, epinephrine must be given every 5 min during resuscitative efforts to maintain therapeutic levels. The beta-adrenergic effects of epinephrine may cause or aggravate myocardial ischemia because of the increased workload and oxygen demand that beta-adrenergic stimulation places on the heart. Therefore, the patient must be adequately ventilated using 100% oxygen to minimize myocardial ischemia. Epinephrine may cause or increase the severity of ventricular ectopic activity. This is of special concern if the patient is taking digitalis, because digitalis causes the heart to become sensitive to the effects of epinephrine. Monitor ECG and vital signs continuously.

Drug Interactions

Beta-adrenergic blocking drugs may block the therapeutic response to epinephrine. The use of epinephrine with oxytocics can cause severe hypertension. Combination of epinephrine with other beta-adrenergic agonists can cause severe arrhythmias.

ESMOLOL

(ES-moe-lole)
Pregnancy Class: C
Brevivloc (Rx)
Classifications: beta blocker, class II antiarrhythmic

Mechanism of Action

Blocks the stimulation of $beta_1$ (myocardial) adrenergic receptors.

Indications

Treatment of sinus tachycardia and supraventricular arrhythmias.

Contraindications

Esmolol should not be used in patients with pulmonary edema, uncompensated CHF, cardiogenic shock or bradycardia.

Precautions

Esmolol should be used with caution in patients with thyrotoxicosis, or in patients with diabetes mellitus, due to possible masking of symptoms. Geriatric patients may have increased sensitivity to esmolol.

Route and Dosage

Adult: 500 mcg/kg loading dose over 1 minute, followed by 50 mcg/kg/min IV infusion for 4 minutes. If no response within 5 minutes, give a second 500 mcg/kg bolus over 1 minute, and increase the infusion to 100 mcg/kg/min for 4 minutes.

Pediatric: 50 mcg/kg/min initially. May be increased q 10 minutes up to 300 mcg/kg/minute.

Adverse Reactions and Side Effects

CNS: fatigue, confusion, dizziness, weakness.
CV: hypotension.
GI: nausea, vomiting.
Local: injection site reactions.

How Supplied

Prediluted solution for injection: 10 mg/mL in 10 mL vials, 20 mg/mL in 5 mL vials.
Solution for injection: 250 mg/mL in 10 mL ampules.
Premixed infusion: 2000 mg/100 mL, 2500 mg/250 mL.

EMS Considerations

Monitor patient's blood pressure, ECG and pulse frequently during treatment. If administration site irritation occurs, stop the infusion and begin at another site.

Drug Interactions

The use of digoxin may cause additive bradycardia effects. Additive hypotensive effects may occur with the additional use of other antihypertensives.

FUROSEMIDE

(fur-OH-she-myd)
Pregnancy Class: C
Lasix (Rx)
Classifications: Loop diuretic, antihypertensive

Mechanism of Action

Inhibits the reabsorption of sodium and chloride from the loop of Henle and distal renal tubule in the kidneys; this results in the excretion of water, sodium, chloride, potassium, calcium, and magnesium. Furosemide also causes vasodilation reducing venous return to the heart. These actions result in reduction of pulmonary edema and decreased blood pressure.

Indications

Management of edema secondary to congestive heart failure. Treatment of hypertension.

Contraindications

Do not administer furosemide to patients with: hypovolemia, hypotension, hypokalemia. Suspect hypokalemia if the patient is on long-term diuretic therapy or if the ECG shows prominent P waves, diminished T waves, or the presence of U waves. Hypersensitivity to furosemide.

Precautions

Patients hypersensitive to sulfonamides or thiazide diuretics may be hypersensitive to furosemide. Administration of furosemide may result in dehydration and hypotension; elderly patients are at increased risk.

Route and Dosage

Adult: 0.5–1.0 mg/kg (20–40 mg) by slow IV bolus over 1–2 minutes. If no response, double the dose to 2 mg/kg over 1–2 minutes.
Pediatric: 1 mg/kg by slow IV bolus over 1–2 minutes. May increase by 1 mg/kg every 2 hours (not to exceed 6 mg/kg).

Adverse Reactions and Side Effects

CNS: Dizziness, headache, blurred vision, vertigo.
Cardiovascular: Hypotension, arrhythmias.
Fluids and electrolytes: Potassium depletion, metabolic alkalosis.
GI: Nausea, vomiting, diarrhea.
GU: Excessive urination.

How Supplied

10 mg/mL.

EMS Considerations

Because of furosemide's diuretic effect, monitor the patient's blood pressure closely. Assess lung sounds before giving furosemide and monitor them closely after administration.

Drug Interactions

Antihypertensive and nitrate drugs may worsen hypotension. Furosemide given with other diuretic drugs may cause severe fluid and electrolyte loss. Severe potassium loss may increase digitalis toxicity in patients taking digoxin.

HEPARIN

(HEP-ah-rin)
Pregnancy Class: C
Hep-Lock, Hep-Lock U/P (Rx)
Classification: Anticoagulant

Mechanism of Action

Potentiates the inhibitory action of antithrombin III on various coagulation factors. Heparin interferes with thrombin formation and prevents the conversion of fibrinogen to fibrin. These actions prevent formation of a blood clot.

Indications

An adjunct to thrombolytic therapy. Prophylaxis and treatment of venous thrombosis, pulmonary embolism, or peripheral arterial embolism. Prophylaxis of postmyocardial infarction thrombi. Treatment of myocardial ischemia in *unstable angina* refractory to treatment.

Contraindications

Hypersensitivity to heparin. Uncontrolled bleeding, severe thrombocytopenia, known bleeding disorders, hemorrhagic cerebrovascular accident.

Precautions

Use with caution in patients with severe liver disease, severe uncontrolled hypertension, peptic ulcer disease, recent surgery, spinal cord or brain trauma.

Route and Dosage

Adults: Initial bolus of 60 international units (IU)/kg. (Maximum of 4000 IU). Followed by a continuous infusion of 12 IU/kg/hr. Maximum of 1000 IU/hr for patients greater than 70 kg.
To prepare infusion: Add 25,000 U heparin (25 mL of 1000 U/mL) to 250 mL D$_5$W or normal saline. Dosages and regimens differ according to local medical protocols.

How Supplied

Solution for injection: 10 U/mL, 100 U/mL, 1000 U/mL, 5000 U/mL, 7500 U/mL, 10,000 U/mL, 20,000 U/mL, 40,000 U/mL.
Premixed solution: 1000 U/500 mL, 2000 U/1000 mL, 12,500 U/250 mL, 25,000 U/250 mL, 25,000 U/500 mL.

Adverse Reactions and Side Effects

GI: GI bleeding.
Miscellaneous: Hypersensitivity, shock, anaphylaxis.
GU: Hematuria.
Dermatologic: Ecchymosis.
Hematologic: Bleeding, anemia, thrombocytopenia.
HEENT: Epistaxis, gingival bleeding.

EMS Considerations

Continuously monitor patient for evidence of bleeding.

Drug Interactions

Risk of bleeding increased with aspirin, non-steroidal anti-inflammatory drugs, other anticoagulants, and thrombolytics.

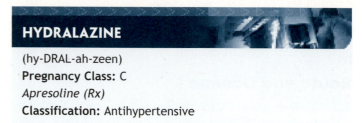

HYDRALAZINE

(hy-DRAL-ah-zeen)
Pregnancy Class: C
Apresoline (Rx)
Classification: Antihypertensive

Mechanism of Action

Hydralazine causes dilation of peripheral arterioles which decreases afterload, and which lowers blood pressure.

Indications

Hydralazine is used to treat moderate to severe hypertension with diuretic therapy. It may be used to treat congestive heart failure that is resistant to more conventional therapy using digitalis glycosides and diuretics.

Contraindications

Do not administer hydralazine to patients with: hypersensitivity to the drug, coronary artery disease, mitral-valve rheumatic heart disease.

Precautions

Use caution in administering hydralazine to patients with: cardiovascular disease, cerebrovascular disease, renal disease.

Route and Dosage

Adult: 5–40 mg by slow IV bolus or IM.
Pediatric: Not recommended for out-of-hospital use.

How Supplied

Injection: 20 mg/mL.

Adverse Reactions and Side Effects

CNS: Headache, dizziness, drowsiness.
CV: Tachycardia, arrhythmias, orthostatic hypotension, chest pain.
GI: Nausea, vomiting.

EMS Considerations

Monitor the patient closely, especially blood pressure and pulse, during and after administration.

Drug Interactions

Use with other antihypertensives and nitrate drugs may produce additive hypotensive effects, which can be particularly severe in the case of diazoxide. Hydralazine may reduce the stimulation and blood-pressure effects of epinephrine.

IBUTILIDE

(ih-BYOU-tih-lyd)
Pregnancy Class: C
Corvert (Rx)
Classification: Antiarrhythmic (Class III)

Mechanism of Action

Delays repolarization, prolongs the action potential duration, and increases refractoriness. These actions result in slowing of the sinus rate and AV conduction.

Indications

Rapid conversion of recent-onset atrial fibrillation or flutter to normal sinus rhythm.

Contraindications

Hypersensitivity to ibutilide.

Precautions

Use cautiously in patients with congestive heart failure or left ventricular dysfunction because of increased risk of serious arrhythmias during infusion. Safety not established in pregnancy, lactation, or age less than 18 years.

Route and Dosage

Adults (Greater than 60 kg): 1 mg IV infused over 10 minutes. If the arrhythmia is not terminated, a second dose may be given 10 minutes after the end of the first infusion.
(Less than 60 kg): 0.01 mg/kg IV infused over 10 minutes. A second dose may be given 10 minutes after the end of the first infusion if the arrhythmia is not terminated. Ibutilide may be given undiluted or diluted in 50 mL of NS or D_5W.

How Supplied

IV solution: 0.1 mg/mL.

Adverse Reactions and Side Effects

CNS: Headache, syncope.
CV: Arrhythmias, hypotension, AV block, bradycardia, congestive heart failure.
GI: Nausea.

EMS Considerations

Continuously monitor vital signs and ECG.

Drug Interactions

Amiodarone or procainamide should not be administered concurrently or within 4 hours of the patient receiving ibutilide because there is an additive effect on refractoriness.

LABETALOL

(lah-BET-ah-lohl)
Pregnancy Class: C
Normodyne, Trandate (Rx)
Classifications: Antianginal, antiarrhythmic, antihypertensive

Mechanism of Action

Decreases blood pressure and heart rate by blocking alpha- and beta-adrenergic receptors.

Indications

Hypertensive urgency or emergency. Second-line agent for the treatment of supraventricular arrhythmias. Patients with suspected myocardial infarction or unstable angina to treat anginal pain, reduce the incidence of ventricular fibrillation, decrease elevated heart rate and blood pressure. May be used with thrombolytics to reduce blood pressure, nonfatal reinfarction, and recurrent ischemia.

Contraindications

Do not administer labetalol to patients with: hypersensitivity to labetalol, bronchial asthma, congestive heart failure, pulmonary edema, cardiogenic shock, bradycardia, heart block. Do not administer labetalol during pregnancy, because its use can result in apnea, low Apgar scores, bradycardia, or hypoglycemia in newborns.

Precautions

Reduce labetalol dosage for patients with diminished renal function. The beta-blocking action of labetalol may cause congestive heart failure in patients with coronary insufficiency. Use caution in administering labetalol to patients with diabetes mellitus because labetalol may mask signs and symptoms of hypoglycemia.

Route and Dosage

Adult (IV Bolus): Administer 20 mg (0.25 mg/kg) over 2 min. Administer subsequent doses of 40–80 mg at 10-min intervals if needed. Total dose should not exceed 300 mg.
Adult (IV Infusion): 2 mg/min.
To prepare IV infusion: Add 200 mg labetalol to 250 mL of D_5W; this results in a drug concentration of 0.8 mg/mL. Run at 150 mgtts/min to yield an infusion rate of 2 mg/min.
Pediatric: Not recommended for out-of-hospital use.

How Supplied

5 mg/mL.

Adverse Reactions and Side Effects

CNS: Fatigue, weakness, depression.
CV: Bradycardia, congestive heart failure, pulmonary edema, hypotension.
Respiratory: Bronchospasm, wheezing.
Eyes: Blurred vision, dry eyes.
GI: Nausea, diarrhea.

EMS Considerations

Monitor patient closely for changes in blood pressure, heart rate and rhythm, and respiratory rate. Patients should remain supine during administration, because labetalol may cause orthostatic hypotension.

Drug Interactions

Use with digitalis glycosides may produce additive bradycardia. Using labetalol with other hypertensive and nitrate drugs may cause additive hypotension. Labetalol may antagonize beta-adrenergic bronchodilator drugs. Concurrent IV administration with calcium channel blockers may result in severe hypotension.

LIDOCAINE

(LYE-doh-kayn)
Pregnancy Class: B
LidoPen, Xylocaine (Rx)
Classification: Antiarrhythmic (Class IB)

Mechanism of Action

Suppresses ventricular ectopy by shortening the refractory period and suppression of automaticity of ectopic foci. In addition, lidocaine increases the ventricular fibrillation threshold.

Indications

An alternative to amiodarone in the treatment for cardiac arrest from ventricular fibrillation/pulseless ventricular tachycardia. To prevent recurrence of ventricular fibrillation/ventricular tachycardia after successful conversion to perfusing rhythm. Stable ventricular tachycardia, wide-complex tachycardias of uncertain origin, and ventricular ectopy in the presence of acute myocardial infarction.

Contraindications

Hypersensitivity to lidocaine. Prophylactic use in AMI. Ventricular ectopy secondary to untreated bradycardia or AV block. Adams-Stokes syndrome. Wolff-Parkinson-White syndrome.

Precautions

Use with caution in patients with liver disease, CHF, patients weighing less than 50 kg, and in the geriatric patient. Infusion should be discontinued if signs of toxicity (CNS symptoms, bradycardia) occur. Use cautiously in the presence of respiratory depression and shock.

Route and Dosage

Adult (cardiac arrest—VF/VT): Initial dose of 1–1.5 mg/kg IV/IO push. Doses of 0.5–0.75 mg/kg IV push may be repeated every 5–10 minutes to a maximum dose of 3 mg/kg. Endotracheal administration is 2–4 mg/kg. When a pulse is restored, a lidocaine infusion should be started at 2–4 mg/min.

Adult (VT with pulse, wide-complex tachycardia of uncertain origin, ventricular ectopy): Initial dose of 1–1.5 mg/kg IV bolus. Lidocaine may be repeated at 0.5–0.75 mg/kg every 5–10 minutes to a maximum dose of 3 mg/kg. Infusion should be initiated at 2–4 mg/min when the arrhythmia has been corrected.

Infusion preparation: Add 2 g of lidocaine to 500 mL of NS or D_5W for a concentration of 4 mg/mL. The dosage rates for this 4:1 infusion are:

- 1 mcg/min–15 gtts/min.
- 2 mcg/min–30 gtts/min.
- 3 mcg/min–45 gtts/min.
- 4 mcg/min–60 gtts/min.

Pediatric: 1 mg/kg per dose. If prolonged therapy is needed, an IV infusion should be started at a rate of 20–50 mcg/kg/min.

Preparation of infusion: Add 120 mg of lidocaine to an amount of D_5W that produces a total volume of solution of 100 mL. An infusion rate of 1–2.5 mL/kg/hr will deliver the required dosage.

Note: Lidocaine can be administered through a catheter that has been passed down and beyond the tip of an established ET tube. The dosage is 2–2.5 times that of the recommended IV bolus dosage and should be diluted in 10 mL of normal saline or distilled water for the adult patient, and diluted in 1–2 mL of NS or 1/2 NS for the pediatric patient.

How Supplied

Injection: 10 mg/mL (1%), 20 mg/mL (2%).
Solution for injection (after further dilution): 40 mg/mL (4%), 100 mg/mL (10%), 200 mg/mL (20%).
Premixed solution for IV infusion (with D_5W): 2 mg/mL, 4 mg/mL, 8 mg/mL.

Adverse Reactions and Side Effects

CNS: Anxiety, drowsiness, confusion, seizures, respiratory arrest.
CV: Hypotension, bradycardia, arrhythmias, cardiac arrest.
GI: Nausea, vomiting.
Other: Anaphylaxis—rare.

EMS Considerations

The therapeutic levels from a bolus dose of lidocaine last approximately 20 min. Once a bolus dose achieves therapeutic levels, an IV infusion of lidocaine is required to maintain the desired therapeutic level. However, the infusion should not be started until the return of spontaneous circulation or the correction of the arrhythmia. Too-rapid administration of lidocaine can result in hypotension, bradycardia, tachycardia, or seizures. If the patient develops seizure activity, discontinue the lidocaine and administer diazepam. Defibrillation causes ventricular irritability, and ventricular irritability can produce ventricular ectopic activity. The administration of lidocaine after a successful defibrillation may be ordered to prevent ventricular ectopic activity. Patients over 70 have a reduced volume of distribution, which makes it necessary to reduce the IV infusion dosage of lidocaine by 50%. When administering lidocaine, closely monitor the patient's cardiac function, respiratory status, and blood pressure.

Some publications have indicated that a contraindication for the use of lidocaine is hypersensitivity to amide-type local anesthetics. Adverse reactions associated with local anesthetics occur rarely (less than 1%). The incidence of adverse reactions may be even less, because most alleged allergic reactions may be caused by an extension of pharmacologic actions or preservatives present in multidose vials (local anesthetic solutions). Life-threatening anaphylactic reactions occur very infrequently. On a practical basis, the incidence of adverse reactions is so rare that there would be a greater risk of withholding lidocaine if the drug is indicated.

Drug Interactions

Simultaneous use of lidocaine and beta-blockers may cause lidocaine toxicity. Lidocaine used simultaneously with phenytoin, procainamide, propranolol, or quinidine can have additive, antagonistic, or toxic effects.

MAGNESIUM SULFATE

(mag-NEE-see-um SUL-fate)
Pregnancy Class: A
Classifications: Electrolyte, Therapeutic: Magnesium supplement, antiarrhythmic

Mechanism of Action

Essential for muscle contraction, some enzyme systems, and nerve transmission. Magnesium sulfate resolves magnesium deficiency which is associated with cardiac arrhythmias.

Indications

Magnesium sulfate is given to correct hypomagnesemia in the following:

1. Torsade de pointes (see Figure 10–6).
2. Severe refractory ventricular fibrillation/pulseless ventricular tachycardia.

Contraindications

Do not administer magnesium sulfate to patients with: hypermagnesemia, hypocalcemia, and heart block.

Precautions

Use with caution in patients with any degree of renal insufficiency and in digitalized patients. Rapid IV administration may cause respiratory or cardiac arrest.

Route and Dosage

Adult (Cardiac arrest): 1–2 gm (2–4 mL of a 50% solution) diluted in 10 mL of D₅W or NS IV push.
Adult (Torsade de pointes): 1–2 gm (2–4 mL of a 50% solution) mixed in 50–100 mL of D₅W or NS IV over 5–60 minutes. Follow with a continuous infusion of 0.5–1 gm/hr, titrate to control arrhythmia.
Pediatric: 25–50 mg/kg IV over 10–20 minutes. May be given faster in patients with Torsades de Pointes.

How Supplied

Injection: 100 mg/mL (10%), 125 mg/mL (12.5%), 250 mg/mL (25%), 500 mg/mL (50%).
Premixed infusion: 1 g/100 mL, 2 g/100 mL, 4 g/50 mL, 4 g/100 mL, 20 g/500 mL, 40 g/1000 mL.

Adverse Reactions and Side Effects

CNS: Drowsiness.
Respiratory: Respiratory depression.
CV: Bradycardia, arrhythmias, hypotension.
Skin: Rash.
Metabolic: Hypothermia, hypocalcemia.

EMS Considerations

An overdose of magnesium sulfate may cause respiratory depression and heart block. To reverse these effects, hyperventilate

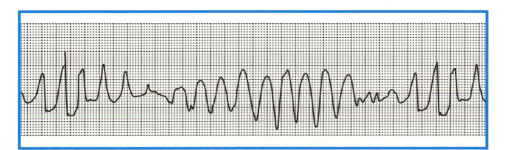

Figure 10–6 Toresade de pointes. (© Delmar/Cengage Learning)

the patient using 100% oxygen and administer an IV bolus of 10% calcium gluconate at 5–10 mEq (10–20 mL). Monitor ECG and vital signs during administration.

Drug Interactions

Cardiac conduction changes may occur if magnesium sulfate is administered with cardiac glycosides.

LISINOPRIL

(lyse-IN- oh-pril)
Pregnancy Class: C (first trimester), D (second and third trimesters)
Prinivil (Rx)
Classification: Angiotensin-converting enzyme (ACE) inhibitor

Mechanism of Action

Lisinopril blocks the conversion of angiotensin I to the vaso-constrictor angiotensin II, which lowers the blood pressure in hypertensive patients.

Indications

Lisinopril can be used alone or with other antihypertensives in the management of patients with hypertension.

Contraindications

Should not be used in patients who are hypersensitive to ACE inhibitors, or in patients who have a history of angioedema with previous use of ACE inhibitors.

Precautions; Should be used with caution (generally lower doses) in patients with renal impairment, hepatic impairment, hypovolemia, or in patients who are on concurrent diuretic therapy.

Route and Dosage

Adults, PO (Hypertension): 10 mg once daily. Can be increased to 20–40 mg/day.
Adults, PO (CHF): 5 mg once daily.
Pediatric >6 yrs, PO (Hypertension): 0.07 mg/kg once daily (Max. dose = 5 mg/day).

How Supplied

Tablets – 2.5 mg, 5 mg, 10 mg, 20 mg, 30 mg, 40 mg.

Adverse Reactions and Side Effects:

CNS: headache, dizziness, vertigo, weakness.
Respiratory: cough, dyspnea.
CV: chest pain, hypotension, edema, tachycardia.
GI: abdominal pain, diarrhea, nausea, vomiting.

Drug Interactions

An increased risk of hypotension may occur with concurrent use of diuretics and other antihypertensives. The antihypertensive response may be reduced by NSAIDs.

MEPERIDINE

(meh-PER-ih-deen)
Pregnancy Class: C
Demerol (C-II) (Rx)
Classification: Opioid analgesic

Mechanism of Action

Binds to opiate receptors in the CNS. Alters the awareness and response to pain and causes generalized CNS depression. Meperidine is synthetically produced and is approximately one-tenth as potent as morphine.

Indications

Meperidine is given for the treatment of moderate to severe pain.

Contraindications

Meperidine should not be given to patients with: hypersensitivity to meperidine or bisulfites, head injury, undiagnosed abdominal pain. Do not use meperidine in patients receiving MAO inhibitors; may cause patient to have a fatal reaction.

Precautions

Use caution in administering meperidine to patients with a history of seizure disorders, because it may cause seizure activity. Use caution in administering meperidine to patients with pulmonary disease, because it may depress respirations.

Route and Dosage

Adult (IV Infusion): 15–35 mg/h. Prepare infusion by adding 50 mg of meperidine to 500 mL of D_5W, making a drug concentration of 0.1 mg/mL.
Adult (IV, IM, SQ): 50–100 mg every 3–4 hours.
Pediatric (IV, IM, SQ): 1–2 mg/kg every 3–4 hours. Maximal single dose is 100 mg.

How Supplied

Injection: 25 mg/mL, 50 mg/mL, 75 mg/mL, 100 mg/mL.

Adverse Reactions and Side Effects

CNS: Headache, confusion, sedation, hallucinations, seizures.
CV: Hypotension, bradycardia.
Respiratory: Respiratory depression.
GI: Nausea, vomiting.

EMS Considerations

Closely monitor the patient for signs of developing respiratory depression. Ensure that naloxone is available to reverse respiratory depression, should it occur.

Drug Interactions

Using meperidine with antihistamines and sedative/hypnotics may cause additive CNS depressant effects.

METOPROLOL

(me-toe-PROH-lohl)
Pregnancy Class: C
Lopressor (Rx)
Classifications: Antianginal, antiarrhythmic, antihypertensive

Mechanism of Action

Blocks stimulation of beta$_1$-adrenergic receptors and results in decreased blood pressure and heart rate.

Indications

Hypertensive urgency or emergency. Second-line agent for the treatment of supraventricular arrhythmias. Patients with suspected MI or unstable angina to treat anginal pain, reduce the incidence of VF, and decrease elevated blood pressure and heart rate. May be used with thrombolytics to reduce nonfatal reinfarction and recurrent ischemia.

Contraindications

Hypersensitivity to metoprolol. Do not administer metoprolol to patients with the following: bronchial asthma, cardiogenic shock, bradycardia, hypotension, cardiac failure, or heart block. Do not administer during pregnancy because it may result in apnea, low Apgar scores, bradycardia, or hypoglycemia in newborns.

Precautions

Use caution in administering metoprolol to patients with coronary insufficiency, because it may cause congestive failure. Use metoprolol cautiously with patients with diabetes mellitus because it may mask the signs and symptoms of hypoglycemia.

Route and Dosage

Adult: 5 mg by slow IV bolus every 2 min for up to 3 doses or as long as vital signs remain stable.
Pediatric: Not recommended for out-of-hospital use.

How Supplied

Injection: 1 mg/mL.

Adverse Reactions and Side Effects

CNS: Weakness, dizziness, depression.
CV: Bradycardia, pulmonary edema, congestive heart failure.
Respiratory: Bronchospasm, wheezing.
Eyes: Blurred vision.
GI: Nausea, vomiting, dry mouth, heartburn.

EMS Considerations

Assess patient vital signs frequently during administration. Side effects can develop rapidly.

Drug Interactions

Use with phenytoin and verapamil may produce additive cardiac depression. Use with digitalis glycosides may cause additive bradycardia. Excessive alpha-adrenergic stimulation may be produced if metoprolol is used with epinephrine.

MORPHINE SULFATE

(MOR-feen)
Pregnancy Class: C
Astramorph, Duramorph, Infumorph, Roxanol (C-II) (Rx)
Classification: Analgesic

Mechanism of Action

Morphine binds to opiate receptors in the CNS and alters the perception of and response to pain, and produces generalized CNS depression. In addition, morphine causes vasodilation that results in decreases in preload and afterload to relieve pulmonary edema.

Indications

Morphine is used to treat pain and anxiety associated with acute MI and in treating acute cardiogenic pulmonary edema.

Contraindications

Do not administer morphine to patients with: hypersensitivity to the drug, hypotension, respiratory depression not associated with pulmonary edema, head injury, undiagnosed abdominal pain. Do not administer to patients who are taking depressant drugs.

Precautions

Use extreme caution in administering morphine to patients with chronic obstructive pulmonary disease, because it may depress respirations and suppress the cough reflex.

Route and Dosage

Adult (Pain): 4–15 mg by slow IV, IO, IM, SQ until it has desired effect. Do not exceed 15 mg in the out-of-hospital setting.

Adult (ACS, CHF, Pulmonary Edema): 2–4 mg slow IV, over 1–5 minutes. May be repeated q 5–15 minutes.
Pediatric (Pain): 0.05–0.2 mg/kg slow IV, IO, IM, SQ.
Pediatric (ACS, CHF, Pulmonary Edema): 0.1–0.2 mg/kg slow IV.

How Supplied

Injection: 1 mg/mL, 2 mg/mL, 4 mg/mL, 5 mg/mL, 8 mg/mL, 10 mg/mL, 15 mg/mL, 25 mg/mL, 50 mg/mL.

Adverse Reactions and Side Effects

CNS: Confusion, sedation, headache.
CV: Hypotension, bradycardia.
Respiratory: Respiratory depression.
Eyes: Dry eyes, blurred vision.
GI: Nausea, vomiting.
Skin: Rashes.

EMS Considerations

Morphine is less likely to cause serious respiratory depression if given slowly and in small amounts. Naloxone should be available in case the patient shows any signs of overdose. Monitor patient vital signs closely after administering morphine.

Drug Interactions

Additive CNS depression may occur when morphine is used with: alcohol, antihistamines, sedative/hypnotics, antidepressants, barbiturates.

NALBUPHINE

(NAL-byou-feen)
Pregnancy Class: C
Nubain (Rx)
Classifications: Analgesic, opioid agonist/antagonist

Mechanism of Action

Binds to opiate receptors in the CNS and alters the perception of and response to pain and produces generalized CNS depression. In addition, nalbuphine produces partial antagonist effects by competitive inhibition at opiate receptors in the CNS. Nalbuphine has similar analgesic potency to morphine.

Indications

Nalbuphine is used to treat moderate to severe pain.

Contraindications

Hypersensitivity to nalbuphine or bisulfites.

Precautions

Use with caution in patients with head trauma, increased intracranial pressure, or in patients with severe renal, hepatic, or pulmonary disease.

Route and Dosage

Adult: 10 mg IV every 3–6 hours as needed. Total single dose should not exceed 20 mg. Total daily dose should not exceed 160 mg.

How Supplied

Injection: 10 mg/mL (1- and 10-mL vials), 20 mg/mL (1- and 10-mL vials), 1-mL syringe.

Adverse Reactions and Side Effects

CNS: Headache, dizziness, vertigo, confusion.
CV: Orthostatic hypotension, hypertension, palpitations.
Respiratory: Respiratory depression.
GI: Nausea, vomiting, dry mouth.

EMS Considerations

Assess the patient's vital signs frequently, because nalbuphine may cause respiratory depression. Note, however, that the respiratory depression does not necessarily worsen with increased doses of the drug.

Drug Interactions

Antihistamines, antidepressants, and sedative/hypnotic drugs may cause additive CNS depression. Simultaneous use with other narcotic agents may diminish nalbuphine's analgesic effects.

NIFEDIPINE

(nye-FED-ih-peen)
Pregnancy Class: C
Adalat, Procardia (Rx)
Classifications: Antianginal, antihypertensive

Mechanism of Action

Inhibits calcium transport into myocardial and vascular smooth muscle cells resulting in systemic and coronary vasodilation. These actions result in decreased blood pressure, decreased afterload, decreased myocardial oxygen demand, and decreased frequency and severity of angina pectoris.

Contraindications

Hypersensitivity to nifedipine. Patients with sick sinus syndrome, second-or third-degree AV block, or hypotension (BP <90 mm Hg). SL nifedipine rapidly lowers blood pressure and may result in cerebral ischemia; do not administer via this route for the management of hypertension.

Precautions

Use caution in administering nifedipine to patients with congestive heart failure (CHF), because it may worsen the heart failure.

Route and Dosage

Adult (PO): 10–30 mg three times daily, not to exceed 180 mg/d.
Adult (SL): 5–10 mg. Repeat every 30–60 min as needed.
Pediatric: Not recommended for out-of-hospital use.

How Supplied

Capsules: 10 mg, 20 mg.
Extended-release tablets: 30 mg, 60 mg, 90 mg.

Adverse Reactions and Side Effects

CNS: Headache, dizziness, nervousness.
Respiratory: Dyspnea, cough, wheezing.
CV: Congestive heart failure, MI, ventricular arrhythmias, hypotension, syncope.
GI: Nausea, abdominal discomfort, diarrhea.

EMS Considerations

Monitor patient blood pressure and pulse both before and during administration. Assess the patient frequently for signs of CHF, which include peripheral edema, rales, dyspnea, and jugular vein distension.

Drug Interactions

Simultaneous use of nifedipine with beta-adrenergic blockers or digoxin increases the risk of cardiac conduction defects or CHF. Severe hypotension may occur if nifedipine is used with beta-adrenergic blockers. Additive hypotension may occur if nifedipine is used with fentanyl, nitrates, or other antihypertensives. Antihypertensive effects may be decreased with concurrent use of NSAIDs.

NITROGLYCERIN

(nye-troh-GLIH-sir-in)
Pregnancy Class: C
Nitro-bid, Nitro-Bid IV, Tridil, Nitrol, Deponit, Minitran, Nitrek, Nitro-Dur, Transderm Nitro, Nitrolingual (Rx)
Classifications: Antianginal, antihypertensive, coronary vasodilator

Mechanism of Action

Nitroglycerin relaxes vascular smooth muscle increasing coronary blood flow and improving collateral flow to ischemic areas. In addition, nitroglycerin decreases ventricular workload, myocardial oxygen demand, and decreases blood return to the heart. These actions result in relief or prevention of anginal attacks, reduction of blood pressure, and relieves congestive heart failure associated with myocardial infarction.

Indications

Prophylaxis and acute treatment of angina pectoris. Adjunct treatment for congestive heart failure and myocardial infarction.

Contraindications

Do not administer nitroglycerin to patients with: hypersensitivity to the drug, head trauma, hypotension, hypovolemia. Do not administer to patients in shock. Do not use in patients with severe bradycardia (<50 beats/min) or tachycardia (>100 beats/min). Nitroglycerin should not be administered to patients taking medications for erectile dysfunction because of the potential of fatal hypotension.

Precautions

Nitroglycerin often causes a rapid decrease in blood pressure. Therefore, patients should remain lying down while taking the drug. Transdermal patches and ointment should be removed prior to defibrillation or cardioversion. Use in pregnancy may compromise fetal blood flow.

Route and Dosage

Adult (Sublingual): 0.3–0.4 mg tablet. Repeat at 5-min intervals as needed to a total dose of 0.9–1.2 mg, (3 doses) if necessary.
Adult (IV Bolus): 12.5–25 mcg , followed by IV infusion.
Adult (IV Infusion): 10 mcg/min. Increase by10 mcg/min every 3–5 min. until desired effect. Maximum dose is 200 mcg/minute.
To prepare infusion: Add 50 mg nitroglycerin to 250 mL D_5W or normal saline in a glass bottle.
Adult (Lingual Spray): 1–2 sprays (0.4 mg/spray), sprayed directly under the tongue; additional one to two sprays every 3–5 minutes for a total of three sprays.
Adult (Ointment): 1–2 in (15–30 mg) every 8 hours, up to 5 in every 4 hours.
Adult (Transdermal Patch): 2.5–15 mg/24 hours.
Pediatric: Not recommended for out-of-hospital use.

How Supplied

SL tablets: 0.3 mg, 0.4 mg, 0.6 mg.
Lingual spray: 0.4 mg/spray in 14.5 gm canister (contains 200 doses).
Transdermal patches: 0.1 mg/hr, 0.2 mg/hr, 0.3 mg/hr, 0.4 mg/hr, 0.6 mg/hr, 0.8 mg/hr.
Injection: 0.5 mg/mL, 5 mg/mL.
Injection solution: 25 mg/250 mL, 50 mg/250 mL, 50 mg/500 mL, 100 mg/250 mL, 200 mg/500 mL.

Adverse Reactions and Side Effects

CNS: Headache, dizziness, weakness, restlessness.
CV: Hypotension, tachycardia, syncope.
EENT: blurred vision.
GI: Nausea, vomiting, dry mouth, abdominal pain.

EMS Considerations

Assess the patient's blood pressure before and after administering nitroglycerin. Nitroglycerin is unstable and may rapidly deteriorate if exposed to the air, light, or temperature extremes. Therefore, it should be stored in a dark, room-temperature area. Nitroglycerin tablets taste bitter and sting the tongue. If the bitter taste is not present, the tablet may have lost its strength. Check the expiration date. Nitroglycerin may cause significant hypotension. Patients with impaired arterial perfusion are more susceptible to this side effect. Severe hypotension may require IV fluid replacement and placement in Trendelenburg position. Standard IV infusion tubing may absorb up to 80% of the nitroglycerin; therefore, you should administer nitroglycerin from glass bottles and use the special tubing provided by the manufacturer.

Drug Interactions

Nitroglycerin may produce additive hypotensive effects in the presence of: alcohol, beta-adrenergic blockers, calcium channel blockers, phenothiazines.

NITROPRUSSIDE

(nye-troh-PRUS-eyed)
Pregnancy Class: C
Nitropress (Rx)
Classifications: Vasodilator, antihypertensive

Mechanism of Action

Nitroprusside has a direct vasodilating effect on both peripheral venous and arterial smooth muscles, which reduces both preload and afterload. Nitroprusside increases the capacity of the venous circulation and reduces blood pressure indications.

Indications

Nitroprusside is used in the treatment of hypertensive crisis. It can also be used to treat acute heart failure and pulmonary edema.

Contraindications

Do not administer nitroprusside to patients with: hypersensitivity to the drug, decreased cerebral perfusion. (According to some local protocols, however, there are no contraindications to nitroprusside in a life-threatening hypertensive crisis.)

Precautions

Use caution in administering nitroprusside to patients with renal or hepatic disease. Geriatric patients may experience an increase in sensitivity to the drug.

Route and Dosage

Adult: Begin IV infusion at 0.1 mcg/kg/min. If necessary, titrate upward q 3–5 minutes to desired effect (usually 5 mcg/kg/min). However, doses of up to 10 mcg/kg/min may be needed.

To prepare infusion: Add 50 mg of nitroprusside dissolved in 2–3 mL of D_5W to 250–500 mL of D_5W. The amount of D_5W depends on the desired concentration ordered. For example:

50 mg added to 250 mL of D_5W yields 200 mg/mL.
50 mg added to 500 mL of D_5W yields 100 mg/mL.

Once the infusion is prepared, immediately wrap the container in aluminum foil or other opaque material to avoid deterioration from exposure to light.

Pediatric: Not recommended for out-of-hospital use.

How Supplied

Injection: 25 mg/mL.

Adverse Reactions and Side Effects

CNS: Headache, dizziness, restlessness.
CV: Palpitations, hypotension.
Respiratory: dyspnea.
EENT: blurred vision, tinnitus.
GI: Nausea, vomiting, abdominal pain.

EMS Considerations

Closely monitor the patient, assessing blood pressure every 3 min. Once the patient is stabilized, assess blood pressure at 5-min intervals. The desired end-point blood pressure can be determined with either of two ways (consult local protocols):

1. Maintain blood pressure between 80–100 mm Hg.
2. Maintain blood pressure at 30–40 mm Hg below previously existing systolic pressure.
3. Monitor ECG continuously. If excessive hypotension occurs, decrease or discontinue infusion; effects last for up to 10 minutes after discontinuation.

Drug Interactions

Use with other antihypertensives may cause additive hypotensive effects.

NITROUS OXIDE-OXYGEN MIXTURE

(NYE-trus-ox-ide)
Pregnancy Class: C
Nitronox, Entonox (Rx)
Classifications: Medicinal gas, analgesic

Mechanism of Action

Inhalation of a 50% mixture of nitrous oxide and oxygen produces CNS depression as well as rapid pain relief. A nitrous oxide-oxygen mixture produces rapid but reversible relief from pain.

Indications

Nitrous oxide-oxygen mixture is used for the relief of moderate to severe pain from any cause.

Contraindications

Do not administer a nitrous oxide-oxygen mixture if any of the following exist:

1. The patient has a decreased level of consciousness.
2. The patient has taken any depressant drug.
3. The patient has sustained thoracic trauma.
4. The patient has respiratory compromise from any cause.
5. Cyanosis develops during administration.
6. The patient is unable to follow simple instructions.
7. The patient has sustained abdominal distension or trauma.
8. The patient is pregnant.

Precautions

Monitor the patient closely during administration. Some patients develop severe nausea and may vomit during administration. Also, patients sometimes pass out while receiving this medication.

Route and Dosage

Adult: 20–50% concentration mixed with oxygen. Self-administration by the patient until the pain is relieved.
Pediatric: Same as the adult.

Adverse Reactions and Side Effects

CNS: Lightheadedness, drowsiness, decreased respirations.
GI: Nausea, vomiting.

EMS Considerations

For patients with respiratory compromise, use 100% oxygen to prevent nitrous oxide from collecting in dead air spaces and further aggravating chest injuries. For patients with myocardial pain, administer oxygen when the nitrous oxide-oxygen mixture is not being given. If intestinal blockage is present, nitrous oxide may collect in the obstructed space, aggravating the blockage. Do not administer a nitrous oxide-oxygen mixture to patients with abdominal pain unless it is certain that intestinal blockage is not present.

Drug Interactions

Administration of a nitrous oxide-oxygen mixture in the presence of other drugs that cause CNS depression can produce additive effects.

NOREPINEPHRINE

(nor-ep-i-NEF-rin)
Pregnancy Class: D
Levophed (Rx)
Classifications: Peripheral vasoconstrictor, inotropic vasopressor

Mechanism of Action

Norepinephrine stimulates primarily alpha-adrenergic receptors to result in potent arterial and venous vasoconstriction. This action increases blood pressure. Norepinephrine stimulates beta$_1$-adrenergic receptors to increase cardiac contractility and cardiac output.

Indications

Norepinephrine is used to treat cardiogenic shock and hemodynamically significant hypotension (SBP <70 mm Hg) with low peripheral resistance.

Contraindications

Do not administer norepinephrine to patients with: hypotension caused by hypovolemia, myocardial ischemia or infarction. Do not administer norepinephrine during pregnancy because of decreased uterine blood flow, presence of thrombosis, hypoxia, hypersensitivity to norepinephrine or bisulfites.

Precautions

Use caution in administering norepinephrine to patients with hypertension or cardiac disease. Norepinephrine increases the heart's oxygen requirements without increasing coronary blood flow. Extravasation causes tissue necrosis.

Route and Dosage

Adult: Begin IV infusion at 0.5–1.0 mcg/min. Increase until there is a therapeutic effect while maintaining blood pressure at 90 mm Hg. The average infusion rate is 2–12 mcg/min. However, patients in refractory shock may need 8–30 mcg/min.
To prepare infusion: Add 4 mg of norepinephrine to 250 mL of D$_5$W or NS, which yields a drug concentration of 16 mcg/mL.
Pediatric: 0.05–2.0 mcg/kg/minute IV. Maximum dose = 2.0 mcg/kg/minute.

How Supplied

Injection: 1 mg/mL in 4-mL ampules.

Adverse Reactions and Side Effects

CNS: Headache, anxiety, dizziness, restlessness.
Cardiovascular: Bradycardia, hypertension, arrhythmias, chest pain, cyanosis of peripheral extremities.

GU: Decreased urine output, renal failure.
Endo: Hypoglycemia.
Respiratory: Dyspnea.
Local: Necrosis at the IV site.

EMS Considerations

Give norepinephrine in the largest vein possible, because infiltration can cause necrosis of the surrounding tissue. If infiltration should occur, the drug phentolamine (Regitine) in doses of 5–10 mg diluted in 10–15 mL of saline solution will minimize tissue necrosis. Monitor ECG and blood pressure constantly. Assess blood pressure every 2–3 min until it stabilizes, then every 5 min thereafter. Do not administer in the same IV line as alkaline solutions.

Drug Interactions

Beta-blockers used concurrently with norepinephrine can result in high elevations in blood pressure or block cardiac stimulation. Administering norepinephrine with atropine blocks reflex bradycardia and enhances norepinephrine's therapeutic effects.

OXYGEN

(OX-ah-gin)
Classification: Medicinal gas

Mechanism of Action

Oxygen is required to enable cells to break down glucose into a usable energy form. Oxygen is a colorless, odorless, tasteless gas, essential to respiration. At sea level, oxygen makes up approximately 10–16% of venous blood and 17–21% of arterial blood. Oxygen is carried from the lungs to the body's tissues by hemoglobin in the red blood cells. The administration of oxygen increases arterial oxygen tension (PaO_2) and hemoglobin saturation. This improves tissue oxygenation when circulation is adequately maintained.

Indications

Oxygen is used:

1. To treat severe chest pain that may be caused by any cardiopulmonary emergency.
2. To treat hypoxemia from any cause.
3. In the treatment of cardiac arrest.

Contraindications

None, for emergency use.

Precautions

Observe a patient closely if there is a history of being dependent on hypoxic respiratory drive (rare). These patients may require initial low flows of oxygen, increased as necessary.

Route and Dosage

Adult (Inhalation): There are several devices used to administer oxygen, including masks, nasal cannulas, positive pressure devices, and volume-regulated ventilators. Some of the more common oxygen devices and their delivery capacities include:

Nasal cannula: O_2 concentrations of 21–44% at flow rates of 1–6 L/min.

Simple face mask: O_2 concentrations of 40–60% at flow rates of 8–10 L/min.

Face mask with oxygen reservoir: O_2 concentration of 60% at a flow rate of 6 L/min. An O_2 concentration of almost 100% can be achieved with a flow rate of 10 L/min.

Venturi mask: 4–12 L/minute giving oxygen concentrations of 24–50%.

Mouth-to-mask: With supplemental O_2 at 10 L/min, O_2 concentration can reach 50%. Without supplemental O_2, concentration reaches only approximately 17%.

Pediatric: Same as the adult.

Adverse Reactions and Side Effects

Respiratory: In some cases of COPD, oxygen administration may reduce respiratory drive (very rare). This is not a reason to withhold oxygen, but be prepared to assist ventilations.

Miscellaneous: Oxygen that is not humidified may dry out or be irritating to mucous membranes.

EMS Considerations

Use humidified oxygen whenever possible. Nonhumidified oxygen may dry and irritate mucous membranes. Oxygen therapy may reduce respiratory drive in patients with COPD. If this should happen, it may be necessary to assist ventilations. If it is indicated, oxygen therapy should never be withheld. Reassure patients who are anxious about face masks but who require high concentrations of oxygen.

Drug Interactions

A 50:50 nitrous oxide-oxygen mixture is an analgesic medicinal gas for use in the out-of-hospital setting for pain relief.

PENTAZOCINE

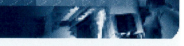

(pen-TAZ-oh-seen)
Pregnancy Class: C
Talwin (C-IV) (Rx)
Classifications: Narcotic agonist-antagonist, analgesic

Mechanism of Action

Pentazocine is a strong analgesic and weak antagonist. It binds to opiate receptors in the CNS, producing CNS depression. Pentazocine alters the awareness of and response to pain.

Indications

Pentazocine is used to treat moderate to severe pain.

Contraindications

Do not administer pentazocine to patients with: hypersensitivity to the drug, head injury, undiagnosed abdominal pain.

Precautions

Use caution in administering pentazocine to patients with pulmonary disease. Use caution in administering pentazocine to older patients, who may also require lower doses. Patients dependent on narcotic analgesics may experience withdrawal.

Route and Dosage

Adult (IV, IM, SQ): 30 mg initially. Repeat the dose every 3–4 hours as needed, not to exceed 360 mg. May be administered without dilution by IV bolus; however it is preferable to dilute each 5 mg with 1 mL of sterile water.
Pediatric: Not recommended for out-of-hospital use.

How Supplied

30 mg/mL.

Adverse Reactions and Side Effects

CNS: Headache, dizziness, sedation, hallucinations, euphoria.
CV: Hypotension or hypertension, palpitations.
Respiratory: Respiratory depression.
GI: Nausea, vomiting, dry mouth.

EMS Considerations

Assess patient vital signs before and frequently after administration.

Drug Interactions

Antihistamines, antidepressants, and sedative/hypnotic agents may cause additive CNS depression. Simultaneous use with other narcotic drugs may diminish the analgesic effect of pentazocine.

PHENYTOIN

(FEN-ih-toyn)
Pregnancy Class: D
Dilantin, Phenytek (Rx)
Classifications: Anticonvulsant, antiarrhythmic (Class 1B)

Mechanism of Action

Phenytoin depresses ventricular automaticity at ectopic pacemaker sites within the heart and atrioventricular conduction.

Indications

Phenytoin is used (unlabeled use) for the treatment of ventricular arrhythmias, especially those caused by digitalis glycoside toxicity.

Contraindications

Do not administer phenytoin to patients with: hypersensitivity to phenytoin or propyene glycol, intolerance of alcohol (present in the IV formulation), bradycardia, sinoatrial or atrioventricular block, Adams-Stokes syndrome.

Precautions

Use caution in administering phenytoin to patients with inadequate cardiac or respiratory function. Use with caution with elderly patients. During pregnancy may result in fetal hydantoin syndrome or hemorrhage in the newborn.

Route and Dosage

Adult: 50–100 mg by slow IV bolus every 10–15 minutes until:
The arrhythmia has been abolished.
Total dose has reached 15 mg/kg.
Toxicity has occurred.
Administer no faster than 50 mg/min.
Pediatric: Not recommended for pediatrics in the out-of-hospital setting.

How Supplied

Injection: 50 mg/mL in 2- and 5-mL ampules, 2- and 5-mL vials, and 2-mL prefilled syringe.

Adverse Reactions and Side Effects

CNS: Poor muscle coordination, drowsiness, dizziness, headache, nervousness, agitation.
CV: Hypotension, tachycardia.
Fluid and electrolytes: Hypocalcemia.
Gastrointestinal: Nausea, vomiting.

EMS Considerations

Slow administration of phenytoin helps prevent toxicity. Elderly patients usually develop toxicity more rapidly. Closely monitor patients for hypotension and for respiratory and cardiac problems.

Drug Interactions

The simultaneous use of phenytoin with dopamine may result in additive hypotension. Phenytoin may increase the metabolism of lidocaine, quinidine, theophylline, and corticosteroids. Barbiturates and alcohol may stimulate the metabolism of phenytoin.

PROCAINAMIDE

(proh-KAYN-ah-myd)
Pregnancy Class: C
Pronestyl (Rx)
Classification: Antiarrhythmic (Class 1A)

Mechanism of Action

Prolongation of the refractory period of the atria, bundle of His-Purkinje system and ventricles. Conduction velocity is slowed, cardiac excitability is decreased and ventricular ectopy and arrhythmias are suppressed.

Indications

Treatment of a wide variety of arrhythmias to include: recurrent VF/VT, PSVT uncontrolled by adenosine and vagal maneuvers if blood pressure stable, stable, wide-complex tachycardia of unknown origin, atrial fibrillation with rapid rate in Wolff-Parkinson-White syndrome.

Contraindications

Procainamide should not be used in patients presenting with preexisting QT prolongation and torsade de pointes (see Figure 10–2), hypersensitivity to procainamide; AV block.

Precautions

Use caution in administering procainamide to patients who may be experiencing: MI, digitalis toxicity, renal failure, CHF, hepatic failure. Geriatric patients.

Route and Dosage

Adult: 20 mg/min by IV infusion until:

1. The arrhythmia has been suppressed.
2. Hypotension develops.
3. The QRS segment widens by 50% of its original width.
4. A total dose of 17 mg/kg has been administered.

Adult (Refractory VF/VT): 20 mg/min IV infusion. In urgent situations, up to 50 mg/min may be given. Total maximum dose = 17mg/kg.
Maintenance infusion: 1–4 mg/min. Dose should be reduced in patients with renal insufficiency.
To prepare infusion: Add 2 mg procainamide to 500 mL D_5W to produce a final concentration of 4 mg/mL. A maintenance infusion may be given at a rate of 1–4 mg/min.
Pediatric: Not recommended for out-of-hospital use.

How Supplied

Injection: 100 mg/mL in 10-mL vials, 500 mg/mL in 2-mL vials.

Adverse Reactions and Side Effects

CNS: Confusion, seizures, dizziness.
CV: Hypotension, ventricular arrhythmias, heart block, asystole.
GI: Nausea, vomiting, diarrhea.

EMS Considerations

Monitor ECG and vital signs closely during administration. Giving procainamide too rapidly increases the probability of severe hypotension or life-threatening arrhythmias. Patient should remain supine during IV infusion because of potential for hypotension.

Drug Interactions

Hypotensive effect may be increased if procainamide is administered with other antihypertensives. Neurologic toxicity may be increased if procainamide is administered with lidocaine.

PROPRANOLOL

(proh-PRAN-oh-lohl)
Pregnancy Class: C
Inderal (Rx)
Classifications: Antianginal, antiarrhythmic (Class II), antihypertensive

Mechanism of Action

Propranolol blocks stimulation of beta$_1$- and beta$_2$-adrenergic receptors. This results in decreased heart rate, decreased cardiac contractility, decreased blood pressure, and decreased myocardial oxygen demand.

Indications

Treatment of hypertension. Second-line treatment for control of rapid supraventricular arrhythmias. Treatment or prevention of angina pectoris. Patients with suspected MI to treat anginal pain, reduce the incidence of VF, decrease elevated heart rate and blood pressure. May be used with thrombolytics to reduce nonfatal reinfarction and recurrent ischemia.

Contraindications

Do not administer propranolol to patients with: depressed cardiac function, congestive heart failure, asthma or chronic obstructive pulmonary disease, hypersensitivity to propranolol, bradycardia, cardiogenic shock, heart block, hypotension, during pregnancy (may result in apnea, low Apgar scores, bradycardia or hyperglycemia in newborns).

Precautions

Stopping propranolol treatment abruptly may cause angina, severe arrhythmias, or an MI. Use caution in administering propranolol to diabetic patients, because it can mask the signs and symptoms of hypoglycemia. Use with caution in patients with renal or hepatic impairment or in patients with pulmonary disease.

Route and Dosage

Adult: 1–3 mg IV. May repeat after 2 minutes.
Pediatric: 10–100 mcg (0.01-0.1 mg) /kg by slow IV.

How Supplied

Injection: 1 mg/mL.

Adverse Reactions and Side Effects

CNS: Weakness, depression, fatigue, anxiety.
CV: Bradycardia, congestive heart failure, hypotension.
Respiratory: Bronchospasm, wheezing.
Endocrine: Hypoglycemia or hyperglycemia.
GI: Nausea, vomiting, diarrhea.

EMS Considerations

Monitor the patient constantly during administration. Propranolol may cause a rapid onset of bradycardia or heart block.

Drug Interactions

Simultaneous use of propranolol with digitalis glycosides may produce an additive bradycardia effect. Use with other antihypertensive drugs may cause severe hypotension. Propranolol may oppose the action of bronchodilators.

RAMIPRIL

(ra-MI-pril)
Pregnancy Class: C (first trimester), D (second and third trimesters)
Altace (Rx)
Classification: angiotensin-converting enzyme (ACE) inhibitor

Mechanism of Action

Block the conversion of angiotensin I to the vasoconstrictor antiotensin II, lowering blood pressure in hypertensive patients.

Indications

Used in the management of hypertension, either alone or with other antihypertensive drugs. Ramipril is also used to treat CHF.

Contraindications

Do not use ramipril in patients who are hypersensitive to the drug, or in patients with a history of angioedema with the previous use of ACE inhibitors.

Precautions

Should be used with caution in patients with renal impairment, hepatic impairment, hypovolemia, hyponatremia, and in patients with concurrent diuretic therapy.

Route and Dosage

PO, Adults (hypertension): initial dose of 2.5 mg once daily.
PO, Adults (CHF): initial dose of 1.25–2.5 mg once daily.
PO, Adult (prevent MI, stroke): initial dose of 2.5 mg once daily.

How Supplied

Capsules, 1.25 mg, 2.5 mg, 10 mg.

Adverse Reactions and Side Effects

CNS: dizziness, fatigue, headache, vertigo, weakness.
CV: hypotension, chest pain, tachycardia, edema.
GI: abdominal pain, diarrhea, nausea, vomiting, taste disturbances.
EMS Considerations: monitor blood pressure and pulse frequently.

RETEPLASE

(REE-teh-place)
Pregnancy Class: C
Retavase (Rx)
Classification: Thrombolytic

Mechanism of Action

Reteplase converts plasminogen to plasmin which degrades fibrin and lyses thrombi in coronary arteries.

Indications

Acute management of MI for improvement of ventricular function, reduction of the incidence of CHF, and reduction of mortality. In addition, used for the treatment of pulmonary emboli.

Contraindications

Active internal bleeding, history of CVA, recent CNS trauma or surgery, neoplasm or arteriovenous malformation, severe uncontrolled hypertension, known bleeding disorders, hypersensitivity to reteplase.

Precautions

Use caution in administering reteplase to patients with cerebrovascular disease, hypertension, severe liver or kidney disease, age greater than 75 years, recent streptococcal infection or previous therapy with anistreplase or streptokinase.

Route and Dosage

Adults: 10 units IV. Repeat 10 units in 30 minutes.

To prepare infusion: Add 10 mL of sterile water to the vial containing the drug. Gently swirl the vial to dissolve the drug. Do not shake.

How Supplied

Powder for injection: 10.8 units (18.8 mg/vial).

Adverse Reactions and Side Effects

CNS: Intracranial hemorrhage, headache.
Respiratory: Bronchospasm, hemoptysis.
CV: Reperfusion arrhythmias, hypotension.
GI: GI bleeding, retroperitoneal bleeding.
GU: Hematuria.
Dermatologic: Ecchymoses, flushing, urticaria.
Local: Hemorrhage at injection site, phlebitits.
HEENT: Epistaxis, gingival bleeding.
Miscellaneous: Allergic reactions including anaphylaxis, fever.

EMS Considerations

Assess vital signs every 15 minutes. ECG should be continuously monitored. Arrhythmias may occur with reperfusion. Assess patient frequently for evidence of bleeding.

Drug Interactions

Aspirin, non-steroidal anti-inflammatory drugs, heparin, and heparin-like drugs increase the risk of bleeding.

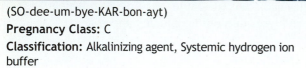

SODIUM BICARBONATE

(SO-dee-um-bye-KAR-bon-ayt)
Pregnancy Class: C
Classification: Alkalinizing agent, Systemic hydrogen ion buffer

Mechanism of Action

Sodium bicarbonate buffers acid buildup in the body caused by severe hypoxia. Severe hypoxia results in anaerobic metabolism, which produces lactic acid and metabolic acidosis. Sodium bicarbonate helps correct metabolic acidosis in conjunction with adequate ventilation, using 100% oxygen to blow off the increasing amounts of carbon dioxide. During cardiac arrest, adequate ventilation with 100% oxygen is the main concern in controlling acid-base balance. Adequate ventilation with oxygen in conjunction with properly performed cardiopulmonary resuscitation (CPR) maintains pH in the coronary and pulmonary circulations very close to, if not at, normal. Therefore, the use of sodium bicarbonate to treat cardiac arrest is not recommended unless there is documented preexisting metabolic acidosis.

Indications

Possibly for the management of metabolic acidosis during prolonged resuscitation (not recommended for the routine use in cardiac arrest). Sodium bicarbonate, however, should only be used after more appropriate treatment has been attempted, such as:

- Adequate ventilations.
- Effective chest compressions (CPR).
- Upon return of spontaneous circulation after a long arrest interval.

Contraindications

None, when used in the treatment of documented metabolic acidosis.

Precautions

In an increasing number of EMS settings, protocols do not include the use of sodium bicarbonate. Sodium bicarbonate administration can result in metabolic alkalosis or sodium overload.

Route and Dosage

Adult: 1mEq/kg by IV bolus to begin, followed by 0.5 mEq/kg every 10 min during the arrest, if ventilations are adequate.
Pediatric: 1 mEq/kg per dose if ventilations are adequate.

How Supplied

4.2% (0.5 mEq/mL) in 2.5-, 5-, and 10-mL prefilled syringes; 7.5% (0.9 mEq/mL) in 50-mL vials and prefilled syringe; 8.4% (1 mEq/mL) in 10- and 50-mL vials and prefilled syringe.

Adverse Reactions and Side Effects

Cardiovascular: Fluid retention, edema.
Fluid and electrolytes: Metabolic alkalosis, hypokalemia, hypocalcemia.
Local: Tissue necrosis at the IV site.

EMS Considerations

Do not let sodium bicarbonate come in contact with catecholamines or calcium agents. Monitor patients closely for the development of fluid overload (rales; peripheral edema; pink, frothy sputum).

Drug Interactions

Sodium bicarbonate may inactivate catecholamines and form a precipitate with calcium agents.

STREPTOKINASE

(strep-toe-KYE-nayz)
Pregnancy Class: C
Kabikinase, Streptase (Rx)
Classification: Thrombolytic

Mechanism of Action

Activates plasminogen, which then acts to dissolve fibrin deposits. Streptokinase dissolves thrombi or emboli, preserving left ventricular function after MI.

Indications

Streptokinase is used to treat coronary thrombosis associated with MI and to treat pulmonary emboli.

Contraindications

Do not administer streptokinase to patients with: hypersensitivity to the drug, active internal bleeding, a cerebrovascular accident (CVA) within 2 mo, uncontrolled severe hypertension.

Precautions

Use caution in administering streptokinase to patients: who have sustained trauma or surgery within the past 2 mo, with cerebrovascular disease, who have had recent streptokinase therapy or streptococcal infection.

Route and Dosage

Adult (MI): 1.5 million International Units (IU) by IV infusion over 60 min.
Adult (Pulmonary Emboli): 250,000 IU by IV infusion over 30 min, followed by 100,000 IU/h for 24 h.
To prepare infusion: Dilute drug to a volume of 90 mL with normal saline or D_5W. Swirl vial gently to dissolve.
Pediatric: Not recommended for out-of-hospital use.

How Supplied

Powder for injection: 250,000 IU, 750,000 IU, 1.5 million IU.

Adverse Reactions and Side Effects

CNS: Intracerebral bleeding.
CV: Arrhythmias due to reperfusion
Respiratory: Bronchospasm, hemoptysis.
HEENT: Epistaxis, gingival bleeding.
GI: GI bleeding, retroperitoneal bleeding.
GU: Hematuria.
Miscellaneous: Anaphylaxis.

EMS Considerations

Assess patient vital signs every 15 minutes. Monitor ECG continuously. Prophylactic IV lidocaine or procainamide may be ordered to control reperfusion arrhythmias.

Drug Interactions

Using streptokinase with anticoagulants or any drug affecting platelet function increases the risk of bleeding.

VASOPRESSIN

(vay-so-PRESS-in)
Pregnancy Class: C
Pitressin (Rx)
Classification: Vasoconstrictor

Mechanism of Action

A nonadrenergic peripheral vasoconstrictor. Administered during CPR, vasopressin increases coronary perfusion pressure, vital organ perfusion, and cerebral oxygen delivery.

Indications

- First-line treatment (alternative to epinephrine) of shock–refractory VF.
- May be useful as an alternative to epinephrine in asystole or PEA.
- Hemodynamic support in vasodilatory shock.

Contraindications

None in cardiac arrest.

Precautions

Vasopressin is not recommended for responsive patients with coronary artery disease because of the potential to induce cardiac ischemia and angina pectoris.

Route and Dosage

Adult (Cardiac arrest): One dose of 40 Units IV/IO in cardiac arrest. NOTE: epinephrine can be given q 3–5 minutes during cardiac arrest.
Pediatrics: Current guidelines do not recommend use.

How Supplied

20 Units/mL in 0.5- and 1-mL ampules and vials.

Adverse Reactions and Side Effects

CNS: Dizziness, "pounding" sensation in head.
CV: MI, chest pain, angina.
GI: Abdominal cramps, nausea, vomiting, diarrhea.
Dermatologic: Paleness, sweating.

EMS Considerations

Vasopressin should be administered as a one-time dose.

VERAPAMIL

(ver-AP-ah-mil)
Pregnancy Class: C
Calan, Isoptin (Rx)
Classifications: Antianginal, antiarrhythmic (class IV), antihypertensive

Mechanism of Action

Verapamil inhibits the transport of calcium into cardiac and vascular smooth muscle, which inhibits cardiac contraction and causes coronary vasodilation, decreased vascular resistance, and a reduction of myocardial oxygen consumption. Verapamil slows conduction in the sinoatrial and atrioventricular nodes and slows ventricular response. The coronary vasodilation effect of verapamil decreases the frequency and the severity of cardiac chest pain.

Indications

Verapamil is used to stop narrow-complex paroxysmal supraventricular tachycardia (PSVT) not requiring cardioversion and not responsive to adenosine. It may also be used for the temporary control of rapid ventricular response caused by atrial fibrillation, management of hypertension, prevention or relief of angina pectoris.

Contraindications

Do not administer verapamil to patients with: hypersensitivity to the drug, sinus bradycardia, severe CHF, high-degree heart block. Verapamil is also contraindicated for patients with Wolff-Parkinson-White syndrome (see Figure 10–1 on p. 128), atrial fibrillation, or atrial flutter, because verapamil may accelerate the heart's ventricular rate.

Precautions

Use caution in administering verapamil to patients with: mild CHF, sick sinus syndrome.

Route and Dosage

Adult: 2.5–5 mg IV given over 2 minutes (3 minutes in geriatric patients.) If necessary, repeat doses of 5–10 mg IV can be administered every 15–30 minutes given over a 2-minute period. The maximum total dose of verapamil should not exceed 20 mg.
Pediatric: Not recommended for the out-of-hospital setting.

How Supplied

Injection: 2.5 mg/mL.
Tablet: 40 mg, 80 mg, 120 mg, 180 mg, 240 mg.

Adverse Reactions and Side Effects

CNS: Dizziness, headache, confusion, nervousness.
CV: arrhythmias, CHF, palpitations, hypotension.
Respiratory: Pulmonary edema, cough, shortness of breath.
Gastrointestinal: Nausea, vomiting, diarrhea, dry mouth.

EMS Considerations

Giving verapamil can cause a decrease in blood pressure. If this should become a concern, calcium chloride can reverse the decreasing blood pressure when 0.5–1 g are given by slow IV. Assess the patient's vital signs frequently and monitor the ECG continuously.

Drug Interactions

There may be additive hypotension if verapamil is used with antihypertensives, nitrates, or quinidine. Verapamil should not be used simultaneously with intravenous beta-adrenergic blockers because of the increased risk of bradycardia, CHF, and arrhythmias.

CONCLUSION

This chapter contains some of the most essential and frequently used medications in the out-of-hospital setting. Additionally, the guidelines, dosages, and drugs used in cardiovascular emergencies are continually changing. While it is a difficult task, EMS providers must attain an in-depth knowledge of these medications and remain current on new drugs, dosages, and guidelines as they evolve.

STUDY QUESTIONS

1. The correct dosage of atropine to be given to the patient with symptomatic bradycardia is:
   a. 1–5 mg by IV initially. This can be repeated every 3–5 min to a total dose of 20 mg.
   b. 0.5 by IV initially. This may be repeated every 3–5 min to a total dose of 2.0 mg.
   c. 0.5– mg IV. This may be repeated every 3–5 min, to a total dose of 0.04 mg/kg (3 mg).
   d. 5 mg by IV. Repeat doses may be given at 10 mg by IV bolus.

2. Propranolol is a nonselective beta-adrenergic blocking agent. Its blocking action reduces the rate and force of heart contractions and blood pressure. Which is *not* an adverse reaction or side effect of propranolol?
   a. Coma
   b. Weakness
   c. Congestive heart failure
   d. Bronchospasm, wheezing

3. Which drug is indicated for the treatment of ventricular fibrillation, ventricular tachycardia, and supraventricular tachycardia?
   a. Lidocaine
   b. Adenosine
   c. Amiodarone
   d. Verapamil

4. Which of the following actions can be attributed to epinephrine when administered during cardiac arrest?
   a. Peripheral vasodilation
   b. Increase in cardiac automaticity
   c. Prolonged refractory period
   d. Decrease in ventricular fibrillation threshold

5. Which of the following is a contraindication to giving lidocaine?
   a. History of seizures
   b. Liver disease
   c. CHF
   d. Sinus bradycardia with PVCs

6. Digoxin:
   a. Is helpful in the treatment of incomplete heart block
   b. Is used in the treatment of bradyarrhythmias
   c. Controls rapid ventricular response caused by atrial fibrillation or atrial flutter
   d. Is used in the treatment of ventricular tachycardia in patients with a pulse who do not respond to more conventional therapy

7. Potential side effects of diltiazem include all of the following *except*:
   a. AV block
   b. Hypotension
   c. CHF
   d. Tachycardia

8. Morphine is contraindicated in patients with:
   a. Acute cardiogenic pulmonary edema
   b. Severe pain associated with myocardial ischemia
   c. Abnormally rapid respirations
   d. Hypotension

9. Dopamine has dose-dependent effects on adrenergic receptors. A dose of 15 mg/kg/min would result in:
   a. Improved blood flow to the kidney
   b. Decreased afterload
   c. Increased blood pressure
   d. Decreased cardiac contractility

10. Adenosine is useful in treating which of the following?
    a. Atrial fibrillation
    b. Second-degree AV block.
    c. PSVT associated with Wolff-Parkinson-White syndrome
    d. Ventricular tachycardia

11. Adverse reactions or side effects of norepinephrine generally include all of the following *except*:
    a. Hypertension
    b. Hypotension
    c. Arrhythmias
    d. Necrosis at the IV site

12. Nitroglycerin relieves anginal attacks by all of the following actions *except*:
    a. Decrease in ventricular work load
    b. Reduction in myocardial oxygen demand
    c. Increase in coronary blood flow
    d. Increase in heart rate

13. Verapamil is used for the treatment of:
    a. Supraventricular tachyarrhythmias
    b. Severe AV heart blocks
    c. Ventricular tachycardia
    d. Bradycardia

14. The correct dosage of vasopressin in ventricular fibrillation is:
    a. 40 units IV every 3–5 minutes
    b. 40 mg IV one time.
    c. 40 units IV one time
    d. 40 units IV, may repeat in 10 minutes if needed

15. Thrombolytic agents, such as reteplase, are absolutely contraindicated in:
    a. Severe hypertension
    b. CHF
    c. Age greater than 75 years
    d. Severe hypotension

▶ EXTENDED CASE STUDY

Ventricular Ectopy Progresses to Ventricular Fibrillation

The initial response: ECG interpretation and treatment remain the same. However, before the patient is transferred to the ambulance, he becomes unconscious and the monitor shows an ECG like that in Figure 10–7. The patient is now unresponsive, pulseless, and has no respirations. The ECG rhythm is interpreted as ventricular fibrillation.

Management: As soon as it has been determined that the patient has no pulse or respirations, CPR should begin while someone is preparing to defibrillate. When ready, defibrillate the patient at 120–200 joules (biphasic defibrillator) or 360 joules (monophasic defibrillator). After defibrillation, immediately resume CPR for five cycles. When five cycles of a CPR have been completed, defibrillate again using the same joules as previously used. After defibrillation, resume CPR.

At this point, medication therapy is initiated. You have two initial drug choices, 1 mg IV every 3–5 minutes, or you may give one dose of vasopressin, 40 units IV to replace the first or second dose of epinephrine. After the medication is given, perform five cycles of CPR.

- Epinephrine: is given due to its $beta_1$-adrenergic (cardiac) effects as well as for its $beta_2$-adrenergic (pulmonary) effects. These two effects produce an increase in blood pressure, an increase in heart rate, and causes bronchodilation when a pulse has been restored.
- Vasopressin: acts as a nonadrenergic peripheral vasoconstrictor. It is used during cardiac arrest to treat refractory shock.

Other antiarrhythmic drugs to be considered during CPR before or after defibrillation include:

- Amiodarone, 300 mg IV one time. Amiodarone inhibits adrenergic stimulation and prolongs the action potential and refractory period of the heart.
- Lidocaine, 1–1.5 mg/kg IV for the first dose, then 0.5–0.75 mg/kg. Lidocaine suppresses automaticity and spontaneous depolarization of the ventricles.

Note: During the course of an actual out-of-hospital emergency such as this, different circumstances and additional information may indicate treatment other than that outlined in this case study. Always follow local protocols and the direction of medical control.

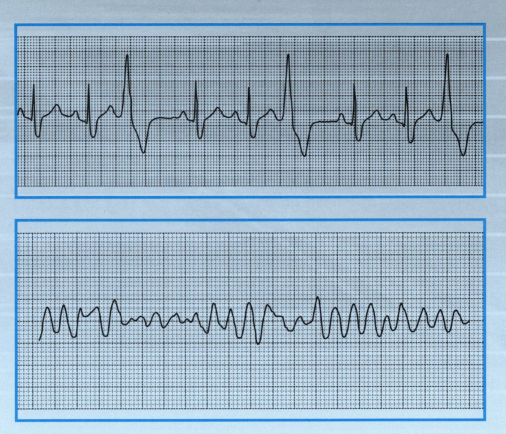

Figure 10–7 From a continuous strip: sinus rhythm with PVC (top) progressing to ventricular fibrillation (bottom). (© Delmar/Cengage Learning)

CHAPTER 11

METABOLIC EMERGENCIES

Therapeutic Classifications of Drugs Used for Metabolic Emergencies

Antidiabetic
Insulin

Antihypoglycemic
Glucagon

Beta adrenergic antagonist
Esmolol

Corticosteroid
Hydrocortisone

Hyperglycemic
Dextrose 50% in water

Vitamin
Thiamine

OBJECTIVES

On completion of this chapter and the study questions, you should be able to:

- Describe in detail the signs and symptoms of hypoglycemia.
- Describe in detail the signs and symptoms of hyperglycemia.
- Describe in detail the out-of-hospital management of hypoglycemia and hyperglycemia.
- Describe in detail the antidiabetic drug, insulin.
- Describe in detail the antihypoglycemic drug, glucagon.
- Describe in detail the beta adrenergic antagonist drug, esmolol.
- Describe in detail the corticosteroid drug, hydrocortisone.
- Describe in detail the hyperglycemic drug, dextrose 50% in water.
- Describe in detail the vitamin, thiamine.

KEY TERMS

Diabetes mellitus
Diabetic ketoacidosis
Glycogen
Glycosuria
Hyperglycemia
Hypoglycemia

Ketones
Korsakoff's syndrome
Kussmaul's respirations
Metabolism
Osmotic diuretic
Polydipsia

Polyphagia
Polyuria
Vitamin
Wernicke's encephalopathy

CASE STUDIES

1. EMS responds to an unconscious, unresponsive man who was found lying in his car. There is nothing to indicate that trauma has occurred. The patient has a patent airway, vital signs are within normal limits, and there are no apparent physical injuries. Several empty beer cans are found on the floor of the car. What is the first drug that medical control might order after you complete your assessment?
   a. $D_{50}W$
   b. Insulin
   c. Thiamine
   d. Glucagon

2. EMS responds to the home of an unconscious, unresponsive female patient. Initial assessment finds the patient presenting with Kussmaul-respirations at 40/min. The ECG monitor shows sinus tachycardia at a rate of 120 beats/min (Figure 11-1). Skin is warm and dry, and the patient has a fruity odor on her breath. Her blood pressure is low. This patient is presenting with classic signs and symptoms of:
   a. Insulin overdose
   b. Ketoacidosis
   c. Metabolic alkalosis
   d. Respiratory acidosis

3. After initial assessment, treatment for the patient in question 2 should include:
   a. IV for volume replacement and insulin
   b. IV and $D_{50}W$
   c. V, thiamine, and $D_{50}W$
   d. IV, $D_{50}W$, and insulin

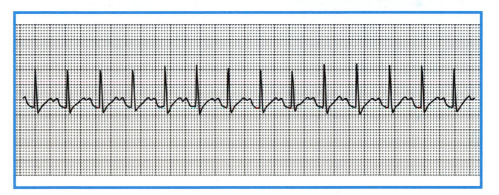

Figure 11–1 Sinus tachycardia. Rate: 120 beats/min. (© Delmar/Cengage Learning)

INTRODUCTION

Hypoglycemia and diabetic ketoacidosis are two emergencies associated with the metabolic disease, diabetes mellitus, that are commonly encountered by EMS providers in the out-of-hospital setting. This chapter presents drugs that are used to treat diabetes mellitus.

Diabetes mellitus is a disorder of carbohydrate metabolism that results from inadequate production or use of insulin. Insulin is a hormone secreted by beta cells in the islets of Langerhans, which are clusters of specialized cells in the pancreas. Insulin enables the body's cells to take in and metabolize glucose to be used by the body for energy.

Type I and Type II Diabetes

Diabetes mellitus is classified into two main types: type I and type II. Type I diabetes mellitus, also known as insulin dependent diabetes mellitus, typically presents at an early age with an acute onset. Individuals with type I diabetes mellitus are at risk for ketoacidosis because of their lack of insulin. These patients require the administration of insulin for the remainder of their lives. Type II diabetes mellitus, also known as non-insulin dependent diabetes mellitus, is caused by tissue resistance to insulin, impaired insulin secretion, and increased hepatic glucose production. Type II diabetes mellitus normally develops in individuals that are at least 40 years of age and has a more gradual onset than type I. Obesity is usually a factor associated with type II diabetes mellitus. Treatment of type II diabetes mellitus may involve just diet and exercise, or oral medications. Some patients do require insulin administration.

Diabetic ketoacidosis occurs when the blood glucose becomes too high (hyperglycemia). Hyperglycemia may occur because the insulin dose is too small, or not administered at all, or the amount of carbohydrates taken in is too large. Ketoacidosis may also occur because of physical or emotional stress, such as infection. Signs and symptoms of diabetic ketoacidosis include: polyuria, polydipsia, polyphagia, nausea and vomiting, tachycardia, Kussmaul's respirations, warm and dry skin, dry mucous membranes, a fruity odor to the breath, fever, abdominal pain, hypotension, and coma. Hyperglycemia results in osmotic diuresis, glycosuria, and polyuria. Dehydration occurs as a result of polyuria and vomiting. Polydipsia occurs as the patient becomes dehydrated. Because of the lack of insulin, the body cannot utilize glucose, and the patient develops polyphagia. Fat is metabolized for energy, which results in the production of acids and ketones. Ketone production may be detected by a fruity odor on the breath. Kussmaul's respirations occur in an attempt to eliminate excess acid through carbon dioxide excretion. As dehydration worsens, the patient may develop tachycardia, hypotension, and dry skin and mucous membranes. Eventually diabetic ketoacidosis may progress to coma. Diabetic ketoacidosis progresses slowly, usually over a period of 12–48 hours. The out-of-hospital treatment of diabetic ketoacidosis includes making a correct assessment of the disorder. The determination of hyperglycemia can be assisted with the use of a *glucose oxidase reagent strip*. In addition, a tube of blood should be collected prior to administration of any medications for later determination of blood glucose concentration. Fluid administration and supportive care are a priority of out-of-hospital treatment of diabetic ketoacidosis. Insulin is the definitive treatment for diabetic ketoacidosis.

Hypoglycemia occurs as a result of too much insulin, too little food, or a combination of both. The brain requires glucose for metabolism. If hypoglycemia develops, the lack of glucose reduces brain metabolism and causes neurologic and psychiatric symptoms. If hypoglycemia is not corrected, permanent brain damage may occur. Hypoglycemia may develop very rapidly. Signs and symptoms of hypoglycemia include: a weak and rapid pulse, cold and clammy skin, weakness and lack of coordination, headache, and irritable or bizarre behavior. Hypoglycemic patients may appear to be intoxicated. In severe cases, patients may develop seizures and coma. The out-of-hospital treatment of hypoglycemia includes a correct assessment of the disorder, which may be assisted with the use of a glucose oxidase reagent strip. A tube of blood should be collected for later determination of the blood glucose concentration. The rapid administration of $D_{50}W$ is necessary to restore adequate blood and brain glucose concentrations. Table 11–1 compares hyperglycemia and hypoglycemia.

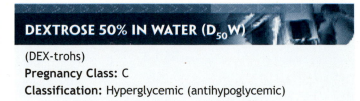

DEXTROSE 50% IN WATER ($D_{50}W$)

(DEX-trohs)
Pregnancy Class: C
Classification: Hyperglycemic (antihypoglycemic)

Table 11-1 Hypoglycemia and Hyperglycemia (Ketoacidosis). (© Delmar/Cengage Learning)

	Hypoglycemia	Hyperglycemia
Definition	Abnormally low level of sugar in the blood	An abnormally high level of sugar in the blood
	Develops rapidly, usually within 30–60 min	Develops slowly, usually over 12–48 h
Precipitating factors	1. Insulin overdose 2. Fasting 3. Increased alcohol intake without increased carbohydrate intake 4. Excessive physical activity without sufficient intake of food	1. Low or nonexistent insulin level 2. Infection (respiratory, urinary, or gastroenteritis)
Signs and Symptoms		
History	Recent insulin injection, inadequate food intake, excessive physical activity after insulin	Often acute infection in the diabetic, inadequate intake of insulin, perhaps no history of diabetes
Skin	Pale, sweating	Flushed, dry
Breath	Normal odor (acetone odor rare)	Acetone odor
Thirst	Absent	Intense
Respirations	Shallow	Deep, rapid (Kussmaul)
Pulse	Full, bounding	Rapid, weak
Blood pressure	Normal	Low
Abdominal pain	Absent	Often acute

Mechanism of Action

Dextrose 50% in water increases circulating blood sugar level to normal. It also acts briefly as an osmotic diuretic.

Indications

Dextrose 50% in water is used to treat patients in coma caused by hypoglycemia and patients in coma of an unknown cause. Patients with an altered level of consciousness whose reagent strip reading indicates less than 45 mg should also be given $D_{50}W$. Some EMS protocols also recommend giving $D_{50}W$ in certain cardiac arrest situations.

Contraindications

Do not administer $D_{50}W$ to patients with intracranial hemorrhage.

Precautions

Use caution in administering $D_{50}W$ to patients with diabetes mellitus or to patients who cannot tolerate carbohydrate agents.

Route and Dosage

Hyperkalemia
Adult: 25 g by slow IV bolus. Repeat if needed.
Pediatric: Dilute 1:1 with sterile water to make a 25% solution ($D_{25}W$) (0.25 mg/mL). 0.5–1.0 g/kg by slow IV bolus.
Hypoglycemia
Adult: 10 to 25 g of $D_{50}W$.

Pediatric (>2 yrs): 2 mL/kg of $D_{50}W$.
Pediatric (<2 yrs): 2 to 4 mL/kg of $D_{10}W$.

How Supplied

Injection: 50% solution, 25 gm/50 mL vial, prefilled syringe.

Adverse Reactions and Side Effects

CNS: May cause neurologic symptoms in the alcoholic patient.
CV: May aggravate hypertension and congestive heart failure in susceptible patients.
Skin: May cause tissue necrosis at the injection site.

EMS Considerations

Before establishing an IV line, take a blood sample for glucose analysis. Establish the IV line in the largest vein possible and run it wide open during slow administration of the $D_{50}W$. Thiamine should be administered before the $D_{50}W$ in the comatose patient. Thiamine is necessary for carbohydrate metabolism. Administering dextrose to an alcohol-dependent patient who is deficient in thiamine can cause Wernicke's encephalopathy or Korsakoff's syndrome (see Thiamine). Remember, it is vital to administer thiamine before dextrose to an alcohol-dependent patient or a patient in coma of unknown cause that may be alcohol related.

Drug Interactions

None, concerning out-of-hospital use.

ESMOLOL

(ES-moe-lole)
Pregnancy Class: C
Brevibloc (Rx)
Classification: Class II Antiarrhythmic, beta blocker

Mechanism of Action

Esmolol blocks the stimulation of $beta_1$ adrenergic (myocardial) receptors.

Indications

Esmolol can be used for the treatment of thyrotoxicosis (hyperthyroidism).

Contraindications

Esmolol should not be used in patients with uncompensated CHF, pulmonary edema, cardiogenic shock, bradycardia, or in patients with known alcohol intolerance.

Precautions

Geriatric patients may have increased sensitivity to esmolol. Even though esmolol can be used to treat hyperthyroidism, it can mask it's symptoms as well. Esmolol may also mask the symptoms of hypoglycemia.

Route and Dosage

Adult: 500 mcg/kg IV over 1 minute. This is followed by a 50 mcg/kg/min IV infusion over 4 minutes. Maximum total dose of 200 mcg/kg.
Pediatric: 500 mcg/kg IV over 1 minute. This is followed by a 25 to 200 mcg/kg/min IV infusion.

How Supplied

Solution for injection (pre-diluted for loading dose) 10 mg/mL in 10 mL vials, 20 mg/mL in 5 mL vials.
Solution for injection (must be diluted for continuous infusion): 250 mg/mL in 10 mL ampules.
Premixed infusion: 2000 mg/100 mL, 2500 mg/250 mL.

Adverse Reaction and Side Effects

CV: hypotension
CNS: dizziness, confusion, weakness, agitation
GI: nausea

EMS Considerations

None

Drug Interactions

Esmolol increases digoxin blood levels, and morphine increases the blood levels of esmolol.

GLUCAGON

(GLOO-kah-gon)
Pregnancy Class: B
Classification: Antihypoglycemic

Mechanism of Action

Glucagon is a hormone excreted by the alpha cells of the pancreas. When released, glucagon increases the level of circulating blood sugar by stimulating the release of **glycogen** from the liver. The glycogen is quickly broken down to become glucose. Glucagon causes an increase in the plasma glucose levels of the circulating blood, causes smooth muscle relaxation, and has positive inotropic and chronotropic effects on the heart.

Indications

Glucagon is given to treat hypoglycemia in the unconscious patient, in the combative patient, or in a patient in which an IV cannot be started.

Contraindications

Do not administer glucagon to a patient who is hypersensitive to the drug.

Precautions

Use caution in administering glucagon to patients with pheochromocytoma. A pheochromocytoma is a catecholamine-secreting tumor that may cause hypertension. Glucagon stimulates the release of catecholamines, which could further increase blood pressure.

Route and Dosage

Hypoglycemia
Adult: 1 mg IM, SC, or IV. If the patient does not respond in about 20 min, administer up to 2 more doses. Glucagon comes in vials that contain 1 mg of powder and 1 mL of diluting solution. Glucagon must by reconstituted before use.
Pediatric: (<20 kg): 0.5 mg IM, IV, or SQ.
Beta-blocker Overdose
Adult: 2 to 5 mg IV over 1 minute.
Pediatric: (<20 kg): 0.5 mg IM, IV, or SQ.

How Supplied

Powder for injection: 1 mg vial.

Adverse Reactions and Side Effects

CNS: Dizziness.
CV: Possible hypertension, tachycardia.
GI: Nausea, vomiting.

EMS Considerations

In emergency situations, $D_{50}W$ is the drug of choice. Use glucagon only if you cannot start an IV and administer glucose. Before administering glucagon, draw a blood sample for glucose determination.

Drug Interactions

A precipitate will form if glucagon is mixed with chloride solutions.

HYDROCORTISONE

(hye-droe-KOR-ti-sone)
Pregnancy Class: C
Cortef, Solu-Cortef (Rx)
Classification: Corticosteroid (short-acting)

Mechanism of Action

Hydrocortisone suppresses inflammation and the normal immune response. It also replaces steroids that are deficient in adrenal insufficiency.

Indications

Hydrocortisone is used in the management of adrenocortical insufficiency.

Contraindications

Hydrocortisone should not be used in patients with active untreated infections, or in patients with known alcohol or bisulfite hypersensitivity.

Precautions

Chronic treatment may lead to adrenal suppression. Therefore, the lowest dose for the shortest period of time must be used. Hydrocortisone should be used with caution in patients with hypothyroidism or cirrhosis.

Route and Dosage

Adult: 100 to 500 mg IV.
Pediatric: 1 to 2 mg/kg IV.

How Supplied

Power for Injection (sodium succinate): 100 mg, 250 mg, 500 mg, and 1 g.

Adverse Reactions and Side Effects

Adverse reactions and side effects are more common when hydrocortisone is used at high doses and for long-term therapy.
CV: hypertension
CNS: headache, restlessness, depression, personality changes
EENT: increased intraocular pressure
GI: anorexia, nausea, vomiting, peptic ulcer formation

EMS Considerations

None

Drug Interactions

Hydrocortisone may cause an increased risk of hypokalemia with the use of diuretics. Hypokalemia may increase the risk of digoxin toxicity. Hydrocortisone may increase the risk of GI effects with the concurrent use with NSAIDs, including aspirin.

INSULIN, REGULAR

(IN-sue-lin)
Pregnancy Class: B
Humulin R, Novolin R (Rx)
Classification: Antidiabetic, Hormone

Mechanism of Action

Insulin lowers blood glucose levels and promotes the conversion of glucose to glycogen. Glycogen is the form in which carbohydrates are stored until they are converted into sugar.

Indications

Insulin is used to treat patients with diabetic ketoacidosis (severe hyperglycemia).

Contraindications

Certain individuals are hypersensitive to beef or pork. Do not administer insulin products derived from these sources to these patients. Another animal-derived insulin to which the patient is not hypersensitive or a biosynthetic insulin should be used in these cases.

Precautions

Use caution in administering insulin, because the effects of a dosage can vary greatly depending on such factors as diet, exercise, stress, and work patterns.

Route and Dosage

The initial dose depends on the patient's blood glucose level, response, as well as many other factors. EMS personnel should refer to local protocols.
Kitoacidosis—regular insulin only (100 units/mL)
Adult (IV): 0.1 U/kg/h by continuous IV infusion.
Pediatric (IV): loading dose of 0.1 unit/kg, followed by a continuous infusion of 0.05 to 0.2 unit/kg/hr.
Maintenance Therapy
Adult and Pediatric (SQ): 0.5 to 1 unit/kg/day.
Hyperkalemia
Adult and Pediatric (SQ, IV): dextrose 0.5 to 1 g/kg combined with insulin (1 unit for every 4 to 5 g dextrose administered.

How Supplied

100 unit/mL vial, cartridge, 500 unit/mL vial.

Adverse Reactions and Side Effects

Local reactions: Itching, swelling, redness.
Endocrine: Hypoglycemia.
Miscellaneous: Allergic reactions, usually to traces of beef or pork protein in the preparation.

EMS Considerations

Only regular insulin can be administered IV. When administering insulin by IV bolus, administer each 50 U over 1 min. Assess patient constantly for signs of hypoglycemia. Keep glucose available.

Drug Interactions

Some of the signs and symptoms of hypoglycemia (such as tachycardia) may be masked by beta-adrenergic blocking drugs. Corticosteroids and thiazide diuretics can cause increases in the insulin required.

Table 11–2 compares some of the common insulin preparations.

THIAMINE (VITAMIN B₁)

(THIGH-ah-min)
Pregnancy Class: A
Betalin S, Biamine (Rx)
Classification: B-complex vitamin

Table 11–2 Comparison of Common Insulin Preparations.
(© Delmar/Cengage Learning)

Insulin	Onset	Peak	Duration
Rapid Acting			
Regular			
Regular Iletin	1/2–1 h	2–4 h	6–8 h
Humulin R*	1/2–1 h	2–4 h	6–8 h
Novolin R	1/2 h	2 1/2–5 h	8 h
Prompt Zinc Suspension			
Semilente	1 1/2 h	5–10 h	16 h
Semilente Ilentin I	1–3 h	3–8 h	10–16 h
Lispro	1/2 h	1/2–1 1/2 h	3–4 h
Intermediate Acting			
Isophane Suspension			
NPH Ilentin	1–4 h	6–12 h	18–26 h
Humulin N*	1–2 h	6–12 h	18–24 h
Insulatard NPH	1 1/2 h	4–12 h	24 h
Novolin N	1 1/2 h	4–12 h	24 h
Zinc Suspension			
Lente Ilentin	2–4 h	6–12 h	18–26 h
Humulin L*	1–3 h	6–12 h	18–21 h
Novolin L	2 1/2 h	7–15 h	22 h
Long Acting			
Protamine Zinc Suspension			
Protamine Zinc Iletin	4–8 h	14–24 h	28–36 h
Extended Zinc Suspension			
Ultralente	4 h	10–30 h	36 h
Glargine	4 h	peakless	24 h

*Humulin insulins have a slightly more rapid onset and a shorter duration of action than animal-derived insulins.

Mechanism of Action

Thiamine is required for the metabolism of carbohydrates and fats. It is necessary for the freeing of energy and the oxidation of pyruvic acid. Without enough thiamine, the cells of the body cannot use most of the energy usually available in glucose. The organ most sensitive to thiamine deficiency is the brain. Administering thiamine when deficiency exists restores the body's supply of the vitamin.

Indications

Thiamine is used to treat patients in a coma of unknown origin, patients in coma caused by alcohol, and patients suffering from delerium tremens.

Contraindications

None.

Precautions

Thiamine deficiency can cause Wernicke's encephalopathy and Korsakoff's syndrome in the alcohol-dependent patient.

Wernicke's encephalopathy: Wernicke's encephalopathy is an acute and reversible disorder associated with chronic alcoholism. It is characterized by poor voluntary muscle coordination, eye muscle weakness, and mental derangement.

Korsakoff's syndrome: Korsakoff's syndrome is a frequent result of chronic alcoholism. It is characterized by disorientation, illusions, hallucinations, and painful extremities; in addition, the patient may have bilateral foot drop.

Route and Dosage

Adult: Before administering $D_{50}W$:

1. Dilute 100 mg of thiamine in 50–100 mL of NS or D_5W and infuse over 15–20 min.
2. Administer 100 mg by slow IV bolus.

NOTE: Too-rapid administration of thiamine may cause hypotension.

Pediatric: Not recommended for out-of-hospital use.

How Supplied

100 mg/mL in 1-mL ampules and prefilled syringes, and 1, 2, 10, and 30-mL vials.

Adverse Reactions and Side Effects

CV: Rapid administration of thiamine may cause vasodilation and hypotension.

Respiratory: Excessive administration of thiamine may cause dyspnea or respiratory failure.

EMS Considerations

Thiamine is necessary for carbohydrate metabolism. The administration of dextrose to an alcohol-dependent patient who is deficient in thiamine may cause Wernicke's encephalopathy or Korsakoff's syndrome. Therefore, it is important to administer thiamine before administering dextrose to an alcohol-dependent patient.

Drug Interactions

N/A.

CONCLUSION

Patients suffering from metabolic disorders can exhibit many different signs and symptoms. Treatment for the diabetic patient depends on accurately assessing the patient. Correct, timely treatment is vital. For example, the brain relies on glucose for its metabolism. If a patient becomes severely hypoglycemic, the brain cannot function properly. If the hypoglycemia is left untreated for an extended period, permanent brain damage could result.

A patient found in a coma needs a rapid, accurate assessment. Drug treatment for these patients is diagnostic in nature as well as potentially life saving. Treatment can include thiamine, glucose, and naloxone.

STUDY QUESTIONS

1. Dextrose 50% in water is indicated for:
   a. Reagent strip reading <45 mg with an altered LOC
   b. Coma of unknown cause
   c. Medical cardiac arrest
   d. All of the above

2. The pediatric dosage for $D_{50}W$ in cases of hyperkalemia is:
   a. 25 g by slow IV bolus
   b. 0.05–0.1 g/kg by slow IV bolus
   c. 0.5–1.0 g/kg by slow IV bolus
   d. 5–10 g/kg by slow IV bolus

3. Before giving glucose to your patient, you should first:
   a. Take a blood sample
   b. Monitor cardiac rhythm
   c. Start an IV of D_5W
   d. Dilute 1:1 with sterile distilled water

4. Insulin is indicated for the treatment of:
   a. Hypoglycemia
   b. Hyperglycemia
   c. Coma of unknown cause
   d. Metabolic acidosis

5. Glucagon causes an increase in the plasma glucose levels of the circulating blood. The adult dose of glucagons in the prehospital setting is:
   a. 0.25–0.5 mg
   b. 0.5–1 mg
   c. 1–1.5 mg
   d. 1.5–2.5 mg

6. The organ most sensitive to the effects of thiamine deficiency is the:
   a. Heart
   b. Liver
   c. Brain
   d. Kidney

7. Thiamine is used as a diagnostic tool in the patient in a coma of unknown cause. The adult dosage of thiamine is:
   a. 50 mg
   b. 75 mg
   c. 100 mg
   d. 1 mg/kg

8. The pancreas is responsible for the production of insulin. Without insulin:
   a. Hypoglycemia will result
   b. A buildup of carbon dioxide produces acidosis
   c. Starches cannot be metabolized into glucose
   d. Glucose cannot pass into the body's cells

Diabetic Emergency—Diabetic Ketoacidosis

Initial Response: EMS responds to the residence of an unconscious woman. On arrival, EMS finds a female patient, about 30, lying on the bedroom floor. A rapid assessment reveals that the patient's breathing is deep and rapid; she has a weak, rapid pulse and responds only to painful stimuli. While placing the patient on oxygen and connecting the ECG monitor, you notice a Medic-Alert bracelet that indicates she has diabetes. There is no evidence of alcohol or drug use.

Additional assessment reveals the following:

Level of consciousness: Unconscious, responds only to pain.
Respirations: Kussmaul, at a rate of 40/min.
Pulse: 120 beats/min and weak. ECG shows sinus tachycardia (Figure 11–2).
Blood pressure: 112/82.
Skin: Warm and dry—dehydrated.

    Management: Differentiating between diabetic ketoacidosis and hypoglycemia can be difficult in the out-of-hospital setting. Therefore, management of the unconscious diabetic patient is generally directed toward treating hypoglycemia, which is the more severe condition. Out-of-hospital management of this patient should proceed as follows:

- Maintain a patent airway; be prepared to intubate and to assist ventilation if necessary.
- Attempt to draw a blood sample for glucose analysis at the hospital.
- Measure glucose level using a glucose reagent strip. However, this may not be accurate. A reading of <45 mg indicates a need for further treatment.
- Begin an IV of D_5W at a keep-open rate.

- Administer 25 g of $D_{50}W$ by slow IV bolus. $D_{50}W$ is a hyperglycemic drug that increases circulating blood sugar levels in the hypoglycemic patient.
- If an IV line cannot be established, administer 0.5–1 mg of glucagons IM. Glucagon elevates blood sugar levels by stimulating the release of glycogen from the liver. Glucagon does not produce results as quickly as $D_{50}W$. $D_{50}W$ shows immediate results, while glucagon may take as long as 20 min.
- Monitor vital signs and cardiac rhythm closely.
- Transport to the nearest appropriate hospital.

Depending on the circumstances at the scene, management can usually take place while the patient is being transported. In this case, the patient's condition does not change during transport. The patient is trying to compensate for metabolic acidosis by creating respiratory alkalosis through the Kussmaul respirations. Diabetic ketoacidosis starves red blood cells of glucose as well as producing a low pH. After arrival at the hospital, treatment will include decreasing serum glucose levels with insulin.

    How would this patient be managed if she were in a coma of unknown cause with no available previous history? After the airway has been appropriately managed, blood drawn, and an IV started, the following treatment should take place:

- If the patient is suspected of being alcohol dependent, administer 100 mg of thiamine by slow IV bolus.
- Administer 25 g of $D_{50}W$ by slow IV bolus.
- If the above treatment is not successful, consider giving naloxone. Naloxone is a narcotic antagonist sometimes used in comas of unknown cause if narcotic drugs are suspected or to rule out narcotic drugs. Chapter 15 has a detailed discussion of naloxone.
- Transport to the nearest appropriate hospital. Depending on the circumstances at the scene, management can usually take place while the patient is being transported.

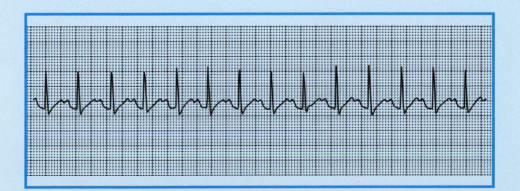

Figure 11–2 Sinus tachycardia. Rate: 120 beats/min. (© Delmar/Cengage Learning)

CHAPTER 12

NEUROLOGIC EMERGENCIES

Therapeutic Classifications of Drugs Used for Neurologic Emergencies

Antianxiety Agents
Diazepam
Lorazepam
Anticonvulsants
Diazepam
Fosphenytoin
Lorazepam
Phenobarbital
Phenytoin
Antihypertensives
Labetolol
Nitroglycerin

Nitroprusside
Antihypoglycemic
Dextrose 50% in Water ($D_{50}W$)
Anti-inflammatory Agents
Dexamethasone
Methylprednisolone
Nonopioid Analgesic
Acetylsalicyclic Acid (aspirin)
Osmotic Diuretic
Mannitol
Sedative-hypnotic Agents
Diazepam

Lorazepam
Phenobarbital
Skeletal Muscle Relaxant
Diazepam
Thrombolytic
Alteplase
Vasodilators
Nitroglycerin
Nitroprusside
Vasopressor
Norepinephrine

OBJECTIVES

On completion of this chapter and the study questions, you should be able to:

- Describe in detail the signs and symptoms of a cerebrovascular accident (CVA).
- Describe in detail the out-of-hospital neurologic assessment of a patient with a suspected CVA.
- Describe in detail the hypertensive management of: patients with ischemic CVA that are thrombolytic candidates, patients with ischemic CVA that are not thrombolytic candidates, and patients with hemorrhagic CVA.
- Describe in detail the following anticonvulsant drugs: diazepam, fosphenytoin, lorazepam, phenobarbital, phenytoin.
- Describe in detail the following antihypertensive drugs: labetolol, nitroglycerin, and nitroprusside.

- Describe in detail the antihypoglycemic drug, $D_{50}W$.
- Describe in detail the following anti-inflammatory drugs: dexamethasone, and methylprednisolone.
- Describe in detail the following nonopioid analgesic drug, acetylsalicyclic acid (aspirin).
- Describe in detail the osmotic diuretic, mannitol.
- Describe in detail the thrombolytic, alteplase.
- Describe in detail the vasopressor, norepinephrine.

KEY TERMS

Antianxiety agent
Anticonvulsant
Anti-inflammatory agent
Cerebrovascular accident (CVA)

Generalized motor seizure
Glucocorticoid
Neurogenic shock
Sedative-hypnotic agent

Skeletal muscle relaxant
Status epilepticus
Stevens-Johnson syndrome

CASE STUDIES

1. EMS responds to the home of a woman "unable to walk and speak." On arrival, a 70-year-old woman is found sitting in a chair at the kitchen table. She is conscious and her eyes follow movements in the room, which indicate she is aware of her surroundings. However, she cannot stand to walk, and she cannot speak. The initial assessment reveals the following:

   Level of consciousness: Conscious, apparently aware of surroundings, but unable to communicate.
   Respirations: 16 breaths/min.
   Pulse: 90 beats/min, irregular. ECG shows atrial fibrillation (Figure 12-1).
   Blood pressure: 152/112.
   Skin: Normal.
   HEENT: Pupils equal and reactive, slight drooling.
   Paralysis: Affecting only the left side of the patient's body.

   The patient's husband states that his wife is currently being treated for high blood pressure, and she has a history of heart disease. His wife appeared normal about 1 hour ago. Immediate treatment for this patient should include:
   a. IV line, verapamil, rapid transport
   b. IV line, rapid transport
   c. Humidified oxygen, rapid transport
   d. Humidified oxygen, precautionary IV line, rapid transport

2. EMS responds to an alley where a man, approximately 50, is found having passed out. There are several empty beer cans and wine bottles in the area. There is no indication that trauma is a factor. Your assessment reveals the following:

   Level of consciousness: Unconscious, responds to pain.
   Respirations: 20 breaths/min, no respiratory difficulty, breath smells of alcohol.
   Pulse: 50 beats/min, irregular. ECG monitor shows a second-degree heart block, Type II (Figure 12-2).

Blood pressure: 196/94.
Skin: Cool, clammy.

There is no medical identification on the patient.

Medical control orders an IV of normal saline started at a keep-open rate. As soon as the IV is established, the patient begins to experience active seizures. The drug of choice to control this seizure activity is:

a. Phenytoin
b. Diazepam
c. Methylprednisolone
d. Dexamethasone

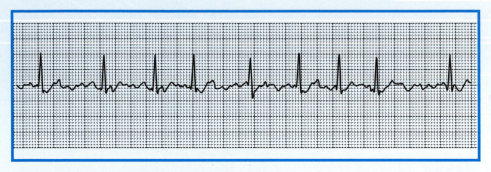

Figure 12–1 Atrial fibrillation. (© Delmar/Cengage Learning)

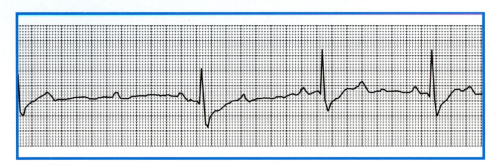

Figure 12–2 Second-degree heart block, Type II. (© Delmar/Cengage Learning)

INTRODUCTION

Neurologic emergencies are often very difficult to manage. Frequently, patients experiencing a neurologic emergency show signs and symptoms that are very subtle, ranging from a headache to coma. The status of a patient experiencing a neurologic emergency may change rapidly, from responding appropriately to unconsciousness. These factors can greatly complicate out-of-hospital treatment.

Neurologic Emergencies

Neurologic emergencies consist of traumatic and nontraumatic disorders. The majority of drug therapy for neurologic emergencies will be utilized in the management of nontraumatic disorders. The most commonly encountered nontraumatic neurologic emergencies include seizures and **CVAs**.

Anticonvulsants are administered for **generalized motor seizures** and the more emergent condition, **status epilepticus**. Anticonvulsants depress abnormal neuron discharges in the central nervous system that may result in seizure activity. Seizures may be a primary disorder or secondary to a number of underlying disorders, such as CVA, hypoglycemia, trauma, and alcohol or drug abuse. Treatment, beyond anticonvulsant therapy, may be required if the seizure is secondary to another disorder. EMS providers should always consider an underlying cause if the patient is not known to have a seizure disorder. Table 12–1 compares the signs and symptoms of CVA, hypoglycemia, and alcohol or drug abuse.

A CVA generally occurs from a clot or hemorrhage in the brain, causing weakness, paralysis, speech impairment, confusion, seizures, and coma. Some signs and symptoms of a CVA are similar to those that occur with hypoglycemia and drug or alcohol abuse, which can make appropriate assessment of the patient's disorder difficult. Treatment of an ischemic CVA has evolved within the last few years, from primarily supportive to very proactive. This evolution in treatment has occurred because of evidence that thrombolytic therapy administered soon after the onset of symptoms significantly affects patient outcome. EMS providers play an important role in the timely treatment of ischemic CVA.

EMS providers are responsible for the correct assessment of signs and symptoms of ischemic CVA, establishing the time of onset, obtaining a comprehensive medical history, providing rapid transport to the hospital, and early communication of the patient's condition to the hospital. Thrombolytic therapy must be administered within 3 hours of onset of the CVA to be effective so this neurologic disorder is now considered a "load and go" situation. Antihypertensive therapy is frequently required in the treatment of CVAs. The following guidelines issued by the American Heart Association for the treatment of hypertension in stroke apply to when an

Table 12-1 Signs and Symptoms of Cerebrovascular Accident (CVA), Hypoglycemia, and Alcohol/Drug Abuse*. (© Delmar/Cengage Learning)

CVA	Hypoglycemia	Alcohol/Drug Intoxication
Headache	Headache	Headache
Confusion	Abnormal behavior—may appear intoxicated	Confusion
Paralysis (usually one side of the body)	Confusion	Profuse perspiration
Facial flacidity, drooling	Convulsions	Abnormal behavior
Impaired speech	Arrhythmias	Elevated or normal blood pressure
Impaired vision	Profuse perspiration	Arrhythmias
Elevated or normal blood pressure	Drooling	Convulsions
Arrhythmias	Normal blood pressure	Coma
Convulsions	Coma	
Coma		

*Some of the signs and symptoms of hypoglycemia often mimic those of CVA or alcohol or drug intoxication.

antihypertensive is administered and which antihypertensive to administer:

1. *Ischemic CVA Nonthrombolytic Candidates*

   For DBP > 140 mm Hg: start nitroprusside at 0.5 mcg/kg/min. Goal is a 10–20% reduction in DBP.

   For SBP > 220 or DBP 121–140 mm Hg: administer 10–20 mg labetolol IV push over 1–2 minutes. May repeat or double dose every 20 minutes up to a maximum dose of 150 mg.

   For SBP < 220 or DBP ≤ 120: antihypertensive therapy is withheld unless aortic dissection, AMI, severe CHF, or hypertensive encephalopathy are present.

2. *Ischemic CVA Thrombolytic Candidates*

   Prethrombolytic treatment:

   For SBP > 185 or DBP > 110 mm Hg: apply 1–2 inches of nitropaste or 1–2 doses of 10–20 mg labetolol IV push. If the BP is not reduced to and maintained at <185/110 mm Hg, the patient should not receive the thrombolytic.

   During and after thrombolytic treatment: monitor BP every 15 minutes for 2 hours, then every 30 minutes for 6 hours, and then every hour for 16 hours.

   For DBP > 140 mm Hg: start nitroprusside at 0.5 mcg/kg/min, IV infusion.

   For SBP > 230 or DBP 121–140 mm Hg: administer 10 mg labetolol IV push over 1–2 minutes. May repeat or double dose every 10 minutes to a maximum dose of 150 mg, or give 10 mg labetolol IV push and then start a labetolol infusion at 2–8 mg/min. If the BP is not controlled by labetolol, start nitroprusside.

   SBP 180–230 or DBP 105–120 mm Hg: administer 10 mg labetolol IV push over 1–2 minutes. May repeat or double dose every 10–20 minutes to a maximum dose of 150 mg, or give labetolol 10 mg IV push and start a labetolol infusion at 2–8 mg/min.

3. *Hemorrhagic Stroke*

   For SBP > 230 or DBP > 120 mm Hg: start nitroprusside at 0.5–10 mcg/kg/min IV or nitroglycerin at 10–20 mcg/min IV.

   For SBP 181–230 or DBP 106–120 mm Hg: administer labetolol 10 mg IV push over 1–2 minutes. May repeat or double dose every 10–20 minutes to a maximum dose of 300 mg, or administer 10 mg labetolol IV push and then start a labetolol infusion at 2–8 mg/min.

   For hypertension relative to prestroke BP: if prehemorrhage BP was considerably lower, then BP should be lowered to prehemorrhage level.

Treatment for traumatic neurologic emergencies is mainly supportive, with rapid transport to the hospital. The primary concerns for patients with traumatic neurologic injury are spinal stabilization, airway maintenance, and treatment of other injuries as needed. However, there are drugs appropriate for out-of-hospital treatment of neurologic trauma, especially when transport times are long. Mannitol and dexamethasone are used to reduce cerebral edema and, therefore, lower intracranial pressure and reduce secondary injury to the brain. Methylprednisolone is administered to patients with spinal injury to improve neurologic outcome, but only when administered within 8 hours of injury. Patients with spinal cord injury may develop **neurogenic shock** caused by autonomic dysfunction. The vasopressor, norepinephrine, may be administered to stabilize the patient's blood pressure.

Individual Drugs

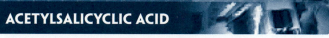

ACETYLSALICYCLIC ACID

(ah-SEE-till-sal-ih-SILL-ick AH-sid)
Pregnancy Class: C
Ascriptin, Aspercin, Aspergum, Aspirtab, Bayer Aspirin, Bufferin, Easprin, Ecotrin, Genacote, Halfprin, Healthprin, St. Joseph Adult Chewable Aspirin, ZORprin
Classification: Antiplatelet, antipyretic, nonopioid analgesic, nonsteroidal anti-inflammatory agent

Mechanism of Action

Antiplatelet activity is produced by decreasing the synthesis of substances that mediate platelet aggregation and cause arteries to constrict.

Indication

Used for prophylaxis to prevent transient ischemic attacks and cerebrovascular accidents.

Contraindications

Hypersensitivity to salicylates. Bleeding disorders or thrombocytopenia. Avoid during pregnancy, especially during the third trimester, because of the potential for adverse effects on the fetus and the mother.

Precautions

Use cautiously in patients with a history of gastrointestinal bleeding or ulcer disease. Use of aspirin in patients with a history as asthma may provoke an acute attack. Avoid use in children or teenagers because of the potential for Reye's syndrome.

Route and Dosage

160 to 325 mg PO as soon as possible when signs/symptoms develop. Thereafter, 80 to 325 mg PO every day.

How Supplied

Chewing gum: 227 mg.
Enteric-coated (delayed release) tablets: 80 mg, 165 mg, 325 mg.
Suppositories: 60 mg, 120 mg, 125 mg, 130 mg, 195 mg, 200 mg, 300 mg, 325 mg.

EMS Considerations

Aspirin should be administered as soon as possible if TIA or CVA are suspected.

Drug Interactions

The risk of bleeding may be increased with warfarin, heparin, heparin-like agents, and thrombolytic agents.

ALTEPLASE (TISSUE PLASMINOGEN ACTIVATOR, TPA)

(AL-teh-playz)
Pregnancy Class: C
Ativase (Rx)
Classification: Thrombolytic

Mechanism of Action

Binds to fibrin in a thrombus, causing the conversion of plasminogen to plasmin, which then degrades fibrin within the clot. Lysis of the clot decreases neurologic deficits associated with a CVA.

Indications

Treatment of acute ischemic stroke, within 3 hours of onset of symptoms, after hemorrhagic stroke has been excluded by CT scan or other diagnostic imaging.

Alteplase is only indicated for patients 18 years of age or older that exhibit a measurable neurologic deficit.

Contraindications

Evidence of intracranial hemorrhage on noncontrast head CT or high clinical suspicion of subarachnoid hemorrhage despite normal CT. Stroke symptoms are minor or rapidly improving. Active internal bleeding or history of GI or GU bleeding within the last 21 days. A known bleeding disorder which may include a platelet count less than 100,000/mm^3, heparin administration within 48 hours, and an elevated aPTT, or recent use of another anticoagulant and elevated INR. Within 3 months of intracranial surgery, serious head trauma, or previous CVA. Within 14 days of major surgery or serious trauma. Recent arterial puncture at a noncompressible site. A lumbar puncture within 7 days. A history of intracranial hemorrhage, arteriovenous malformation, or aneurysm. A witnessed seizure at stroke onset. A recent MI. If on repeated measurements, the SBP remains greater than 185 mm Hg or DBP remains greater than 110 mm Hg at the time treatment with alteplase should start, or if aggressive antihypertensive treatment was required to reduce the BP to these limits.

Precautions

Use cautiously in patients greater than 75 years of age. Severe liver or kidney disease.

Route and Dosage

Adults: 0.9 mg/kg IV (maximum dose 90 mg), with 10% of the dose given as a bolus. The remainder of the dose given as an infusion over 60 minutes.

To prepare alteplase: Reconstitute with sterile water for injection without preservatives immediately prior to use. Once reconstituted, the preparation contains 1 mg/mL. The reconstituted solution may be further diluted in an equal volume of normal saline to yield a concentration of 0.5 mg/mL. Dilution should be performed by gently swirling the solution. Do not shake.

How Supplied

Powder for injection: 2 mg/vial, 50 mg/vial, 100 mg/vial.

Adverse Reactions and Side Effects

CNS: Intracranial bleeding, headache.
Respiratory: Bronchospasm, hemoptysis.
CV: Reperfusion arrhythmias, hypotension.
GI: GI bleeding, retroperitoneal bleeding.
Miscellaneous: Allergic reactions including anaphylaxis, fever.
GU: Hematuria.
Dermatologic: Ecchymoses, flushing, urticaria.
Hematologic: Bleeding.
Local: Hemorrhage at injection site, phlebitis at IV site.

EMS Considerations

Assess vital signs every 15 minutes. ECG should be continuously monitored. Assess patient frequently for signs of bleeding; if the patient deteriorates, stop the infusion immediately.

Drug Interactions

Patients should not receive aspirin, heparin, warfarin, heparin-like drugs, or other antithrombotic or antiplatelet drugs during the first 24 hours of treatment.

DEXAMETHASONE

(dex-ah-METH-ah-zohn)
Pregnancy Class: C
Decadron, Solurex (Rx)
Classification: Anti-inflammatory, Corticosteroid (long-acting)

Mechanism of Action

A long-acting **glucocorticoid** that suppresses inflammation and decreases cerebral edema.

Indications

Treatment of cerebral edema.

Contraindications

None for a single out-of-hospital dose.

Precautions

Use caution in administering dexamethasone to patients with: hypertension, diabetes mellitus, seizures, CHF, glaucoma.

Route and Dosage

Adult (cerebral edema): Initial dose of 10 mg by slow IV bolus over 1 minute. Then 4 mg IV every 6 hours. As edema improves, dose may be decreased to 2 mg IV every 8–12 hours.

Pediatric: Not recommended for out-of-hospital use.

How Supplied

Solution for injection (dexamethasone sodium phosphate): 4 mg/mL, 10 mg/mL.

Adverse Reactions and Side Effects

CNS: Headache, depression, restlessness, euphoria, psychoses.

CV: Hypertension.

GI: Peptic ulceration, nausea, vomiting.

Miscellaneous: Allergic reactions, increased susceptibility to infection.

Dermatologic: Decreased wound healing, ecchymoses, petechiae.

Hematologic: Thromboembolism, thrombophlebitis.

Endocrine: Adrenal suppression, hyperglycemia.

Fluids and electrolytes: Fluid retention, hypokalemia.

EMS Considerations

Only dexamethasone sodium phosphate may be administered IV. Do not administer dexamethasone acetate IV.

Drug Interactions

Additive hypokalemia may occur with thiazide and loop diuretics.

Hypokalemia may increase the risk of digoxin toxicity.

DEXTROSE 50% IN WATER (D$_{50}$W)

(DEX-trohs)

Pregnancy Class: C

Classifications: Hyperglycemic (antihypoglycemic)

Mechanism of Action

Dextrose 50% in water increases circulating blood sugar level to normal. It also acts briefly as an osmotic diuretic.

Indications

Dextrose 50% in water is used to treat hypoglycemia, altered level of consciousness, coma of unknown etiology, seizure of unknown origin, and status epilepticus.

Contraindications

Dextrose 50% in water should not be given to patients with known intracranial hemorrhage.

Precautions

Use caution in administering D$_{50}$W to patients with diabetes mellitus or to patients who cannot tolerate carbohydrate agents.

Route and Dosage

Adult: 12.5–25 g by slow IV bolus. May repeat dosage if necessary.

Pediatric: 0.5–1.0 g/kg by slow IV bolus.

How Supplied

Injection: 50% solution, 25 g/50 mL vial, prefilled syringe.

Adverse Reactions and Side Effects

CV: May aggravate hypertension and CHF in susceptible patients.

CNS: May cause neurologic symptoms in the alcoholic patient.

Skin: May cause tissue necrosis at the injection site.

EMS Considerations

Before establishing an IV line, take a blood sample for glucose analysis. Establish the IV line in the largest vein possible and run it wide open during the slow administration of the D$_{50}$W. Thiamine should be administered before the D$_{50}$W in the comatose patient. Thiamine is necessary for carbohydrate metabolism.

Drug Interactions

None, concerning out-of-hospital use.

DIAZEPAM

(dye-AYZ-eh-pam)

Pregnancy Class: D

Valium (C-IV) (Rx)

Classifications: Antianxiety agent, anticonvulsant, sedative-hypnotic, skeletal muscle relaxant

Mechanism of Action

Causes CNS depression, producing relief of anxiety and sedation.

Diazepam produces skeletal muscle relaxation by inhibition of spinal pathways. Decreases seizure activity caused by enhanced presynaptic inhibition.

Indications

Treatment of generalized motor seizures and status epilepticus. It can also be used as a skeletal muscle relaxant in treating orthopedic injuries.

Contraindications

Do not administer diazepam to patients with: hypersensitivity to diazepam, benzodiazepines, or propylene glycol, preexisting CNS depression, acute narrow-angle glaucoma, or pregnancy and lactation.

Precautions

Use caution in administering diazepam to patients with a history of psychosis or drug addiction. Administer lower than usual adult doses to elderly patients because they are more sensitive to the drug's CNS effects. Use with caution in patients with hepatic dysfunction, as effects may be more intense and prolonged.

Route and Dosage

Adults (seizures/status epilepticus): 5–10 mg slow IV bolus. May repeat every 10–15 minutes as needed to a total of 30 mg. May be administered IM if unable to obtain IV access.

Adults (skeletal muscle relaxant): 5–10 mg slow IV bolus or IM. Elderly or debilitated (skeletal muscle relaxant): 2–5 mg slow IV bolus or IM.

Pediatric (seizures/status epilepticus): >5 years: 1 mg slow IV bolus or IM every 2–5 minutes to a total dose of 10 mg. <5 years: 0.2–0.5 mg slow IV bolus or IM every 2–5 minutes to a maximum dose of 5 mg.

Pediatric (skeletal muscle relaxant): 0.2–0.5 mg/kg slow IV bolus or IM. Maximum doses: >5 years: 10 mg. <5 years: 5 mg.

How Supplied

Injection: 5 mg/mL.

Adverse Reactions and Side Effects

CNS: Dizziness, drowsiness, mental depression, headache.
Respiratory: Respiratory depression.
CV: Hypotension.
Local: Pain with IM injection; phlebitis with IV administration.
HEENT: Blurred vision, intraocular pressure in patients with narrow-angle glaucoma.

EMS Considerations

Diazepam may cause respiratory arrest if administered too rapidly or in excess doses. Do not mix diazepam with any other drug. Diazepam may react with the IV tubing; to minimize this, administer diazepam at the IV site, not higher in the tubing. Thoroughly flush the IV line before administering diazepam if other drugs have already been administered through the line. Assess the patient's vital signs continuously.

Drug Interactions

Additive CNS depression may occur if diazepam is administered with other CNS depressants, such as antihistamines, tricyclic antidepressants, alcohol, narcotics, or other sedatives or hypnotics.

FOSPHENYTOIN

(FOS-fen-ih-toyn)
Pregnancy Class: D
Cerebyx (Rx)
Classification: Anticonvulsant

Mechanism of Action

Fosphenytoin is converted to phenytoin after administration. It then acts to decrease seizure activity by altering ion transport and decreasing synaptic transmission.

Indications

Treatment of generalized motor seizures and status epilepticus.

Contraindications

Hypersensitivity to fosphenytoin or phenytoin. Pregnancy because of the potential for fetal deformities. Sinus bradycardia, SA node block, second- or third-degree AV block, or Adams-Stokes syndrome.

Precautions

Dosage should be reduced in severe hepatic disease. Safety in pediatric patients has not been established.

Route and Dosage

Adults (seizures/status epilepticus): Loading dose of 15–20 mg PE/kg IV given at a rate of 100–150 mg PE/min. or IM. Dilute fosphenytoin dose in D_5W or NS to produce a concentration of 1.5–25 mg PE/mL.

NOTE: Doses of fosphenytoin are expressed as phenytoin sodium equivalents (PE = phenytoin sodium equivalents). Adjustments in the recommended doses should not be made when substituting fosphenytoin for phenytoin sodium or vice versa.

How Supplied

Injection: 50 mgPE/mL.

Adverse Reactions and Side Effects

CNS: Dizziness, drowsiness, nystagmus, vertigo, stupor.
CV: Hypotension, tachycardia, vasodilation.
GI: Nausea, vomiting.
Dermatologic: Pruritis, rash.

EMS Considerations

Do not use IM fosphenytoin to treat status epilepticus because therapeutic phenytoin concentrations may not be reached as quickly as with IV administration. During IV administration, monitor ECG, BP, and respirations.

Drug Interactions

Phenytoin levels and risk of toxicity are increased by acute ingestion of alcohol, amiodarone, cimetidine, and diazepam. Chronic alcohol use and carbamazepine may decrease phenytoin levels and, therefore, phenytoin effectiveness. Phenobarbital and valproate may increase or decrease phenytoin levels. Phenytoin may decrease the effectiveness of oral contraceptives, warfarin, and theophylline.

LABETOLOL

(lah-BET-ah-lohl)
Pregnancy Class: C
Trandate (Rx)
Classification: Antihypertensive

Mechanism of Action

Decreases BP by blocking alpha-adrenergic receptors.

Indications

To treat hypertension in CVA patients.

Contraindications

Cardiogenic shock, cardiac failure, bronchial asthma, bradycardia, second- or third-degree AV block.

Precautions

Use with caution during lactation, in chronic bronchitis and emphysema. Labetolol may mask the signs and symptoms of hypoglycemia, so use caution in patients with diabetes mellitus.

Route and Dosage

Adults (ischemic CVA nonthrombolytic candidates): If SBP > 220 or DBP 121–140 mm Hg, administer 10–20 mg IV push over 1–2 minutes. May repeat or double dose every 20 minutes to a maximum dose of 150 mg.
Adults (ischemic CVA thrombolytic candidates): If SBP > 230 or DBP 121–140 mm Hg during or after thrombolytic treatment, administer 10 mg IV push over 1–2 minutes.

May repeat or double dose every 10 minutes to a maximum dose of 150 mg, or give 10 mg IV push, then start a labetolol infusion at 2–8 mg/min. If SBP 180–230 or DBP 105–120 mm Hg during or after thrombolytic treatment, administer 10 mg IV push over 1–2 minutes every 10–20 minutes to a maximum dose of 150 mg, or give 10 mg IV push and then start a labetolol infusion at 2–8 mg/min.
Adults (hemorrhagic CVA): If SBP 181–230 or DBP 106–120 mm Hg, administer 10 mg IV push over 1–2 minutes. May repeat or double dose every 10–20 minutes to a maximum dose of 300 mg, or give 10 mg IV push, then start a labetolol infusion at 2–8 mg/min. Labetolol may be administered undiluted or diluted with D_5W or NS.

How Supplied

Injection: 5 mg/mL.

Adverse Reactions and Side Effects

CNS: Fatigue, drowsiness, headache.
Respiratory: Dyspnea, bronchospasm.
CV: Arrythmias, hypotension, bradycardia, CHF.
GI: Nausea, vomiting.

EMS Considerations

Monitor vital signs and ECG continuously.

Drug Interactions

Labetolol is not compatible with sodium bicarbonate. Do not infuse through the same IV line. Additive hypotension may occur when concurrently administered with other antihypertensives.

LORAZEPAM

(lor-AYZ-eh-pam)
Pregnancy Class: D
Ativan (C-IV) (Rx)
Classifications: Antianxiety, anticonvulsant, sedative-hypnotic

Mechanism of Action

Causes CNS depression, producing relief of anxiety and sedation. Decreases seizure activity caused by enhanced presynaptic inhibition.

Indications

Treatment of generalized motor seizures and status epilepticus.

Contraindications

Hypersensitivity to lorazepam or other benzodiazepines. Preexisting CNS depression. Acute narrow-angle glaucoma. Do not administer in pregnancy or lactation.

Precautions

Use caution in administering lorazepam to patients with a history of psychosis or drug addiction. Administer lower than usual adult doses to elderly patients because they are more sensitive to the drug's CNS effects. The dosage of IV lorazepam has not been established in children less than 18 years of age. Use cautiously in the presence of hepatic dysfunction.

Route and Dosage

Adults (seizures/status epilepticus): 0.05 mg/kg IV bolus (maximum dose of 4 mg). Do not administer faster than 2 mg/min. The initial dose may be repeated after 10–15 minutes. Do not exceed 8 mg/12 hours.
To administer: Dilute with an equal amount of sterile water for injection, NS, or D_5W.

How Supplied

Injection: 2 mg/mL, 4 mg/mL.

Adverse Reactions and Side Effects

CNS: Dizziness, drowsiness, mental depression, headache.
Respiratory: Respiratory depression.
CV: Hypotension.
Local: Phlebitis.
HEENT: Blurred vision, increased intraocular pressure in patients with narrow-angle glaucoma.

EMS Considerations

May cause respiratory arrest if administered too rapidly or in excess doses. Do not mix with any other drug. Thoroughly flush the IV line before administering lorazepam if other drugs have already been administered. Assess the patient's vital signs continuously.

Drug Interactions

Additive CNS depression may occur if lorazepam is administered with other CNS depressants, such as antihistamines, tricyclic antidepressants, alcohol, narcotics, or other sedatives or hypnotics.

MANNITOL

(MAN-nih-tol)
Pregnancy Class: C
Osmitrol, Resectisol (Rx)
Classification: Osmotic diuretic

Mechanism of Action

Increases osmotic pressure in the glomerular filtrate. This inhibits the reabsorption of water and electrolytes, which causes their excretion in the urine. The diuretic action of mannitol causes a decrease in cerebral edema and intracranial pressure.

Indications

Used to relieve excessive intracranial pressure.

Contraindications

Do not administer mannitol to patients with: hypersensitivity to mannitol, preexisting dehydration, active intracranial bleeding, or pulmonary edema.

Precautions

Use caution in administering mannitol to patients with a tendency to CHF, because mannitol may cause a sudden expansion of extracellular fluid, which could bring on CHF.

Route and Dosage

Adult: 0.25–2 g/kg of a 15–25% solution by IV infusion, using an in-line IV filter. Infuse over 30–60 minutes.
Pediatric: 1–2 g/kg of a 15–20% solution over 30–60 minutes.

How Supplied

5%, 10%, 15%, 20%, and 25% solution.

Adverse Reactions and Side Effects

CNS: Headache, confusion.
Respiratory: Pulmonary edema.
CV: Tachycardia, chest pain, CHF, edema, hypotension, or hypertension.
GI: Nausea, vomiting.
HEENT: Blurred vision.
Fluids and electrolytes: Dehydration.

EMS Considerations

Monitor patients closely for any signs of dehydration, including: hypotension, thirst, decreased skin turgor, dry skin and mucous membranes, or decreased urine output. Slow infusion if signs of pulmonary edema occur, including: dyspnea, cyanosis, rales, or frothy sputum. Mannitol has a tendency to crystallize at temperatures below 45 degrees Fahrenheit. Use an in-line filter when administering mannitol to filter any crystals out of the solution.

Drug Interactions

Additive CNS depression can result if mannitol is administered with other CNS depressants. Additive adrenergic effects and anticholinergic effects may occur when administered with CNS depressants.

METHYLPREDNISOLONE

(meth-ill-pred-NISS-oh-lohn)
Pregnancy Class: C
A-methapred, Solu-medrol (Rx)
Classification: Anti-inflammatory

Mechanism of Action

Methylprednisolone is a glucocorticoid that suppresses inflammation of tissue. It is believed to protect nerve fibers and inhibit swelling, ischemia, nerve cell death, and electrolyte imbalance to the spinal cord caused by traumatic injury. Methylprednisolone may improve muscle and sensory function following traumatic injury to the spinal cord.

Indications

Treatment of patients who have sustained traumatic spinal cord injury and demonstrate a loss of motor function or sensation.

Contraindications

None, during emergency use.

Precautions

Use caution in administering methylprednisolone to patients with: hypertension, diabetes mellitus, and CHF.

Route and Dosage

Adults: 30 mg/kg by IV bolus over 15 minutes. Follow with NS at kvo for 1 hour. Then follow with an IV infusion of methylprednisolone of 5.4 mg/kg/h over 23 hours.
To prepare infusion: Mix 25 g methylprednisolone in 500 mL NS for a final concentration of 50 mg/mL.
Pediatric: Same as the adult dose.

How Supplied

Methylprednisolone acetate injection: 20 mg/mL, 40 mg/mL, 80 mg/mL.
Methylprednisolone sodium succinate powder for injection: 40 mg, 125 mg, 500 mg, 1 g, 2 g.

Adverse Reactions and Side Effects

CNS: Depression, euphoria, headache, psychoses, restlessness.
CV: Hypertension.
GI: Peptic ulceration, nausea, vomiting.
Miscellaneous: Increased susceptibility to infection.
Dermatologic: Decreased wound healing, ecchymoses, petechiae.
Hematologic: Thromboembolism, thrombophlebitis.
Endocrine: Adrenal suppression, hyperglycemia.
Fluids and electrolytes: Hypokalemia, fluid retention.
HEENT: Increased intraocular pressure.

EMS Considerations

For methylprednisolone to be effective, treatment should begin within 8 hours of the injury.

Drug Interactions

Additive hypokalemia may occur if administered with diuretics. Hypokalemia increases the risk of digoxin toxicity.

NITROGLYCERIN

(nye-troh-GLIH-sir-in)
Pregnancy Class: C
Nitro-Bid IV, Nitroglycerin in 5% Dextrose, Tridil, Nitro-Bid, Nitrol (Rx)
Classifications: Antihypertensive, Vasodilator

Mechanism of Action

Produces vasodilation and reduces blood pressure.

Indications

Hypertension in acute stroke patients.

Contraindications

Hypersensitivity to nitroglycerin. Pericardial tamponade or constrictive pericarditis. Concurrent use of sildenafil (Viagra Rx).

Precautions

Use cautiously in head trauma, glaucoma, cardiomyopathy, severe hepatic impairment, hypovolemia. Use in pregnancy may compromise maternal or fetal circulation.

Route and Dosage

Adults (ischemic CVA thrombolytic candidates): As a pretreatment to thrombolytics if SBP > 185 or DBP > 110 mm Hg, apply 1–2 inches of nitroglycerin ointment.
(Hemorrhagic CVA): For SBP > 230 or DBP > 120 mm Hg, administer nitroglycerin by continuous infusion at 10–20 mcg/min. Titrate to desired BP.
To prepare infusion: Dilute 50 mg nitroprusside to a volume of 250 mL with D_5W or NS. Nitroglycerin should be prepared in a glass bottle and administered with the set provided by the manufacturer.

How Supplied

Transdermal ointment: 2%.
Injection: 0.5 mg/mL, 5 mg/mL.
Injection solution: 25 mg/250 mL, 50 mg/250 mL, 50 mg/500 mL, 100 mg/250 mL, 200 mg/500 mL.

Adverse Reactions and Side Effects

CNS: Dizziness, headache, restlessness, weakness, syncope.
CV: Hypotension, tachycardia, flushing.
GI: Nausea, vomiting.
Dermatologic: Contact dermatitis with ointment.
HEENT: Blurred vision.

EMS Considerations

Monitor vital signs and ECG continuously during infusion. If hypotension occurs, decrease or discontinue infusion or administer additional IV fluids and place patient in

Trendelenburg position. Nitroglycerin IV requires gradually tapering dose to avoid adverse effects.

Drug Interactions

Concurrent use of nitrates with sildenafil (Viagra Rx) is contraindicated because of the risk of potentially fatal hypotension. Additive hypotension may occur with other antihypertensive agents, acute alcohol ingestion, or phenothiazines.

NITROPRUSSIDE

(nye-troh-PRUS-eyed)
Pregnancy Class: C
Nitropress (Rx)
Classifications: Antihypertensive, vasodilator

Mechanism of Action

Directly acts on vascular smooth muscle, causing peripheral vasodilation of arteries and veins. This action lowers the blood pressure.

Indications

Hypertension in acute stroke.

Contraindications

Hypersensitivity to nitroprusside.

Precautions

Use cautiously in the elderly and patients with renal or hepatic disease.
   Safety not established in pregnancy or lactation.

Route and Dosage

Adults (ischemic CVA nonthrombotic candidates): If DBP > 140 mm Hg, infuse nitroprusside at 0.3 mcg/kg/min. Titrate for a 10–20% reduction in BP.
Adults (ischemic CVA thrombolytic candidates): If DBP > 140 mm Hg during or after thrombolytic treatment, or if SBP > 230 or DBP 121–140 mm Hg and patient fails to respond to labetolol, infuse nitroprusside at 0.5 μg/kg/min.
Adults (Hemorrhagic CVA): If SBP > 230 or DBP > 120 mm Hg, infuse nitroprusside at 0.5–10 mcg/kg/min.
To prepare infusion: Dissolve 50 mg in 2–3 mL of D_5W, then further dilute in 250–1000 mL D_5W. The solution bag and tubing must be wrapped with aluminum foil or brown plastic bag during infusion.

How Supplied

Injection: 25 mg/mL.
Powder for injection: 50 mg.

Adverse Reactions and Side Effects

CNS: Dizziness, headache, restlessness.
Respiratory: Dyspnea.
CV: Hypotension, palpitations.
GI: Nausea, vomiting.
Local: Phlebitis at IV site.
HEENT: Blurred vision, tinnitus.

EMS Considerations

Monitor vital signs and ECG continuously during infusion. Monitor BP and titrate infusion to desired BP. If hypotension occurs, decrease or discontinue infusion.

Drug Interactions

Increased hypotensive effects occur with concurrent use of other antihypertensives.

NOREPINEPHRINE

(nor-ep-i-NEF-rin)
Pregnancy Class: C
Levophed (Rx)
Classification: Vasopressor

Mechanism of Action

Stimulates alpha-adrenergic receptors causing constriction of blood vessels and reverses vasodilation and hypotension associated with neurogenic shock.

Indications

Neurogenic shock.

Contraindications

Hypersensitivity to norepinephrine or bisulfites. Hypotension caused by hypovolemia. May reduce uterine blood flow in pregnancy.

Precautions

Use cautiously in patients with cardiovascular disease, and history of hypertension.

Route and Dosage

Adults: 0.5–1 mcg/min IV and titrate from 2–12 mcg/min to desired BP.
To prepare infusion: Add 4 mg to 500 mL D_5W or NS.
Pediatrics: 0.1 mcg/kg/min IV; titrate up to 1 mcg/kg/min to achieve desired BP.
To prepare infusion for pediatrics:

$$\frac{6 \times weight\ (kg) \times desired\ dose\ (\mu g/kg/min)}{IV\ infusion\ rate\ (mL/h)} = \begin{array}{l} mg\ of\ drug\ to\ be\ added \\ to\ 100\ mL\ of\ IV\ fluid \end{array}$$

NOTE: Norepinephrine dosage is stated in terms of norepinephrine base and IV formulation is norepinephrine bitartrate. Norepinephrine bitartrate 2 mg = norepinephrine base 1 mg.

How Supplied

Injection as bitartrate: 1 mg/mL, 4 mg/mL vials.

Adverse Reactions and Side Effects

CNS: Dizziness, headache, restlessness, tremor.
Respiratory: Dyspnea.
CV: Arrhythmias, bradycardia, chest pain, hypertension.
GU: Decreased urine output, renal failure.
Local: Phlebitis at IV site.
Endocrine: Hyperglycemia.
Fluids and electrolytes: Metabolic acidosis.

EMS Considerations

Monitor vital signs and ECG continuously during infusion. Monitor IV site for extravasation. Administer through a large vein. If extravasation occurs, inject phentolamine into affected area.

Drug Interactions

Norepinephrine is incompatible with sodium bicarbonate; do not administer through the same IV line. Concurrent use with digoxin may result in increased myocardial irritability. Use with monoamine oxidase inhibitors or tricyclic antidepressants may result in severe hypertension. Beta-adrenergic blockers may potentiate hypertension.

PHENOBARBITAL

(fee-no-BAR-bih-tal)
Pregnancy Class: D
Luminal (C-IV) (Rx)
Classifications: Anticonvulsant, sedative-hypnotic

Mechanism of Action

Produces generalized CNS depression, decreases motor activity, and inhibits transmission in the CNS. This inhibition raises the seizure threshold and suppresses seizure activity.

Indications

Treatment of generalized motor seizures and status epilepticus, hypertensive crisis.

Contraindications

Hypersensitivity to phenobarbital and other barbiturates. Preexisting CNS depression. Pregnancy and lactation. Respiratory depression.

Precautions

Use caution in administering phenobarbital to patients: with severe liver or kidney dysfunction, or who are drug-dependent. Elderly patients are more likely to experience side effects of phenobarbital so they should receive 66–75% of the usual dose.

Route and Dosage

Adults (anticonvulsant): 200–320 mg slow IV bolus or IM. May repeat in 6 hours if needed.
Adults (status epilepticus): 15–20 mg/kg IV administered slowly over 10–15 minutes. Dose may be repeated if needed.
Adults (hypertensive crisis): 5–10 mg IV or IM.
Pediatrics (anticonvulsant): 10–20 mg/kg by slow IV bolus over 10–15 minutes.
Pediatrics (status epilepticus): 15–20 mg/kg by slow IV bolus over 10–15 minutes.
Pediatrics (hypertensive crisis): Not recommended.

How Supplied

Injection: 30 mg/mL, 60 mg/mL, 65 mg/mL, 130 mg/mL.

Adverse Reactions and Side Effects

CNS: Drowsiness, headache, vertigo, possible paradoxic excitation.
Respiratory: Bronchospasm, laryngospasm, respiratory depression.
CV: Hypotension.
GI: Nausea, vomiting.
Dermatologic: Rash.

EMS Considerations

Assess patients frequently for respiratory status, pulse, and blood pressure. Advanced airway equipment should be readily available in the event severe respiratory depression occurs.

Drug Interactions

Phenobarbital may cause additive CNS depression if used with other CNS depressants including: alcohol, antidepressants, antihistamines, narcotics, and other sedative-hypnotics.

PHENYTOIN

(FEN-ih-toyn)
Pregnancy Class: C
Dilantin (Rx)
Classification: Anticonvulsant

Mechanism of Action

Phenytoin causes an increase in the transport of sodium out of motor cortex cell neurons. This increase helps to limit cell depolarization, thus preventing the spread of seizure activity.

Indications

To prevent or treat generalized motor seizures and status epilepticus.

Contraindications

Hypersensitivity to phenytoin, or propylene glycol. Phenytoin decreases AV conduction and should not be administered to patients with bradycardia, heart block, or Adams-Stokes syndrome.

Precautions

Use caution in administering phenytoin to: elderly patients, patients with severe cardiac, hepatic dysfunction, or respiratory problems. Use in pregnancy may result in fetal deformities.

Route and Dosage

Adults: 15–20 mg/kg by slow IV bolus, no faster than 50 mg/min. Initial dose should be followed by 100 mg IV every 6–8 hours.
Pediatrics: 15–20 mg/kg by slow IV bolus at a rate of 1–3 mg/kg/min.

How Supplied

Injection: 50 mg/mL.

Adverse Reactions and Side Effects

CNS: Ataxia, agitation, dizziness, headache, drowsiness.
CV: Hypotension, tachycardia, vasodilation.
GI: Nausea, vomiting, hepatitis, altered taste.
Miscellaneous: Allergic reactions including **Stevens-Johnson syndrome**.
Dermatologic: Rash, exfoliative dermatitis, pruritis.
Local: Phlebitis at IV site.
HEENT: Double vision, nystagmus, tinnitus.

EMS Considerations

Slow administration of phenytoin helps prevent toxicity. Elderly patients may develop toxic effects more rapidly than younger patients. Monitor the patients closely for developing hypotension and respiratory and cardiac problems. Administer phenytoin through an IV established in a large vein. Do not use veins in the hands.

Drug Interactions

Phenytoin may cause additive CNS depression if administered with other CNS depressants, including alcohol, antidepressants, antihistamines, narcotics, and other sedative/hypnotics. Phenytoin is not compatible with dextrose solutions; a precipitate will form.

CONCLUSION

The neurologic emergencies presented in this chapter are frequently encountered in the out-of-hospital setting. Drug therapy used for neurologic emergencies plays a secondary role to initial stabilization, rapid transport, detailed assessment of patients, and early notification to the hospital.

STUDY QUESTIONS

1. The initial recommended adult dosage of diazepam for the patient experiencing status epilepticus is:
   a. 2–5 mg by slow IV bolus
   b. 5–10 mg by slow IV bolus
   c. 10–20 mg by slow IV bolus
   d. 20–30 mg by slow IV bolus

2. A potentially life-threatening side effect of diazepam is:
   a. Cardiac arrhythmia
   b. Hypotension
   c. Respiratory arrest
   d. Anaphylaxis

3. Alteplase should not be administered in which of the following situations?
   a. Age > 18 years
   b. SBP < 185 and DBP < 110 mm Hg
   c. Onset of symptoms 6 hours prior to admission to hospital
   d. Hemorrhagic CVA ruled out by head CT

4. Which of the following situations demands caution in the use of mannitol?
   a. Active intracranial bleeding
   b. Preexisting dehydration
   c. Hypersensitivity
   d. Tendency to develop congestive heart failure

5. Methylprednisolone may improve muscle function and sensation following traumatic injury to the spinal cord. A patient estimated to weigh 180 pounds should receive _____ mg of methylprednisolone by IV bolus, followed by an IV infusion of _____ mg/h.
   a. 5400 mg; 972 mg
   b. 2700 mg; 486 mg
   c. 2460 mg; 443 mg
   d. 1230 mg; 222 mg

6. A contraindication for the use of phenobarbital sodium is:
   a. Kidney dysfunction
   b. Elderly patient
   c. Pediatric patient
   d. Hypersensitivity to barbiturates

7. The pediatric dose of phenytoin for the treatment of a generalized motor seizure is:
   a. 0.5–1.5 mg/kg
   b. 15–20 mg/kg
   c. 20–30 mg/kg
   d. 150–250 mg

8. A contraindication for the use of phenytoin is:
   a. Heart block
   b. Elderly patient
   c. Respiratory problem
   d. Headache

9. Norepinephrine is indicated for the treatment of neurogenic shock. Which of the following is a contraindication to the administration of norepinephrine?
   a. Hypotension secondary to hypovolemia
   b. Cardiovascular disease
   c. Renal failure
   d. Hyperglycemia

10. A benefit of fosphenytoin over phenytoin is:
    a. Fewer adverse effects
    b. May be administered to patients with heart block
    c. No dosage adjustment required for patients with hepatic dysfunction
    d. May be administered IM

EXTENDED CASE STUDY

Status Epilepticus

Initial Response: EMS responds to the home of a man "having a seizure." On arrival, EMS finds a man, who appears to be approximately 40, experiencing active seizures. His extremities are outstretched, his jaw is clenched, and he is drooling. As EMS approaches, seizure activity appears to be slowing down. However, just as the patient is placed on oxygen, seizures begin again. Family members state he has been going from one seizure to another.

This patient is experiencing status epilepticus. Status epilepticus is considered a major emergency because the patient may aspirate, become extremely hypoxic, fracture long bones including the spinal column, or sustain myocardial damage caused by cardiac ischemia. Hyperthermia and exhaustion can result from prolonged seizures and cause death.

Management: Patients experiencing status epilepticus are very difficult to manage. This is a life-threatening situation, however, so rapid treatment is essential.

Maintain the patient's airway with the administration of high flow rates of high concentrations of oxygen. Assist ventilations if necessary. Monitor cardiac function. It may be difficult to keep ECG leads attached or to record an accurate strip because of seizure activity. If possible, establish an IV line of normal saline at a keep-open rate. Normal saline is the fluid of choice in case phenytoin is administered. Phenytoin is not compatible with D_5W, because a precipitate forms when phenytoin comes in contact with dextrose. Phenytoin causes an increase in the transport of sodium out of motor cortex cell neurons to limit cell depolarization, thus preventing the spread of seizure activity. The suggested route and dosage of phenytoin is 15–20 mg/kg by slow IV bolus.

Once an IV has been established, there are two out-of-hospital agents of choice: diazepam and $D_{50}W$. Diazepam is a CNS depressant with anticonvulsant properties. The suggested route and dosage for diazepam in this case is 5–10 mg by slow IV bolus initially, repeated if necessary, but not to exceed a total dose of 30 mg. Dextrose 50% in water increases circulating blood sugar levels to normal in hypoglycemic states. Hypoglycemia may be a factor in treating status epilepticus. The suggested route and dosage of $D_{50}W$ for an adult is 25 g by slow IV bolus, repeated as necessary.

Status epilepticus is a true emergency. Rapid transport to the nearest appropriate emergency facility is essential.

CHAPTER 13

DRUGS USED TO TREAT GASTROINTESTINAL EMERGENCIES

Therapeutic Classifications of Drugs Used for Gastrointestinal Emergencies

Anticholinergics
Diphenhydramine
Hydroxyzine
Promethazine
Antidote, Adsorbent
Activated Charcoal

Antiemetics
Diphenhydramine
Hydroxyzine
Promethazine
Antihistamines
Diphenhydramine

Hydroxyzine
Promethazine
Emetic
Syrup of ipecac

OBJECTIVES

On completion of this chapter and the study questions, you should be able to:
- Describe in detail the adsorbent antidote, activated charcoal.
- Describe in detail the following antiemetic drugs: diphenhydramine, hydroxyzine, and promethazine.

KEY TERMS

Anticholinergic
Antidote, adsorbent

Antiemetic
Antihistamine

Chemoreceptor trigger zone

CASE STUDIES

1. EMS responds to an overdose of acetamino-phen. The patient is a 29-year-old male who took a bottle of acetaminophen approximately 15 minutes prior to calling EMS. He is fully conscious. What is the appropriate action to take?
   a. Administer activated charcoal
   b. Administer syrup of ipecac 30 mL PO followed by 240 mL of water
   c. Administer activated charcoal in milk to make the taste more acceptable to the patient
   d. Administer promethazine to prevent vomiting

2. En route to the hospital, the patient has vomited several times, and the contents of the stomach appear to be completely emptied. The most appropriate action to take at this time is:
   a. Administer promethazine
   b. Administer a second dose of activated charcoal
   c. Administer a second dose of syrup of ipecac
   d. Administer diphenhydramine

INTRODUCTION

Various gastrointestinal emergencies may be encountered in the out-of-hospital setting. Gastrointestinal emergencies may include traumatic injuries and nontraumatic illnesses. Traumatic gastrointestinal injuries may include blunt or penetrating trauma. The primary responsibility of EMS providers in traumatic gastrointestinal emergencies is initial stabilization and rapid transport to the hospital.

The majority of nontraumatic gastrointestinal emergencies (such as *aortic aneurysm*, gastrointestinal bleeding, *appendicitis, pancreatitis, and peritonitis*) are managed in the out-of-hospital setting with stabilization and rapid transport to the hospital. Few gastrointestinal emergencies require drug therapy in the out-of-hospital setting. Drug overdose and poisonings may be treated with syrup of ipecac and activated charcoal.

Toxicologic emergencies are discussed in detail in Chapter 15. The remainder of drug therapy discussed in this chapter is for the management of nausea and vomiting caused by a variety of conditions.

Individual Drugs

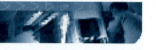

ACTIVATED CHARCOAL

(CHAR-kole)
Pregnancy Class: C

Acta-Char Liquid-A, Actidose-Aqua,, CharcoAid 2000, , Insta-Char, Insta-Char Aqueous Suspension, Liqui-Char, SuperChar Aqueous
Classifications: Antidote, adsorbent

Mechanism of Action

Adsorbs toxic substances or irritants, inhibiting gastrointestinal absorption. Sorbitol is added to some formulations to cause hyperosmotic laxative action and promote elimination of the toxic substance.

Indications

Acute management of many oral poisonings, following emesis and/or lavage.

Contraindications

No known contraindications.

Precautions

Activated charcoal may cause vomiting, which is hazardous in petroleum distillate and caustic ingestions. Therefore, use with caution in poisonings due to cyanide, corrosives, ethanol, methanol, petroleum distillates, organic solvents, mineral acids, or iron.

Route and Dosage

Charcoal in water: Single dose.
Adults: 30–100 g PO.
Infants (< 1 year): 1 g/kg PO.
Children (1–12 years): 1–2 g/kg PO.

How Supplied

Capsule: 260 mg.
Liquid: 12.5 g (60 mL), 25 g (120 mL), 15 g (75 mL), 30 g (120 mL), 30 g (240 mL), 50 g (240 mL).
Liquid with propylene glycol: 12.5 g (60 mL), 25 g (120 mL).
Powder for suspension: 15 g, 30 g, 40 g, 120 g, 240 g.

Adverse Reactions and Side Effects

GI: Black stools, constipation, diarrhea , nausea/vomiting.

EMS Considerations

When using syrup of ipecac with activated charcoal, induce vomiting with ipecac before administering activated charcoal. Charcoal binds ipecac, rendering it ineffective.

Drug Interactions

Do not administer with syrup of ipecac. Milk, ice cream, or sherbet will decrease the ability of charcoal to adsorb other agents.

DIPHENHYDRAMINE

(dye-fen-HY-drah-meen)
Pregnancy Class: B

AllerMax, Allermed, Banophen Caplets, Benadryl, Compoz, Diphenhist, Genahist, Hyrexin-50, Siladryl (OTC and Rx)
Classifications: Anticholinergic, antiemetic, antihistamine

Mechanism of Action

Significant CNS depressant, anticholinergic, and antiemetic effects. Antagonizes the effects of histamine at histamine-receptor sites.

Indications

Treatment or prevention of nausea and vomiting. Prevention of motion sickness. Relief of acute dystonic reactions. Treatment of hypersensitivity reactions.

Contraindications

Hypersensitivity to diphenhydramine, acute asthma attacks, and lactation.

Precautions

Dosage reductions recommended in the elderly because of increased susceptibility to adverse effects. Use cautiously in severe liver disease. May increase intraocular pressure in patients with narrow-angle glaucoma.

Route and Dosage

Adult: 25–50 mg IV or IM every 2–3 hours as needed. Patients may require up to 100 mg/dose. Do not exceed 400 mg/day.
Pediatric: 1 to 1.25 mg/kg IV or IM every 6 hours as needed. Do not exceed 300 mg/day. May be administered IV undiluted. Do not administer faster than 25 mg/min.

How Supplied

Injection: 10 mg/mL, 50 mg/mL.

Adverse Reactions and Side Effects

CNS: Drowsiness, dizziness, headache, paradoxic excitation in children.
Resp.: Chest tightness, wheezing, thickening of bronchial secretions.
CV: Hypotension, palpitations.
GI: Anorexia, dry mouth, constipation.
GU: Urinary retention.
Local: Pain at IM site.
HEENT: Blurred vision, tinnitus.

EMS Considerations

Monitor blood pressure following IV administration.

Drug Interactions

Additive CNS depression may occur: with other antihistamines, alcohol, narcotic analgesics, and sedative-hypnotics.

HYDROXYZINE

(hy-DROX-ih-zeen)
Pregnancy Class: C
Atarax, Vistaril, Hyzine-50 (Rx)
Classifications: Anticholinergic, antiemetic, antihistamine

Mechanism of Action

Has antiemetic, anticholinergic, and antihistaminic effects. Acts as a CNS depressant.

Indications

Treatment of anxiety and treatment or prevention of nausea and vomiting. Treatment of hypersensitivity reactions.

Contraindications

Hypersensitivity to hydroxyzine and pregnancy (potential for congenital defects).

Precautions

Dosage reduction is recommended in elderly patients because of increased susceptibility to adverse effects. Use caution in patients with severe liver disease. Safety not established in lactation.

Route and Dosage

Adult: 25–100 mg IM every 6 hours as needed.
Pediatrics: 0.5–1 mg/kg/dose IM every 6 hours as needed.

How Supplied

Injection: 25 mg/mL, 50 mg/mL.

Adverse Reactions and Side Effects

CNS: Drowsiness, agitation, ataxia, dizziness, headache, weakness.
Resp.: Wheezing.
GI: Dry mouth, constipation.
Miscellaneous: Chest tightness.
GU: Urinary retention.
Dermatologic: Flushing.
Local: Pain at IM site, abscesses at IM site.

EMS Considerations

Hydroxyzine should not be administered IV.

Drug Interactions

Additive CNS depression may occur with other CNS depressants including: alcohol, antidepressants, antihistamines, narcotic analgesics, and sedative-hypnotics.

PROMETHAZINE

(proh-METH-ah-zeen)
Pregnancy Class: C
Promethacon (Rx)
Classifications: Anticholinergic, antiemetic, antihistamine

Mechanism of Action

Blocks the effects of histamine. Antiemetic effects are caused by inhibition of the **chemoreceptor trigger zone** (CTZ). Also, effective in motion sickness because of its central anticholinergic effect which inhibits the **vestibular apparatus**, the integrative **vomiting center**, and the CTZ.

Indications

Treatment and prevention of nausea and vomiting. Treatment of motion sickness. Treatment of hypersensitivity reactions.

Contraindications

Hypersensitivity to promethazine or phenothiazines. Comatose patients. May increase intraocular pressure in patients with narrow-angle glaucoma.

Precautions

Use cautiously in patients with a history of seizure disorders. Avoid chronic use in pregnancy. Safety not established in lactation.

Route and Dosage

Adult: 12.5–25 mg PO, Rectal, IM or IV every 4 hours as needed. Initial PO dose should be 25 mg.

Pediatrics (2–12 years): 0.25 to 1 mg/kg (not to exceed 25 mg) PO, Rectal, IM or IV every 4 hours as needed. Must be diluted to 25 mg/mL for IV administration. Do not administer at a rate faster than 25 mg/min.

How Supplied

Tablets: 12.5 mg, 25 mg.
Suppositories: 12.5 mg, 25 mg, 50 mg.
Injection: 25 mg/mL, 50 mg/mL.

Adverse Reactions and Side Effects

CNS: Neuroleptic malignant syndrome, confusion, sedation, dizziness, extrapyramidal reactions, paradoxical excitation in children.
CV: Bradycardia or tachycardia, hypotension.
GI: Dry mouth, constipation.
GU: Urinary retention.
Local: Thrombophlebitis.
HEENT: Blurred vision, tinnitus.

EMS Considerations

Do not administer to children less than two years of age.

Drug Interactions

Additive CNS depression may occur with other CNS depressants including: alcohol, other antihistamines, narcotic analgesics, and sedative-hypnotics.

CONCLUSION

Very few gastrointestinal emergencies require drug treatment in the out-of-hospital setting. However, EMS providers should be familiar with drugs administered for poisonings, overdoses, and nausea and vomiting. This chapter has presented the common drugs used by EMS providers for these conditions.

STUDY QUESTIONS

1. Activated charcoal should not be administered for which of the following ingestions?
   a. Phenobarbital
   b. Gasoline
   c. Aspirin
   d. Acetaminophen

2. The appropriate dose of diphenhydramine to treat nausea and vomiting in a 10-year-old is:
   a. 0.5 mg/kg IV or IM every 6 hours as needed
   b. 2.5 mg/kg IV or IM every 6 hours as needed
   c. 1–1.25 mg/kg IV or IM every 6 hours as needed
   d. 5 mg/kg IV or IM every 6 hours as needed

3. Hydroxyzine is contraindicated in all of the following *except*:
   a. Intravenous administration
   b. Elderly patients
   c. Pregnancy
   d. Hypersensitivity

4. An adverse effect of promethazine is:
   a. Diarrhea
   b. Insomnia
   c. Drooling
   d. Drowsiness

EXTENDED CASE STUDY

Response: EMS responds to a 23-year-old female complaining of vomiting every 2 hours for the past 24 hours. Upon questioning, the patient reveals that she is 6 weeks pregnant. **Physical examination reveals the following:**

> *Level of consciousness:* alert and oriented.
> *Respirations:* 24/min.
> *Blood pressure:* 110/70 mm Hg.
> *Pulse:* regular, rate of 110 beats/min.
> *Skin:* dry, poor turgor.

Questioning of medical history reveals that the patient has a history of seizures.

Management: The patient appears to be dehydrated because of excessive vomiting over a prolonged time period and lack of PO intake. The initial management of this patient should include initiation of IV access with administration of NS to provide rehydration. An antiemetic should be administered to prevent further vomiting and loss of fluids. The most appropriate antiemetic to administer is diphenhydramine at a dose of 10–50 mg IV every 2–3 hours as needed. Diphenhydramine has a pregnancy classification of B; although, safety has not been fully established in pregnancy, it has been used safely. Other antiemetics, hydroxyzine, and promethazine, are not the best choice for this patient. Hydroxyzine is contraindicated in pregnancy and promethazine should be used with caution in patients with a history of seizures.

CHAPTER 14

DRUGS USED TO TREAT OBSTETRIC AND GYNECOLOGIC EMERGENCIES

Therapeutic Classifications of Drugs Used in Obstetric and Gynecologic Emergencies

Antianxiety Agent
Diazepam

Anticonvulsants
Diazepam
Magnesium sulfate

Antihypertensive
Hydralazine

Bronchodilator
Terbutaline

Oxytocic
Oxytocin

Skeletal Muscle Relaxant
Diazepam

Tocolytic
Terbutaline

OBJECTIVES

On completion of this chapter and the study questions, you should be able to:

- Describe in detail the out-of-hospital management of preterm labor.
- Describe in detail the out-of-hospital management of postpartum hemorrhage.
- Describe in detail the out-of-hospital management of preeclampsia and eclampsia.
- Describe in detail the following anticonvulsant drugs: diazepam and magnesium sulfate.
- Describe in detail the antihypertensive drug hydralazine.
- Describe in detail the oxytocic drug, oxytocin.
- Describe in detail the tocolytic drug, terbutaline.

KEY TERMS

Eclampsia
Oxytocic
Preeclampsia

Preterm labor
Postpartum
   hemorrhage

Tocolytic
Toxemia of
   pregnancy

CASE STUDIES

1. EMS is dispatched to the home of a "woman having chest pain." On arrival, EMS finds a 24-year-old patient who says that she is 8 months pregnant. She also reports that she has had a headache for the past 2 days, and today has developed chest pain. Further history and physical examination identify the chest pain as epigastric pain. Initial assessment reveals the following:

   Level of consciousness: Alert, oriented.
   Respirations: 18 breaths/min, lungs clear bilaterally.
   Pulse: 96 beats/min, regular.
   Blood pressure: 164/110.
   Skin: Pale, edematous.

   The patient says that this is her first pregnancy. She has no history of high blood pressure or any other illness.

   All signs and symptoms indicate this patient is preeclamptic. Preeclampsia can lead to true eclampsia. Do not delay transport to the emergency department. Headache and epigastric pain in this situation could be signs of impending seizure activity.

   The drug of choice for the prevention of seizure activity in the preeclamptic patient is:
   a. Diazepam
   b. Oxytocin
   c. Mannitol
   d. Magnesium sulfate

2. EMS is called to the home of a woman "having seizures." On arrival, EMS finds a woman in her late twenties who is experiencing active seizures. The patient's mother says that her daughter is 7 months pregnant. She also reports this is her daughter's second seizure since she called for help. Earlier in the day, the patient had complained of severe headache, dizziness, nausea, chest pain, and spots before her eyes. Seizure control for this patient should begin with:
   a. Diazepam
   b. Calcium gluconate
   c. Magnesium sulfate
   d. Oxytocin

INTRODUCTION

For most out-of-hospital emergency care professionals, the opportunity to assist in the delivery of a baby is one of the most exciting and fulfilling events in their careers. Most out-of-hospital deliveries occur without complications. During and after delivery, out-of-hospital treatment for both the mother and infant is usually supportive. In some cases, however, out-of-hospital emergency care providers encounter a potentially fatal obstetric emergency, such as: preterm labor, postpartum hemorrhage, and preeclampsia or eclampsia.

Preterm labor occurs between the beginning of the 21st week and the end of the 37th week of pregnancy. Preterm labor occurs in approximately 5—15% of pregnancies and is the most common complication that occurs during the 3rd trimester. The exact cause of preterm labor is unknown in the majority of cases, but may be initiated by an underlying maternal, fetal, or placental problem. Tocolytics, such as terbutaline, are used to decrease or inhibit uterine contraction. The goal is to extend the pregnancy until the fetus is mature enough to survive outside the womb. The following criteria are used to determine if tocolytic therapy is appropriate: the fetus is alive with a gestational age of less than 35 weeks, the fetal weight is less than 2500 g, the membranes are unruptured, cervical dilation is less than 4 cm, effacement is less than 80% complete, and there are no maternal or fetal problems that require immediate delivery. Terbutaline is very effective in terminating preterm labor, and decreasing the mortality and morbidity associated with preterm birth.

Postpartum hemorrhage is the loss (by the mother) of more than 500 mL of blood within 24 hours after delivery. It is important to frequently assess the patient's clinical appearance and vital signs in order to determine blood loss. The initial treatment for severe postpartum hemorrhage is the same as for anyone experiencing hypovolemia caused by hemorrhage. This treatment includes maintaining an adequate airway, using supplemental oxygen, and administering intravenous volume expanders. If out-of-hospital pharmacologic therapy is needed, the drug of choice in treating postpartum hemorrhage is oxytocin. If this treatment is delayed, a life-threatening situation could rapidly develop.

Preeclampsia is a toxemia of pregnancy characterized by increasing blood pressure, headaches, and edema of the lower extremities. If left untreated, preeclampsia may develop into true eclampsia. Eclampsia generally occurs during the last trimester of pregnancy. The cause of eclampsia is unknown. However, it is associated with preexisting hypertension (blood pressure exceeding 140/90), renal disease, and diabetes; it is more prevalent in women experiencing their first pregnancy. Eclampsia is characterized by hypertension, diffuse edema, seizures, and possibly coma. It develops in approximately 1 out of 200 patients and is usually fatal if untreated. The drugs used for the out-of-hospital treatment of eclampsia are magnesium sulfate and diazepam.

Individual Drugs

DIAZEPAM

(dye-AYZ-eh-pam)
Pregnancy Class: D
Diastat, Valium, (Rx)
Classifications: Antianxiety agent, anticonvulsant, skeletal muscle relaxant

Mechanism of Action

Causes CNS depression, producing relief of anxiety and sedation. Diazepam produces skeletal muscle relaxation by inhibition of spinal pathways. Decreases seizure activity caused by enhanced presynaptic inhibition.

Indications

Treatment of generalized motor seizures associated with eclampsia.

Contraindications

Do not administer diazepam to patients with hypersensitivity to diazepam, benzodiazepines, or propylene glycol. Diazepam should not be used in patients with severe pulmonary impairment, severe hepatic dysfunction, pre-existing CNS depression, and narrow-angle glaucoma because it may increase intraocular pressure.

Precautions

Use caution in administering diazepam to patients with a history of psychoses or drug addiction. Use with caution in patients with mild/moderate hepatic dysfunction; the effects may be more intense and prolonged.

Route and Dosage

5–10 mg by slow IV bolus. May repeat every 10–15 minutes as needed, to a total of 30 mg.

How Supplied

Injection: 5 mg/mL.

Adverse Drug Reactions and Side Effects

CNS: Dizziness, drowsiness, mental depression, headache.
Respiratory: Respiratory depression.
CV: Hypotension.
Local: Phlebitis.
HEENT: Blurred vision.

EMS Considerations

Diazepam may cause respiratory arrest if administered too rapidly or in excess doses. Do not mix diazepam with any other drug. Diazepam may react with the IV tubing; to minimize this, administer diazepam at the IV site, not higher in the tubing. Thoroughly flush the IV line before administering diazepam if other drugs have already been administered through the line. Assess the patient's vital signs continuously.

Drug Interactions

Additive CNS depression may occur if diazepam is administered with other CNS depressants, such as: antihistamines, tricyclic antidepressants, alcohol, narcotic analgesics, or other sedatives or hypnotics.

HYDRALAZINE

(hye-DRAL-a-zeen)
Pregnancy Class: C
Apresoline (Rx)
Classification: Antihypertensive

Mechanism of Action

Hydralazine is a direct-acting peripheral arteriolar vasodilator.

Indications

Moderate to severe hypertension associated with pre-eclampsia and eclampsia.

Contraindications

Hypersensitivity. Should also be avoided in patients with known intolerance to tartrazine.

Precautions

Use cautiously in patients with cardiovascular, cerebrovascular, and several renal and hepatic disease.

Route and Dosage

Hypertension: 5–40 mg IM or IV. Repeat as necessary.
Eclampsia: 5 mg q 15–20 minutes up to a maximum dose of 20 mg.

How Supplied

20 mg/mL.

Adverse Reactions and Side Effects

CV: tachycardia, arrhythmias, angina, edema, orthostatic hypotension.
CNS: headache, dizziness, drowsiness.
GI: diarrhea, nausea, vomiting.

EMS Considerations

None.

Drug Interactions

There may be an increased chance of hypotension if used with other antihypertensives, nitrates, or MAO inhibitors.

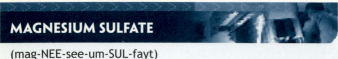

MAGNESIUM SULFATE

(mag-NEE-see-um-SUL-fayt)
Pregnancy Class: A
(Rx)
Classification: Anticonvulsant

Mechanism of Action

Causes CNS depression and controls seizures by blocking release of acetylcholine at the myoneural junction. Magnesium also decreases the sensitivity of the motor end plate to acetylcholine and decreases the excitability of the motor membrane.

Indications

Management of preeclampsia and eclampsia.

Contraindications

Do not administer in toxemia of pregnancy during the 2-hour period prior to delivery. Do not administer to patients with heart block or myocardial damage. Do not administer to patients with hypermagnesemia or hypocalcemia.

Precautions

Use caution in administering to patients with decreased renal function, because toxicity may occur.

Route and Dosage

4–5 g by IV infusion, concurrently with up to 5 g IM in each buttock; then follow with 1–2 g/hr continuous infusion. Do not exceed 40 g/day.

How Supplied

Injection: 10%, 12.5%, 25%, 50%.

Adverse Reactions and Side Effects

CNS: Drowsiness.
Respiratory: Respiratory depression.
CV: Arrhythmias, bradycardia, hypotension.
GI: Nausea, vomiting.
Dermatologic: Flushing, sweating.

EMS Considerations

Rapid IV injection of magnesium sulfate may cause respiratory or cardiac arrest. Before administering magnesium sulfate, be sure that the patient's respiratory rate is at least 16 breaths/min. An overdose of magnesium sulfate may cause respiratory depression and heart block. To reverse these effects, hyperventilate the patient using 100% oxygen and administer an IV bolus of 10% calcium gluconate at 5–10 mEq (10–20 mL). Constant monitoring of the blood pressure is extremely important. The patient's blood pressure must not fall below 130/80 to prevent inadequate blood supply to the fetus.

Drug Interactions

Additive CNS effects may occur when magnesium sulfate is administered with: alcohol, narcotic analgesics, barbiturates, antidepressants, sedative-hypnotics, and antipsychotics. Concurrent administration with digoxin may cause cardiac conduction changes.

OXYTOCIN

(OX-eh-TOE-sin)
Pregnancy Class: X
Pitocin, Syntocinon (Rx)
Classification: Oxytocic agent, hormone

Mechanism of Action

A synthetic compound identical to a naturally produced pituitary hormone. Stimulates uterine muscle contraction and contraction of uterine blood vessels to reduce postpartum bleeding.

Indications

Control of postpartum hemorrhage after delivery of the placenta.

Contraindications

Hypersensitivity to oxytocin.

Precautions

Do not administer oxytocin until the mother has delivered both the fetus and the placenta.

Route and Dosage

IV: 10 units infused at 20–40 milliunits/minute.
IM: 10 units after delivery of the placenta.

How Supplied

Injection: 10 units/mL.

Adverse Reactions and Side Effects

CNS: Coma, seizures.
CV: Hypotension.
Miscellaneous: Painful uterine contractions.
Fluids and electrolytes: Hypochloremia, hyponatremia, water intoxication.

EMS Considerations

If possible, place the newborn at the mother's breast. The baby's sucking action promotes the secretion of oxytocin, which will also aid in controlling postpartum hemorrhage. Oxytocin overdose can cause uterine rupture; continuously monitor the patient's vital signs. Magnesium sulfate should be available for administration to relax the uterus in the event of titanic uterine contractions.

Drug Interactions

Concurrent use of oxytocin with vasoconstrictors may cause severe hypertension.

TERBUTALINE

(ter-BYOU-tah-leen)
Pregnancy Class: B
Brethaire, Brethine, Bricanyl (Rx)
Classifications: Beta$_2$-adrenergic agonist, bronchodilator, tocolytic agent

Mechanism of Action

Stimulates beta$_2$-adrenergic receptors, which results in relaxation of uterine smooth muscle, relaxation of vascular smooth muscle, and bronchodilation.

Indications

Management of premature labor.

Contraindications

Hypersensitivity to terbutaline and other adrenergic amines.

Precautions

Safety in lactation not established. Use cautiously in patients with: cardiac disease, hypertension, hyperthyroidism, diabetes, and glaucoma.

Route and Dosage

250 mcg every hour subcutaneously until contractions stop. Do not exceed 500 mcg within a 4-hour period, or 10 mcg/min infusion IV.

How Supplied

Injection: 1 mg/mL.

Adverse Reactions and Side Effects

CNS: Nervousness, restlessness, tremor, headache, insomnia.
CV: Angina, arrhythmias, hypertension, tachycardia.
GI: Nausea, vomiting.
Endocrine: Hyperglycemia.

EMS Considerations

Monitor vital signs and ECG continuously.

Drug Interactions

Concurrent use with other adrenergic agonists will have additive adrenergic side effects. Use with monoamine oxidase inhibitors may lead to hypertensive crisis. Beta-adrenergic blockers may prevent the effectiveness of terbutaline.

CONCLUSION

Most out-of-hospital obstetric and gynecologic emergencies do not require pharmacologic intervention. The out-of-hospital professional can manage the majority of these emergencies by maintaining an adequate airway, using supplemental oxygen, and administering intravenous volume expanders, if needed. If out-of-hospital pharmacologic intervention is needed in preterm labor, terbutaline should be used. If out-of-hospital pharmacologic intervention is needed to treat severe cases of postpartum hemorrhage, the drug of choice is oxytocin; to treat preeclampsia, the drug of choice is magnesium sulfate; to treat seizures caused by eclampsia, diazepam and magnesium sulfate should be used.

In treating out-of-hospital obstetric and gynecologic emergencies, medical control may order other drugs in place of or in addition to the drugs presented in this chapter. For example, the physician may order an antihypertensive drug to treat hypertension associated with the obstetric patient. Other obstetric and gynecologic out-of-hospital emergencies may call for other kinds of flexibility in treatment. It is important that EMS providers be knowledgeable about local protocols so that they are ready to carry out treatment orders from medical control.

STUDY QUESTIONS

1. The out-of-hospital indication for oxytocin is for the:
   a. Control of seizures
   b. Treatment of hypertension
   c. Control of postpartum hemorrhage
   d. Treatment of severe bronchospasm

2. A major concern in a patient with eclampsia is seizures. The out-of-hospital drug of choice in the treatment of severe eclampsia is:
   a. Oxytocin
   b. Magnesium sulfate
   c. Diazepam
   d. Labetalol

3. The out-of-hospital dosage for magnesium sulfate is:
   a. 3–10 U IV
   b. 1 mg/kg IV
   c. 2–5 mg IV
   d. 4–5 g IV

4. The dose of diazepam for a patient having seizures caused by eclampsia is:
   a. 2–5 mg
   b. 5–10 mg
   c. 10–20 mg
   d. 30 mg

5. All of the following are adverse effects of terbutaline except:
   a. Hypotension
   b. Tremor
   c. Tachycardia
   d. Nervousness

OB/GYN Emergency

Initial Response: EMS is dispatched to a "woman in labor." On arrival, a 32-year-old patient is found who is experiencing strong uterine contractions every 2 minutes, each lasting approximately 1 minute. The patient tells you that this is her second child, but it is not due for another 3 weeks. On visual examination, you notice that the baby's buttocks are visible, which indicates that delivery is imminent. Preparations for delivery are quickly made.

Place the mother on 100% oxygen. If delivery complications arise, it is important to increase oxygen content and oxygen delivery to the tissues.

As the baby emerges, the buttocks and legs come out smoothly, but the head remains in the birth canal. In this situation, an adequate airway must be provided, because the baby may attempt to begin spontaneous respirations. You form an airway at the bottom of the birth canal*, but there is no evidence of respirations. After approximately 2 minutes, the baby's head delivers. Initial assessment of the baby reveals the following:

Level of consciousness: Unconscious.
Respirations: None.
Pulse: None.
*While wearing gloves, fingers are inserted into the birth canal to form a space, making a temporary airway for the baby.

Management: Immediately use suction to clear the baby's airway and ventilate, with 100% oxygen using a bag-valve mask and chest compressions. There is a risk that 100% oxygen will have toxic effects on the baby's lungs and eyes, but oxygen should never be withheld from an infant during an emergency.

Assessment of ventilations reveals good breath sounds over the chest and gastric area. It is now a good idea to place an ET tube in the baby for airway protection and administration of emergency drugs if necessary. Vascular access in a newborn is difficult at best, so in most cases ET access for drug administration is preferable. The ECG monitor shows asystole.

Once the ET is in place and adequate ventilations are achieved, administer approximately 0.1 mg (0.04 mL) epinephrine in a 1:1000 solution down the ET tube. The dosage of epinephrine is 0.01 mg/kg IV of a 1:10,000 solution or 0.1 mg/kg of a 1:1000 solution via the ET tube. (The average normal birthweight of a newborn is 4–5 kg.) When administering epinephrine ET, it is best to dilute the drug with normal saline solution.

Epinephrine is a natural catecholamine that stimulates both alpha-adrenergic and beta-adrenergic receptors. It elevates perfusion pressure during cardiac compressions, improves cardiac contractions, and stimulates spontaneous contractions in asystole. In this case, the newborn responds to the epinephrine and ventilations with a heart rate beginning at 40 beats/min and gradually increasing to a normal sinus rhythm. In the newborn, a heart rate less than 80 beats/min is considered bradycardia, and it does not produce adequate perfusion. Therefore, chest compressions are necessary until the epinephrine and ventilation gradually increase the newborn's heart rate to normal.

The key to successful resuscitation of a newborn is adequate airway maintenance and ventilation using supplemental oxygen. Medical control may call for medications if the patient does not respond to ventilation and chest compressions. In this case, the newborn now has a sinus rhythm at a rate of 144 beats/min, with a good pulse and adequate respirations.

While attention is focused on the baby, another member of the team begins having problems with the mother. She complained of severe abdominal pain after delivery of the placenta and soon began hemorrhaging.

Hemorrhage after delivery calls for several out-of-hospital management techniques. Immediately one of the team begins massaging the patient's fundus while another team member starts an IV lifeline of lactated Ringer's or normal saline. The patient should remain on high-flow 100% oxygen. If massaging the fundus does not control the hemorrhage, the drug of choice used for out-of-hospital hemorrhage control is oxytocin. Oxytocin is a hormone secreted by the pituitary gland that stimulates uterine contractions. In this out-of-hospital emergency, oxytocin is used to contract uterine blood vessels, thus reducing postpartum hemorrhage. If possible, the newborn should be placed at the mother's breast. The sucking action of the baby will promote the secretion of oxytocin, also aiding in controlling hemorrhage. However, in this case the baby should be closely monitored while en route to the emergency department because of its potentially unstable condition. The oxytocin dosage is 10–40 units added to lactated Ringer's or normal saline at a rate adjusted to the severity of the hemorrhage.

CHAPTER 15

DRUGS USED TO TREAT TOXICOLOGIC EMERGENCIES

Therapeutic Classifications of Drugs Used for Toxicologic Emergencies

Antianginal
Nitroglycerin
Anticonvulsant
Diazepam
Antidotes
Acetylcysteine (to acetaminophen)
Activated charcoal
Atropine (to cholinesterase inhibitors)

Physostigmine (antimuscarinic)
Pralidoxime (to cholinesterase inhibitors)
Antihypertensive
Phentolamine
Benzodiazepine Antagonist
Flumazenil
Cyanide Poisoning Adjuncts
Amyl nitrite
Sodium nitrite

Sodium thiosulfate
Hydrogen Ion Buffer
Sodium bicarbonate
Medicinal Gas
Oxygen
Narcotic Antagonists
Nalmefene
Naloxone
Urine Alkalinizer
Sodium bicarbonate

OBJECTIVES

On completion of this chapter and the study questions, you should be able to:
- Describe in detail the assessment of the poisoned patient.
- Describe in detail the common toxins encountered in the out-of-hospital setting.
- Describe in detail the antianginal drug, nitroglycerin.
- Describe in detail the anticonvulsant, diazepam.
- Describe in detail the following antidotes: acetylcysteine, activated charcoal, atropine, physostigmine, and pralidoxime.

- Describe in detail the antihypertensive drug, phentolamine.
- Describe in detail the benzodiazepine antagonist, flumazenil.
- Describe in detail the following cyanide poisoning adjuncts: amyl nitrite, sodium nitrite, and sodium thiosulfate.
- Describe in detail the hydrogen ion buffer and urine alkalinizer, sodium bicarbonate.
- Describe in detail the following narcotic antagonists: nalmefene and naloxone.

KEY TERMS

Anticholinesterase agent	Cholinergic agent	Poison
Antidote	Organophosphates	Withdrawal symptoms
Antimuscarinic agent	Overdose	

CASE STUDIES

1. EMS is dispatched to a farm and upon arrival is directed to a cotton field. A male patient is found lying on the ground, shivering. The patient's son says that his father was spraying malathion on the cotton crop when he started "acting funny" just before he collapsed. Initial patient assessment reveals the following:

   Level of consciousness: Depressed, responds to pain, in obvious distress.
   Respirations: 36/min, shallow.
   Pulse: 42/min, regular.
   Blood pressure: 60 systolic.
   Skin: Diaphoretic.
   Eyes: Watering, constricted pupils.

   The patient is also salivating and has a watering nose. His shivering is caused by virtually all his skeletal muscles twitching simultaneously.

   A. This patient is probably suffering from:
      (1) Cerebrovascular accident
      (2) Organophosphate poisoning
      (3) Cyanide poisoning
      (4) Narcotic overdose
   B. Pharmacologic treatment for this patient will probably include:
      (1) Atropine and physostigmine
      (2) Amyl nitrite and sodium nitrite
      (3) Naloxone and pralidoxime
      (4) Atropine and pralidoxime

2. EMS responds to the home of a known cocaine abuser. On arrival, the patient is found to be a 21-year-old man, lying unresponsive in a closet. He has a pair of panty hose tied around his right upper arm. There are obvious "tracks" on both arms. The patient's roommate says the patient had been high on cocaine and suddenly became unconscious. Further assessment reveals:

   Level of consciousness: Unconscious; responds to painful stimuli by occasional tonic and clonic jerking movements and incoherent speech.
   Respirations: 28/min, shallow.
   Pulse: 124 beats/min, irregular.
   Blood pressure: 190/102.
   Skin: Warm and moist.
   Pupils: Dilated, slow to react.

   Medical control instructs you to start an IV of normal saline at a keep-open rate. The first drug ordered in this case will probably be:
   a. Diazepam
   b. Naloxone
   c. Atropine
   d. Pralidoxime

INTRODUCTION

Out-of-hospital toxicologic emergencies include the management of overdoses and poisonings. An overdose is the intake of a drug in sufficient quantity to cause harm to the body. The drugs involved in overdoses are commonly drugs of abuse, but may also consist of prescription medications, over-the-counter medications, herbals, or home remedies. Acute reactions from overdoses may range from excessive excitement to coma and may progress to death. A poison is any substance that irritates, damages, or impairs the activity of the body's tissues. Poisons may be absorbed through the skin, inhaled, or ingested. There is a wide variety of substances that are potential poisons. Out-of-hospital management of toxicologic emergencies includes immediate stabilization of the patient, identifying the substance, attempting to slow or stop the absorption of the substance, and administering an antidote. The drugs used in the treatment of toxicologic emergencies include specific antidotes, emetics, drug antagonists, oxygen, anticonvulsants, and alkalinizing agents.

Assessing the Poisoned Patient

Initial assessment of the poisoned patient should begin with assessment of ABCs. The secondary assessment should include unusual skin color (i.e., cherry red skin with carbon monoxide poisoning), and assessment of patient's breath for odors that may indicate what substance was involved in the poisoning (i.e., bitter almonds with cyanide poisoning). Obtaining a history of the poisoning should include: determining what substance and how much was involved in the poisoning, when the poisoning occurred, any attempt to treat the poisoning, whether the poisoning was accidental or a suicide gesture, and any significant medical history of the patient. Signs and symptoms should be continually assessed to assist in identifying the poison.

Common Toxic Agents

Common toxic agents that are ingested or injected may include drugs such as: narcotics, benzodiazepines, amphetamines, hallucinogens, aspirin, acetaminophen, tricyclic antidepressants, and barbiturates. Other common toxic agents that are ingested include: strong acids (i.e., toilet bowl cleaners, hydrochloric acid, etc.), strong alkaloids (i.e., drain cleaner, ammonia, household bleach, etc.), petroleum products (i.e., kerosene, gasoline, furniture polish, etc.), methanol, antifreeze, cyanide, strychnine, arsenic, and organophosphates (i.e., pesticides, insecticides). The management of ingested poisons varies according to the specific substance ingested. Some poisonings by ingestion should be treated with induction of emesis and administration of antidotes. Vomiting should never be induced in the following situations: comatose or seizing patients; patients with a decreased level of consciousness; pregnant patients;

ingestions involving corrosives, petroleum products, iodides, silver nitrate, cyanide, or strychnine.

Common toxic agents that may be absorbed through the skin include cyanide or organophosphates. Management of absorbed poisonings should include decontamination of the skin and administration of specific antidotes.

Common toxic agents that may be inhaled include: carbon monoxide, freon, glue, solvents (i.e., cleaning fluids, paint thinner, gasoline, etc.), propellants and fluorocarbons from aerosol cans, paint, cyanide, or organophosphates. Management of inhaled poisonings should include: optimizing ventilation, and providing specific antidotes, when indicated.

Cyanide compounds are among the most common and most deadly poisons known. Fortunately, cyanide poisoning is relatively rare. When cyanide is inhaled, symptoms usually occur within seconds to minutes. Cyanide inhibits cellular respirations, which causes cellular hypoxia and death. Symptoms generally begin with giddiness and progress rapidly to headache, palpitations, vomiting, unconsciousness, seizures, and death. Cyanide poisoning may cause the patient's breath to smell like "bitter almonds." However, this odor should not be relied on for diagnosis. Treatment for cyanide poisoning should be immediate. Drug therapy consists of a three-step protocol, beginning with amyl nitrite, followed by sodium nitrite, and sodium thiosulfate.

Organophosphates are a major component of many insecticides. The manifestations of organophosphate poisoning include nausea, profuse sweating, epigastric and substernal tightness, abdominal cramps, profuse salivation, and muscle twitching. Severe cases of organophosphate poisoning may produce seizures and respiratory arrest. Pharmacologic treatment for severe cases of organophosphate poisoning includes the administration of atropine followed by pralidoxime.

Individual Drugs

ACETYLCYSTEINE
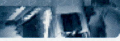

(ah-see-til-SYS-tay-een)
Pregnancy Class: B
Acetadote (Rx)
Classification: Antidote (acetaminophen)

Mechanism of Action

Decreases the buildup of a hepatotoxic metabolite in acetaminophen overdose to prevent liver damage.

Indications

Management of potentially hepatotoxic overdose of acetaminophen.

Contraindications

Hypersensitivity to acetylcysteine.

Precautions

Use with caution in patients with severe respiratory insufficiency, asthma, elderly patients, and patients with a history of gastrointestinal bleeding. Safety has not been established in pregnancy or lactation.

Route and Dosage

Adults and Pediatrics (PO): 140 mg/kg initially PO then 70 mg/kg every 4 hours for 17 additional doses.
Adults and Pediatrics (IV): Loading dose: 150 mg/kg over 10 minutes. *Maintenance dose:* 50 mg/kg over 4 hours.

How Supplied

Solution: 10%, 20%.
Injection: 20% in 30 mL vials.

Adverse Reactions and Side Effects

CNS: Drowsiness.
Respiratory: Bronchoconstriction, chest tightness, increased secretions.
GI: Nausea, vomiting.
Dermatologic: Clamminess, urticaria.
HEENT: Rhinorrhea.
Miscellaneous: Chills, fever.

EMS Considerations

The odor of the solution is very unpleasant, but will become less noticeable with continuing treatment. Be prepared for vomiting. Acetylcysteine increases secretions. Monitor respiratory status. Acetylcysteine should be administered as soon as possible after acetaminophen ingestion.

Drug Interactions

Activated charcoal may adsorb acetylcysteine and decrease its effectiveness. Do not administer together.

ACTIVATED CHARCOAL

(CHAR-kole)
Pregnancy Class: C
Acta-Char Liquid-A, Actidose-Aqua, , Charcoaid 2000, , Inst-Char, SuperChar (OTC)
Classifications: Antidote, adsorbent

Mechanism of Action

Adsorbs toxic substances or irritants, inhibiting gastrointestinal absorption. Sorbitol is added to some formulations to cause hyperosmotic laxative action and promote elimination of the toxic substance.

Indications

Acute management of many oral poisonings, following emesis and/or lavage.

Contraindications

Not effective for the following ingestions: cyanide, mineral acids, caustic alkalis, organic solvents, iron, ethanol, methanol, or lithium. Do not use charcoal with sorbitol in children less than one year of age.

Precautions

Activated charcoal may cause vomiting, which is hazardous in petroleum distillate and caustic ingestions.

Route and Dosage

Charcoal in water: Single dose.
Adults: 25–100 g PO.
Infants (< 1 year): 1 g/kg PO.
Children (1–12 years): 25–50 g/kg PO.

How Supplied

Powder for suspension: 15 g, 30 g, 40 g, 120 g, 240 g.

Adverse Reactions and Side Effects

GI: Black stools, constipation, diarrhea with sorbitol formulations, vomiting.

EMS Considerations

When using syrup of ipecac with activated charcoal, induce vomiting with ipecac before administering activated charcoal. Charcoal binds ipecac rendering it ineffective.

Drug Interactions

Do not administer with syrup of ipecac. Milk, ice cream, or sherbet will decrease the ability of charcoal to adsorb other agents.

AMYL NITRITE

(AM-ill NY-tryt)
Pregnancy Class: X
Amyl Nitrite Aspirols, Amyl Nitrite Vaporole (Rx)
Classification: Cyanide poisoning adjunct

Mechanism of Action

Amyl nitrite converts hemoglobin into methemoglobin. Methemoglobin reacts with cyanide and chemically binds it, which prevents it from having any toxic effect.

Indications

Immediate treatment of cyanide poisoning.

Contraindications

None in cyanide poisoning.

Precautions

Use caution in administering to patients with: hypersensitivity to amyl nitrite, head trauma, cerebral hemorrhage, increased intracranial pressure, hypotension, or glaucoma.

Route and Dosage

Adult: 1–2 ampules crushed. Inhale for 15–30 seconds of each minute until sodium nitrite is prepared or administer for 30–60 seconds every 5 minutes until patient is conscious. Then repeat at longer intervals for 24 hours.
Pediatrics: 1 ampule crushed. Inhale for 15–30 seconds of each minute until sodium nitrite is prepared or administer for 30–60 seconds every 5 minutes until the patient is conscious. Then repeat at longer intervals for 24 hours.

How Supplied

Ampules for inhalation: 0.3 mL.

Adverse Reactions and Side Effects

CNS: Headache, dizziness, syncope, weakness.
Respiratory: Shortness of breath.
CV: Hypotension, tachycardia.
Dermatologic: Cyanosis of lips, fingernails, or palms (indicates methemoglobinemia).

EMS Considerations

Assess vital signs frequently. The patient should remain lying or sitting down during and after amyl nitrite administration because of the potential for hypotension to develop. Amyl nitrite administration is the first step in a three-step treatment protocol for cyanide poisoning. After administering amyl nitrite, administer sodium nitrite, then sodium thiosulfate.

Drug Interactions

Additive hypotension may occur with antihypertensive agents, acute ingestion of alcohol, phenothiazines, or beta-blockers.

ATROPINE

(AH-troh-peen)
Pregnancy Class: C
Atro-Pen (Rx)
Classifications: Antidote (Organophosphate poisoning or mushroom poisoning caused by muscarine), anticholinesterase inhibitor

Mechanism of Action

Atropine blocks the action of acetylcholine in the parasympathetic nervous system, aiding in the treatment of anticholinesterase poisoning from organophosphate pesticides. Table 15–1 lists some of the more common organophosphate pesticides with which an individual may come in contact.

Indications

Treatment of organophosphate poisoning or muscarine mushroom poisoning.

Contraindications

None, when used in severe cases of organophosphate poisoning.

Precautions

Use cautiously in infants, small children, and the elderly because they are more prone to adverse effects with atropine administration. Use caution in administering atropine to patients with chronic renal disease, cardiac disease, or pulmonary disease.

Route and Dosage

Adults (Organophosphates): 2 mg IM initially. Then 2 mg q 10 minutes as needed up to 3 total doses.
Adults (Mushroom poisoning): 1–2 mg IV or IM every hour until respiratory effects decrease.
Pediatrics (Organophosphates)
6 mo to 4 yrs (IM): 0.5 mg.
4–10 years (IM): 1 mg.
>10 years (IM): 2 mg.
Pediatrics (IV): 0.02–0.05 mg/kg q 10 minutes until therapeutic effects seen.

How Supplied

Injection: 0.05 mg/mL, 0.1 mg/mL, 0.3 mg/mL, 0.4 mg/mL, 0.5 mg/mL, 0.8 mg/mL, 1 mg/mL.

Adverse Reactions and Side Effects

CNS: Drowsiness, confusion, paradoxic excitation in children.
CV: Tachycardia, palpitations.
GI: Dry mouth, constipation.
GU: Urinary retention.
HEENT: Blurred vision, dry eyes.
Miscellaneous: Decreased sweating.

EMS Considerations

Initial stabilization should include: obtaining and maintaining a patent airway, administration of oxygen, and obtaining IV access. Assess the patient frequently for adverse effects, monitor vital signs and ECG continuously. Severe cases of organophosphate poisoning may require the administration of pralidoxime in addition to atropine.

Drug Interactions

Additive anticholinergic effects may occur with concurrent administration of antihistamines, tricyclic antidepressants, and quinidine.

DIAZEPAM

(dye-AYZ-eh-pam)
Pregnancy Class: D
Diastat, Valium (Rx)
Classifications: -Antianxiety agent, anticonvulsant, sedative-hypnotic, skeletal muscle relaxant

---

Mechanism of Action

Causes CNS depression producing relief of anxiety and sedation. Diazepam produces skeletal muscle relaxation by inhibition of spinal pathways. Decreases seizure activity

Table 15-1 Organophosphate Pesticides.
(© Delmar/Cengage Learning)

High Toxicity	Moderate Toxicity	Mild Toxicity
Demeton	Coumaphos	Chlorthion
Disulfoton	Diazinon	Dimethoate
OMPA	Dichlorvos	Malathion
Parathion		
Phosdrin		
Schradon		
TEPP		

caused by enhanced presynaptic inhibition. Diazepam controls CNS overstimulation.

Indications

Prevention or treatment of seizures caused by poisoning or overdoses from various substances. Control of advancing CNS overstimulation caused by cocaine overdose.

Contraindications

Do not administer diazepam to patients with: hypersensitivity to diazepam, benzodiazepines, or propylene glycol; pre-existing CNS depression; acute narrow-angle glaucoma; or pregnancy and lactation.

Precautions

Use caution in administering diazepam to patients with a history of psychosis or drug addiction. Administer lower than usual adult doses to elderly patients because they are more sensitive to the drug's CNS effects. Use with caution in patients with hepatic dysfunction, as effects may be more intense and prolonged.

Route and Dosage

Adult (Advancing CNS Overstimulation): 2.5–5 mg IV bolus.
Adult (Seizures): 5–10 mg by slow IV bolus over 2–3 minutes. Repeat every 10–15 minutes as needed, to a maximum of 30 mg.
Pediatric: Not recommended for out-of-hospital use for cocaine overdose.
Pediatric (Seizures): > 5 years: 1 mg slow IV bolus or IM every 2–5 minutes to a total dose of 10 mg.
(Seizures): < 5 years: 0.2–0.5 mg slow IV bolus or IM every 2–5 minutes to a total dose of 5 mg.

How Supplied

Injection: 5 mg/mL.

Adverse Reactions and Side Effects

CNS: Dizziness, drowsiness, mental depression, headache.
Respiratory: Respiratory depression.
CV: Hypotension.
Local: Pain with IM injection; phlebitis with IV administration.
HEENT: Blurred vision, intraocular pressure in patients with narrow-angle glaucoma.

EMS Considerations

Diazepam may cause respiratory arrest if administered too rapidly or in excess doses. Do not mix diazepam with any other drug. Diazepam may react with the IV tubing. To minimize this, administer diazepam at the IV site, not higher in the tubing. Thoroughly flush the IV line before administering diazepam if other drugs have already been administered through the line. Assess the patient's vital signs continuously.

Drug Interactions

Additive CNS depression may occur if diazepam is administered with other CNS depressants, such as antihistamines, tricyclic antidepressants, alcohol, narcotics, or other sedatives or hypnotics.

FLUMAZENIL

(floo-MAZ-eh-nill)
Pregnancy Class: C
Romazicon (Rx)
Classification: Benzodiazepine antagonist, antidote

Mechanism of Action

Antagonizes the effects of benzodiazepines by inhibiting their action at the benzodiazepine receptor.

Indications

Management of benzodiazepine overdose.

Contraindications

Hypersensitivity to flumazenil or benzodiazepines; patients receiving benzodiazepines for life-threatening medical disorders, such as status epilepticus or increased intracranial pressure; serious cyclic antidepressant overdose, because of risk of seizures and arrthymias.

Precautions

Administration of flumazenil may result in seizures in certain high-risk patients, such as: concurrent sedative-hypnotic drug withdrawal, recent use of repeated doses of benzodiazepines, or a history of seizures; patients with mixed CNS depressant overdosage. The effects of the other agents may emerge when the effects of the benzodiazepine are reversed. Use with caution in patients with head injuries; flumazenil may increase the risk of intracranial pressure and seizures. Safety not established in pregnancy, lactation, or children less than 2 years.

Route and Dosage

Adults: 0.2 mg IV over 30 seconds. Additional doses of 0.5 mg may be given at 1-minute intervals. Maximum total dose of 3 mg.
For resedation: Repeated doses may be given every 20 minutes at no more than 0.5–1 mg/min. No more than 3 mg/h should be administered.
Pediatric: 0.01 mg/kg IV (maximum dose of 0.2 mg) over 30 seconds. Maximum cumulative dose of 1 mg.

How Supplied

Injection: 0.1 mg/mL.

Adverse Reactions and Side Effects

CNS: Seizures, dizziness, agitation, confusion, headache.
CV: Arrhythmias, chest pain, hypertension.
GI: Nausea, vomiting, hiccups.
Dermatologic: Flushing, sweating.
Local: Phlebitis.
HEENT: Abnormal hearing, blurred vision.
Miscellaneous: Rigors, shivering.

EMS Considerations

The smallest effective dose should be used. If the patient has not responded 5 minutes after receiving a cumulative dose of 5 mg, the major cause of sedation is probably not from benzodiazepines. Additional doses are likely to have no effect. The duration of effect of a benzodiazepine may exceed that of flumazenil; observe closely for resedation and redose if needed. Before administering flumazenil, have a secure airway and IV access. Patients should be awakened gradually. Be prepared for patients attempting to remove airway or IV access while awakening.

Drug Interactions

None.

NALOXONE

(nal-OX-ohn)
Pregnancy Class: B
Narcan (Rx)
Classification: Narcotic antagonist

Mechanism of Action

Combines with narcotic receptors and blocks or reverses the action of narcotic analgesics, including CNS and respiratory depression.

Indications

Treatment of symptomatic narcotic overdose. May be administered as a diagnostic tool in coma of unknown origin.

Contraindications

Hypersensitivity to naloxone.

Precautions

Use cautiously in patients with: cardiovascular disease; physical dependence on narcotics, because **withdrawal symptoms** may occur; head injury, or increased intracranial pressure; history of seizures, because naloxone may cause seizures; neonates of narcotic-dependent mothers.

Route and Dosage

Adult: 0.4–2 mg by slow IV bolus, IM, ET, or SQ. Can be *given intra-nasally at 2 mg. Pediatric (<5 years):* 0.1 mg/kg IV,

ET, IM, or SQ. May be repeated q 2–3 minutes. Pediatric (>5 years): 2 mg IV, ET, IM, or SQ.

How Supplied

Injection: 0.02 mg/mL, 0.4 mg/mL, 1 mg/mL.

Adverse Reactions and Side Effects

CV: Hypertension or hypotension, ventricular tachycardia, ventricular fibrillation.
GI: Nausea, vomiting.

EMS Considerations

The duration of action of naloxone is shorter than that of narcotics; repeated doses of naloxone may be necessary. Monitor vital signs and ECG continuously. Naloxone may be administered IM, SC, or by ETT if IV access cannot be obtained.

Drug Interactions

May precipitate withdrawal symptoms in patients physically dependent on narcotics. Larger than usual doses may be required to reverse the effects of buprenorphine, butorphanol, nalbuphine, pentazocine, or propoxyphene.

NITROGLYCERIN

(nye-tro-GLIH-ser-in)
Pregnancy Class: C
Nitro-Bid, Nitro-Dur, Nitromist, NitroQuick, Nitrostat (Rx)
Classification: Antianginal

Mechanism of Action

Increases coronary blood flow by dilating coronary arteries. Reduces myocardial oxygen consumption.

Indications

Given for myocardial ischemia associated with cocaine intoxication.

Contraindications

sensitivity to nitrates or patients taking medications for erectile dysfunction.

Precautions

Use cautiously in patients with head trauma or cerebral hemorrhage, glaucoma, or severe liver impairment.

Route and Dosage

Adults:
  SL Tablets: 0.3 to 0.4 mg (1 tablet) q 5 minutes to a maximum of 3 doses.
  Translingual spray: 0.4 mg (1 spray) q 5 minutes to a maximum of 3 sprays.

IV Bolus: 12.5 to 25 mcg.
IV Infusion: 5 mcg/minute. Rate may be increased by 5 to 10 mcg/min q 5 to 10 minutes as necessary.
Pediatric IV Infusion: Initial infusion is 0.25 to 0.5 mcg/kg/minute. This may be adjusted by medical control as necessary.

How Supplied

SL tablets: 0.3 mg, 0.4 mg, 0.6 mg.
Translingual spray: 400 mcg/spray.
Injection: 5 mg/mL
Premixed solution: 25 mg/250 mL, 50 mg/250 mL, 50 mg/500 mL, 100 mg/250 mL, 200 mg/500 mL.

Adverse Reactions and Side Effects

CV: hypotension, tachycardia, syncope.
CNS: headache, dizziness, restlessness, weakness.
GI: abdominal pain, nausea, vomiting.

EMS Considerations

Administration to a patient with right ventricular MI may result in hypotension.

Drug Interactions

Concurrent use with nirates in any form may result in serious or fatal hypotension. Additive hypotensive effects may occur if given in patients taking antihypertensives, beta-blockers, or calcium channel blockers.

OXYGEN

(OX-ah-gin)
Classification: Medicinal gas

Mechanism of Action

Oxygen is required to enable cells to break down glucose into a usable energy form. Oxygen is a colorless, odorless, tasteless gas, essential to respiration. At sea level, oxygen makes up approximately 10–16% of venous blood and 17–21% of arterial blood. Oxygen is carried from the lungs to the body's tissues by hemoglobin in the red blood cells. The administration of oxygen increases arterial oxygen tension and hemoglobin saturation. This improves tissue oxygenation when circulation is adequately maintained. Oxygen is administered in carbon monoxide poisoning to displace carbon monoxide molecules from hemoglobin.

Indications

Treatment of various poisonings and overdosages to prevent or treat hypoxemia.

Contraindications

None, for emergency use.

Precautions

May depress respirations in patients with chronic obstructive pulmonary disease.

Route and Dosage

Adults and Pediatrics (Inhalation): There are several devices used to administer oxygen, including masks, nasal cannulas, positive pressure devices, and volume-regulated ventilators. Some of the more common oxygen devices and their delivery capabilities include:

- *Nasal cannula:* Oxygen concentrations of 24–44% at flow rates of 1–6 L/min.
- *Simple face mask:* Oxygen concentrations of 40–60% at flow rates of 8–10 L/min.
- *Face mask with oxygen reservoir:* Oxygen concentrations of 60% at a flow rate of 6 L/min. An oxygen concentration of almost 100% can be achieved with a flow rate of 10 L/min.
- *Venturi mask:* Oxygen concentrations of 24% at 4 L/min, 28% at 4 L/min, 35% at 8 L/min, 40% at 8 L/min.
- *Mouth-to-mask:* With supplemental oxygen at 10 L/min, oxygen concentration can reach 50%. Without supplemental oxygen, concentration reaches only approximately 17%.

How Supplied

As a compressed gas in cylinders of varying size.

Adverse Reactions and Side Effects

Respiratory: In some cases of chronic obstructive pulmonary disease, oxygen administration may reduce respiratory drive. This is not a reason to withhold oxygen, but be prepared to assist ventilations.

Miscellaneous: Oxygen that is not humidified may dry or irritate mucous membranes.

EMS Considerations

Use humidified oxygen whenever possible. Oxygen therapy may reduce respiratory drive in patients with chronic obstructive pulmonary disease. Be prepared to assist ventilations. If it is indicated, oxygen therapy should never be withheld. Reassure patients who are anxious about face masks but who require high concentrations of oxygen.

Drug Interactions

None.

PHENTOLAMINE

(fen-TOLE-a-meen)
Pregnancy Class: C
Oraverse, Regitine (Rx)
Classification: Alpha-adrenergic blocker, Antihypertensive

Mechanism of Action

Causes hypotension by direct relaxation of vascular smooth muscle and by alpha blockade.

Indications

Hypertensive emergencies caused by pheochromocytoma, or cocaine-induced vasospasm of the coronary arteries.

Contraindications

Do not use in patients with coronary or cerebral arteriosclerosis or in patients with renal impairment.

Precautions

Use cautiously in patients with peptic ulcer disease.

Route and Dosage

Hypertensive Emergency
    Adults: 5–15 mg IV or IM.
    Pediatric: Not recommended.
Cocaine-induced Vasospasm
    Adult: 5 mg IV or IM.
    Pediatric: Not recommended.

How Supplied

Powder for Injection: 5 mg/vial.

Adverse Reactions and Side Effects

CV: hypotension, angina, arrhythmias.
CNS: cerebrovascular spasm, weakness, dizziness.
GI: abdominal pain, diarrhea, nausea, vomiting.

EMS Considerations

None.

Drug Interactions

Antagonizes the effects of alpha-adrenergic stimulant drugs.

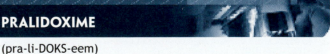

PRALIDOXIME

(pra-li-DOKS-eem)
Pregnancy Class: C
Protopam (Rx)
Classifications: -Antidote (organophosphate poisoning), anticholinesterase inhibitor

Mechanism of Action

Reactivates cholinesterase that has been inactivated by organophosphate poisoning or anticholinesterase overdose. Results in reversal of respiratory paralysis and paralysis of skeletal muscle.

Indications

Pralidoxime is administered after atropine in severe cases of organophosphate poisoning and for the treatment of anticholinesterase overdose.

Contraindications

Hypersensitivity to pralidoxime. Do not administer to patients who have been poisoned by inorganic phosphates.

Precautions

Use cautiously in patients with myasthenia gravis, because it may precipitate myasthenic crisis. Dosage reduction may be necessary for patients with impaired renal function, because the drug may accumulate to toxic concentrations.

Route and Dosage

Adults (Organophosphates): 1–2 g by IV infusion over 30–60 minutes after atropine administration. Dose may be repeated in one hour if muscle paralysis is still present. Additional doses may be given every 3–8 hours. Administer 600 mg IM if IV access cannot be obtained. May be repeated twice at 15-minute intervals if needed.
Anticholinesterase overdose: 1–2 g by IV infusion over 30–60 minutes. Then 250 mg every 5 minutes as needed.
Pediatrics (Organophosphates): 20–40 mg/kg by IV infusion over 30–60 minutes. Dose may be repeated in one hour if muscle paralysis is still present. Additional doses may be given every 3–8 hours. May administer IM or SC if IV access cannot be obtained.

How Supplied

Powder for injection: 1 g/20 mL vial.
Auto-injector (for IM use): 600 mg/2 mL.

Adverse Reactions and Side Effects

CNS: Dizziness, drowsiness, headache.
Respiratory: Laryngospasm, hyperventilation.
CV: Tachycardia.
GI: Nausea.
Dermatologic: Rash.
Local: Pain with IM injection.
HEENT: Blurred vision, double vision.
Miscellaneous: Muscle rigidity, muscle weakness, neuromuscular blockade.

EMS Considerations

Rapid administration may cause tachycardia, laryngospasm, or muscle rigidity. Draw a blood sample for red blood cell and cholinesterase evaluation before giving pralidoxime.

Drug Interactions

Avoid concurrent use with succinylcholine, morphine, aminophylline, theophylline, and respiratory depressants, including: barbiturates, narcotic analgesics, and sedative-hypnotics.

SODIUM BICARBONATE

(SO-dee-um bye-KAR-bon-ayt)
Pregnancy Class: C
Classifications: Hydrogen ion buffer, urine alkalinizer

Mechanism of Action

Buffers excess acid to assist returning the blood to a physiologic pH, in which normal metabolic processes work more effectively. Sodium bicarbonate is excreted in the urine resulting in an alkalinized pH of the urine that causes increased urinary elimination of some drugs, such as barbiturates and aspirin.

Indications

Treatment of metabolic acidosis in certain poisonings or overdoses, such as ethylene glycol (antifreeze), aspirin, and methanol. To promote urinary excretion of some drugs taken in overdoses such as barbiturates and aspirin.

Contraindications

Should not be administered to patients with metabolic or respiratory alkalosis, hypocalcemia, excessive chloride loss, as an antidote following ingestion of strong mineral acids, untreated hypokalemia, or patients who cannot tolerate high sodium loads.

Precautions

Use with caution in patients with congestive heart failure and renal failure.

Route and Dosage

Adults: 2–5 mEq/kg by IV infusion over 4–8 hours.
Pediatrics: Same.

How Supplied

Solution for injection: 4.2% (0.5 mEq/mL), 5% (0.6 mEq/mL), 7.5% (0.9 mEq/mL), 8.4% (1 mEq/mL).

Adverse Reactions and Side Effects

CV: Edema.
Local: Irritation at IV site.
Fluids and electrolytes: Metabolic alkalosis, hypernatremia, hypocalcemia, hypokalemia, sodium and water retention.

EMS Considerations

Monitor the patient closely for the development of fluid overload (rales, peripheral edema, pink and frothy sputum).

Drug Interactions

Sodium bicarbonate may inactivate catecholamines. Sodium bicarbonate will form a precipitate with calcium agents. Do not mix together.

SODIUM NITRITE

(SO-dee-um NY-tryt)
Pregnancy Class: X
Classification: Cyanide poisoning adjunct

Mechanism of Action

Sodium nitrite reacts with hemoglobin to form methemoglobin. Methemoglobin reacts with cyanide causing the cyanide to be chemically bound, which prevents it from having any toxic effect. Subsequent administration of sodium thiosulfate produces thiocyanate, which is excreted in the urine, thereby detoxifying the body. Sodium nitrite degrades cyanide in cases of cyanide poisoning.

Indications

Sodium nitrite is the second of a 3-step treatment protocol for cyanide poisoning. It should be preceded by amyl nitrite and followed by sodium thiosulfate.

Contraindications

None.

Precautions

Sodium nitrite is a strong vasodilator. If administered too rapidly, it could cause significant hypotension.

Route and Dosage

Adult: 300 mg (one 10-mL ampule of a 3% solution) after amyl nitrite inhalation. Administer either by slow IV bolus over 5 min or by diluting the 300 mg in 50–100 mL of normal saline and infusing slowly, monitoring blood pressure closely.
Pediatric: 0.15–0.33 mL/kg by slow IV bolus.

How Supplied

Injection: 3% (300 mg/10 mL) solution.

Adverse Reactions and Side Effects

Cardiovascular: Hypotension, tachycardia, fainting.
Gastrointestinal: Nausea, vomiting.

EMS Considerations

Monitor blood pressure during the administration of sodium nitrite. Excessive doses of sodium nitrite may cause methemoglobinemia and death. Methemoglobinemia occurs when more than 1% of the hemoglobin in the blood has been oxidized to the ferric form. Oxidized hemoglobin is incapable of transporting oxygen. Signs of methemoglobinemia include cyanosis, vomiting, shock, and coma.

Drug Interactions

Not applicable.

SODIUM THIOSULFATE

(SO-dee-um thye-oh-SUL-fate)
Pregnancy Class: C
Classification: Cyanide poisoning adjunct

Mechanism of Action

Sodium thiosulfate converts cyanide to the less toxic thiocyanate. The thiocyanate is then excreted in the urine and the body is detoxified.

Indications

Sodium thiosulfate is the third of a 3-step treatment protocol for cyanide poisoning. It should be preceded by amyl nitrite and sodium nitrite.

Contraindications

None.

Precautions

None.

Route and Dosage

Adult: 12.5 g by slow IV bolus (one 50 mL ampule of a 25% solution).
Pediatric: 1.65 mL/kg of a 25% solution by slow IV bolus.

How Supplied

Injection: 25% (12.5 g/50 mL) solution.

Adverse Reactions and Side Effects

None have been reported.

EMS Considerations

If the clinical response to treatment is inadequate, administer a second dose of both sodium nitrite and sodium thiosulfate at half the initial doses, 30 min after the initial doses.

Drug Interactions

Not applicable.

CONCLUSION

Toxicologic emergencies are becoming more and more common in out-of-hospital emergency care. Patients who are experiencing either poisoning or overdose emergencies should be treated symptomatically. The initial out-of-hospital management of toxicologic emergencies should include management of the ABCs, the administration of oxygen, the establishment of an IV line, and placing the patient on a cardiac monitor.

Management of poisoning emergencies includes identifying the poison, attempting to slow or stop the absorption process, and administrating an antidote. Management of overdose emergencies is aimed at stabilizing the ABCs and in some cases antidotes.

STUDY QUESTIONS

1. Amyl nitrite is indicated in the treatment of:
   a. Organophosphate poisoning
   b. Cyanide poisoning
   c. Narcotic overdose
   d. Anticholinergic poisoning

2. The initial adult dose for amyl nitrite is:
   a. 1–2 mL
   b. 0.5–1 mL
   c. 0.3–0.6 mL
   d. 0.1–0.3 mL

3. Activated charcoal is used in the treatment of certain cases of poisoning and overdoses. The use of activated charcoal is contraindicated if the patient has taken:
   a. Aspirin
   b. Phenytoin
   c. Acetaminophen
   d. Cyanide

4. The two main uses for atropine in the out-of-hospital setting are to treat symptomatic bradycardia and to treat:
   a. Narcotic overdose
   b. Organophosphate poisoning
   c. Cyanide poisoning
   d. Ethanol poisoning

5. Medical control has ordered you to administer 1 mg of atropine by IV bolus to an adult patient suffering from organophosphate poisoning. If there is no improvement, the repeat dosage of atropine is:
   a. 1/2 the original dose
   b. 1 mg
   c. 2–5 mg
   d. 5–10 mg

6. Naloxone is classified therapeutically as a(n):
   a. Emetic
   b. Cyanide poisoning adjunct
   c. Cholinesterase poisoning antidote
   d. Narcotic antagonist

7. The initial dose for naloxone to treat a patient in a coma of unknown cause is:
   a. 10 mg
   b. 2–4 mg
   c. 0.4–2 mg
   d. 0.4 mg/kg

8. If a patient is overdosed with physostigmine during treatment, _____ can be used as an antidote.
   a. Naloxone
   b. Pralidoxime
   c. Syrup of ipecac
   d. Atropine

9. Your pediatric patient is suffering from a severe case of organophosphate poisoning. Medical control instructs you to give the patient atropine. While you are en route to the emergency department, medical control instructs you to administer pralidoxime. How would you administer the pralidoxime?
   a. 1–2 g by IV infusion over 30–60 min
   b. 20–40 mg/kg by IV infusion over 30–60 min
   c. 1 mg by IV bolus. Repeat every 2–3 min as needed
   d. 20–40 g/kg by IV infusion over 30–60 min

10. Which of the following is a potential adverse effect of acetylcysteine?
    a. Increased respiratory secretions
    b. Insomnia
    c. Diarrhea
    d. Hypotension

11. Flumazenil is used in the treatment of:
    a. Phenobarbital overdose
    b. Narcotic overdose
    c. Aspirin overdose
    d. Benzodiazepine overdose

12. Your patient has overdosed on an unknown amount of cocaine. She is experiencing severe chest pain. The physician orders you give your patient phentolamine. The initial dose is:
    a. 5–15 mg IV
    b. 5 mg IV or IM
    c. 15 mg IV or IM
    d. 15 mg SQ

EXTENDED CASE STUDY

Overdose

Initial Response: EMS is dispatched to a "possible overdose." On arrival, an anxious mother directs EMS to her 17-year-old son's room. The patient is found on the bedroom floor; his level of consciousness is depressed and he is unable to speak coherently. His mother says that she has not noticed anything unusual concerning her son lately. In a rapid survey of the patient's room, you notice 4 empty beer cans and an empty medication bottle labeled "Tofranil-PM, 50 mg. Take two tablets at bedtime."

Initial assessment of the patient reveals the following:
Level of consciousness: Conscious, disoriented, slurred speech.
Respirations: 16/min, shallow.
Pulse: 124 beats/min, regular.
Blood pressure: 122/84.
Skin: Warm, dry.
Pupils: Equal, do not respond to light.

Tofranil-PM is a tricyclic antidepressant (TCA) prescribed for various forms of depression, often in conjunction with psychotherapy. It has significant anticholinergic properties and increases the effect of norepinephrine. Tofranil-PM is often used in suicide attempts. Adverse reactions and side effects of Tofranil-PM include sedation, drowsiness, confusion, hypotension, convulsions, life-threatening cardiac arrhythmias, and coma.

The evidence of alcohol ingestion in conjunction with a TCA overdose means that this is truly an emergency situation. It is necessary to maintain the patient's airway and to administer oxygen. Establish an IV line using D_5W at a keep-open rate.

Do not administer syrup of ipecac to any patient who has taken an overdose of tricyclic drugs, even an alert patient.

An overdose of a TCA is sure to lead to a depressed level of consciousness, often very rapidly, even before the syrup of ipecac can have an effect.

Place the patient in the ambulance at this point, and continue treatment while en route to the emergency department.

On the way to the hospital, the patient develops seizure activity. EMS administers the drug of choice in this situation, physostigmine, while en route.

Indications for physostigmine in a TCA overdose include anticholinergic seizures, severe anticholinergic delirium, and severe anticholinergic movement disorders. Physostigmine is a cholinesterase inhibitor that can reverse the toxic effects of anticholinergic and tricyclic drugs. It produces generalized cholinergic responses, including bronchial constriction and bradycardia. In this case, the adult dose of physostigmine is 0.5–2 mg by slow IV bolus. If you cannot establish an IV, administer the drug IM. If the patient shows signs of physostigmine toxicity, you can administer atropine as an antidote.

While en route to the emergency department, medical control orders 2 mg of physostigmine. The only noticeable result of this dose is a decrease in the patient's heart rate to 100 beats/min. The lack of improvement in the patient's condition could be caused by his blood alcohol level, the possible ingestion of another drug, or hypoglycemia. It would not be inappropriate to administer 25 g (50 mL) of $D_{50}W$ to reverse possible hypoglycemia while still en route.

Out-of-hospital treatment of TCA overdose is symptomatic. Toxic symptoms such as cardiac arrhythmias, seizures, and congestive failure can occur rapidly. The patient must be transported rapidly to the emergency department.

CHAPTER 16

DRUGS USED TO TREAT BEHAVIORAL EMERGENCIES

Therapeutic Classifications of Drugs Used for Behavior Emergencies

Antianxiety Agents
Diazepam
Droperidol
Hydroxyzine

Antipsychotics
Chlorpromazine
Droperidol
Fluphenazine
Haloperidol

Sedatives
Droperidol
Hydroxyzine

Sedative/Hypnotic
Diazepam

OBJECTIVES

On completion of this chapter and the study questions, you should be able to:

- Describe in detail the basic principles to follow when treating a patient with a behavior emergency.
- Describe in detail the following antianxiety drugs: diazepam, droperidol, and hydroxyzine.
- Describe in detail the following antipsychotic drugs: chlorpromazine, droperidol, fluphenazine, and haloperidol.
- Describe in detail the following sedative drugs: droperidol and hydroxyzine.
- Describe in detail the sedative/hypnotic drug: diazepam.

KEY TERMS

Antipsychotic
Anxiety
Psychosis

CASE STUDIES

1. At 5:30 AM, EMS is called to the home of a man "not breathing." On arrival it is determined that the individual has been down too long, and resuscitative efforts should not be initiated. When the wife is told, she becomes hysterical. Attempts are made to calm her down, but nothing seems to help. After calming efforts fail, medical control is called and the situation is explained. The physician orders sedation and transport. Which drug(s) should the physician order for sedation?
   a. Chlorpromazine
   b. Haloperidol
   c. Diazepam
   d. Hydroxyzine

2. EMS is called to the home of an individual who has previously experienced psychotic episodes and seizures. On arrival, the patient is displaying bizarre and aggressive behavior. The more attempts are made to calm him down, the more aggressive he seems to become. Medical control is familiar with this patient, and instructs EMS to give him 25 mg of chlorpromazine to treat his psychosis. In this situation, what other drug should be readily available?
   a. Haloperidol
   b. Diazepam
   c. Hydroxyzine
   d. $D_{50}W$

INTRODUCTION

Many out-of-hospital emergency care professionals feel most uncomfortable and unprepared when treating patients in behavior emergencies. As a result, many EMS professionals are uncertain when faced with behavior emergencies. This uncertainty stems in part from the lack of behavior protocols for out-of-hospital use and in part from the knowledge that the outcome of a behavior emergency is not as predictable as that of trauma or other medical emergencies. The behavior emergency presents us with the most unpredictable scenarios and patient outcomes.

There are no definite presenting signs or symptoms for individuals with a behavior disorder. Basically a behavior "emergency" call is a result of anxiety or panic on the part of the patient, the patient's family, or bystanders. The problem for the responder is that abnormal behavior may stem from mental illness or some other condition. For example, drug or alcohol abuse, cerebrovascular accident, infection, and metabolic disorders—each can cause symptoms that appear to indicate a behavior or mental problem.

These are the basic principles to follow when treating an individual who shows signs of psychological or emotional disorder:

1. Clearly identify yourself, being as calm and direct as possible.
2. If possible, interview the patient alone, letting the individual tell his or her own story.
3. Provide honest reassurance, maintaining a nonjudgmental attitude.
4. Take a definite plan of action. This will help to relieve the patient's anxiety.
5. Never leave the patient alone, and never assume it is impossible to talk with the patient unless you have tried.

Only rarely do the most progressive EMS systems use pharmacologic interventions when treating behavior emergencies. Patient management is generally directed at supportive measures and the attempt to give the patient a feeling of friendly and secure surroundings.

There are, however, six drugs used in some out-of-hospital emergency care systems to treat patients in behavior emergencies: chlorpromazine, diazepam, droperidol, fluphenzaine, haloperidol, and hydroxyzine.

Individual Drugs

CHLORPROMAZINE

(klor-PROH-mah-zeen)
Pregnancy Class: C
Thorazine, (Rx)
Classification: Antipsychotic

Mechanism of Action

Blocks the effects of dopamine in the CNS; this results in decreasing the signs and symptoms of psychosis.

Indications

Treatment of acute psychotic episodes and mild alcohol withdrawal.

Contraindications

Hypersensitivity to chlorpromazine, phenothiazines, or sulfites. Do not use in patients with: narrow-angle glaucoma, severe cardiac disease, CNS depression, or patients who have taken hallucinogens.

Precautions

Chlorpromazine may lower the seizure threshold; use caution in administering to patients with seizure disorders.

Route and Dosage

Adult: psychoses or alcohol withdrawal: 25–50 mg IM initially. May be repeated in 1 hour.
Pediatric: psychoses: 0.55 mg/kg IM.

How Supplied

Injection: 25 mg/mL.

Adverse Reactions and Side Effects

CNS: Neuroleptic malignant syndrome, sedation, extrapyramidal reactions.
CV: Hypotension, tachycardia.
GI: Constipation, dry mouth.
GU: Urinary retention.
HEENT: Dry eyes, blurred vision.

EMS Considerations

Assess vital signs frequently, especially mental status, blood pressure, pulse, and respirations.

Drug Interactions

Additive hypotension may develop if chlorpromazine is used simultaneously with antihypertensives. Additive depression may develop if chlorpromazine is used with other CNS depressants. Additive anticholinergic effects may occur if chlorpromazine is used with other anticholinergic drugs.

DIAZEPAM

(dye-AYZ-eh-pam)
Pregnancy Class: D
Valium (Rx)
Classifications: Anticonvulsant, antianxiety agent, sedative/hypnotic

Mechanism of Action

Causes CNS depression producing relief of anxiety and sedation. Decreases seizure activity caused by enhanced presynaptic inhibition.

Indications

Treatment of generalized motor seizures and status epilepticus. Used as a sedative for out-of-hospital emergency treatment of severe anxiety.

Contraindications

Do not administer diazepam to patients with: hypersensitivity to diazepam, benzodiazepines, or propylene glycol; preexisting CNS depression; acute narrow-angle glaucoma; or pregnancy and lactation.

Precautions

Use caution in administering diazepam to patients with a history of suicide attempt or drug addiction. Administer lower than usual adult doses to elderly patients, because they are more sensitive to the drug's CNS effects. Use with caution in patients with hepatic dysfunction; effects may be more intense and prolonged.

Route and Dosage

Adults (antianxiety) IM or IV: 2–10 mg.
Adults (seizures/status epilepticus): 5–10 mg slow IV bolus. May repeat every 10–15 minutes as needed, to a total of 30 mg. May be administered IM if unable to obtain IV access.
Pediatric (antianxiety) IM or IV: 0.04–0.3 mg/kg/dose.
Pediatric (seizures/status epilepticus): >5 years: 1 mg slow IV bolus or IM every 2–5 minutes to a total dose of 10 mg. < 5 years: 0.2–0.5 mg slow IV bolus or IM every 2–5 minutes to a maximum dose of 5 mg.

How Supplied

Injection: 5 mg/mL.

Adverse Reactions and Side Effects

CNS: Dizziness, drowsiness, mental depression, headache.
Respiratory: Respiratory depression.
CV: Hypotension.
Local: Pain with IM injection. Phlebitis with IV administration.
HEENT: Blurred vision.

EMS Considerations

Diazepam may cause respiratory arrest if administered too rapidly or in excess doses. Do not mix diazepam with any other drug. Diazepam may react with the IV tubing; to minimize this administer diazepam at the IV site, not higher in the tubing. Thoroughly flush the IV line before administering diazepam if other drugs have already been administered through the line. Assess the patient's vital signs continuously.

Drug Interactions

Additive CNS depression may occur if diazepam is administered with other CNS depressants, such as antihistamines, tricyclic antidepressants, alcohol, narcotics, or other sedatives or hypnotics.

DROPERIDOL

(droe-PAIR-ih-dohl)
Pregnancy Class: C
Inapsine (Rx)
Classifications: Antianxiety agent, antipsychotic, sedative

Mechanism of Action

Blocks the effects of dopamine in the CNS; this decreases the signs and symptoms of psychoses and relieves anxiety and causes sedation.

Indications

Treatment of acute psychotic episodes. Used as a sedative for out-of-hospital emergency treatment of severe anxiety.

Contraindications

Hypersensitivity to droperidol or phenothiazines. Do not administer to patients with narrow-angle glaucoma, CNS depression, severe cardiac disease, or patients who have taken hallucinogens.

Precautions

Use caution when administering droperidol to patients with seizure disorders, because it may lower the seizure threshold.

Route and Dosage

Adults: 2.5 mg IM.
Pediatrics: Not recommended for out-of-hospital use.

How Supplied

Injection: 2.5 mg/mL.

Adverse Reactions and Side Effects

CNS: Seizures, extrapyramidal reactions, confusion, dizziness, sedation, hallucinations, mental depression.
Respiratory: Bronchospasm, laryngospasm.
CV: Hypotension, tachycardia.
GI: Constipation, dry mouth.
HEENT: Blurred vision, dry eyes.

EMS Considerations

Frequently assess vital signs.

Drug Interactions

Additive hypotension may occur with antihypertensive agents. Additive CNS depression may occur with other CNS depressants. Additive anticholinergic effects may occur with other anticholinergic drugs.

FLUPHENAZINE

(floo-FEN-a-zeen)
Pregnancy Class: C
Prolixin Decanoate (Rx)
Classification: Antipsychotic

Mechanism of Action

Alters the effects of dopamine in the CNS. Also has an anticholinergic and an alpha-adrenergic blocking effect.

Indications

Acute and chronic psychoses.

Contraindications

Known hypersensitivity, severe CNS depression, and concurrent use of medications that prolong the QT interval.

Precautions

Use with caution in patients with cardiovascular disease, Parkinson's disease, Angle-closure glaucoma, Myasthenia gravis, BPH, and seizure disorders.

Route and Dosage

Adults: 12.5–25 mg IM.
Pediatrics: Not recommended for out-of-hospital use.

How Supplied

25 mg/mL

Adverse Reactions and Side Effects

CV: hyper or hypotension, tachycardia.
CNS: sedation, extrapyramidal reactions.
EENT: blurred vision, dry eyes.
GI: anorexia, constipation, dry mouth, nausea.

EMS Considerations

None.

Drug Interactions

Concurrent use with antiarrhythmics should be avoided. May be additive CNS depression if used with other antidepressants.

HALOPERIDOL

(hah-low-PAIR-ih-dohl)
Pregnancy Class: C
Haldol (Rx)
Classification: Antipsychotic

Mechanism of Action

Blocks the effects of dopamine in the CNS; this decreases the signs and symptoms of psychoses.

Indications

Treatment of acute and chronic psychoses.

Contraindications

Hypersensitivity to haloperidol or phenothiazines. Do not administer to patients with CNS depression, severe cardiac disease, or narrow-angle glaucoma.

Precautions

Use caution in administering haloperidol to patients with seizure disorders, because the drug may lower the seizure threshold.

Route and Dosage

Adult: 2–5 mg IM, or 0.5–5 mg IV.
Pediatric: Haloperidol is not recommended for pediatric patients in the out-of-hospital setting.

How Supplied

Injection: 5 mg/mL.

Adverse Reactions and Side Effects

CNS: Seizures, sedation, confusion, restlessness, extrapyramidal reactions, neuroleptic malignant syndrome.
Respiratory: Respiratory depression.
CV: Hypotension, tachycardia.
GI: Constipation, dry mouth.
GU: Urinary retention.
Local: Pain with IM injection.

EMS Considerations

Assess patient's mental status, blood pressure, pulse, and respirations before and frequently after drug administration.

Drug Interactions

Haloperidol use with antihypertensives or nitrates may produce additive hypotension. Use with other CNS depressants may cause additive CNS depression. Using haloperidol with anticholinergics may cause additive anticholinergic effects. Phenobarbital may decrease the effectiveness of haloperidol.

HYDROXYZINE

(hy-DROX-ih-zeen)
Pregnancy Class: C
Vistaril (Rx)
Classifications: Antianxiety agent, sedative

Mechanism of Action

Causes CNS depression through suppression of activity at the subcortical levels in the brain. Relieves anxiety and causes sedation.

Indications

Treatment of anxiety.

Contraindications

Hypersensitivity to hydroxyzine. Do not use in pregnancy.

Precautions

Use caution when administering hydroxyzine to elderly patients; use less than adult dosages.

Route and Dosage

Adult: 25–100 mg deep IM.
Pediatric: 0.5–1.0 mg/kg deep IM.

How Supplied

Injection: 25 mg/mL, 50 mg/mL.

Adverse Reactions and Side Effects

CNS: Drowsiness, dizziness, weakness, headache.
Respiratory: Wheezing, chest tightness.
GI: Dry mouth, nausea.
GU: Urinary retention.
Dermatologic: Flushing.
Local: Pain with IM injection, abscess at IM site.

EMS Considerations

Administer hydroxyzine deep into well-developed muscle to prevent subcutaneous tissue infiltration. Inadvertent injection into the subcutaneous tissue may cause tissue damage.

Drug Interactions

Additive CNS depression may occur if hydroxyzine is used with other CNS depressants, antidepressants, antihistamines, narcotics, or sedative/hypnotics. Additive anticholinergic effects may occur if hydroxyzine is used with other drugs that have anticholinergic properties.

CONCLUSION

Patients who present with irrational behavior may do so because of disease or injury process, not because of mental illness. For example, head injury, drug abuse, or a severe diabetic episode can lead to behavior suggestive of a psychotic disorder. If possible, the patient who presents with psychotic behavior should be assessed for other medical or physical causes. For example, giving an antipsychotic drug to an individual suffering from an overdose of crack cocaine would not help and could be harmful. If the patient's problem is in fact of psychiatric origin, treat the patient appropriately.

It is more appropriate to give antipsychotic drugs in the hospital setting, which is a more controlled environment. However, there may be occasions when out-of-hospital antipsychotic drug therapy is ordered before transport to an emergency facility is complete. As with any emergency situation, follow local protocols.

STUDY QUESTIONS

1. Chlorpromazine, droperidol, fluphenazine, and haloperidol are classified as antipsychotics, and their use is contraindicated for patients:
   a. In mild alcohol withdrawal
   b. With CNS depression
   c. With a history of acute psychotic episodes
   d. With a history of seizure disorders

2. The recommended adult dose for chlorpromazine is:
   a. 10–15 mg
   b. 15–20 mg
   c. 25–50 mg
   d. 50–100 mg

3. What dose of haloperidol would you expect medical control to order for an 11-year-old patient suffering from chronic psychosis?

   a. 0.55 mg/kg
   b. 2–5 mg
   c. 25 mg
   d. Not recommended

4. You have a pediatric patient who weighs 46 lb. Medical control instructs you to administer hydroxyzine to this patient for the treatment of anxiety. What dose of hydroxyzine would you give?
   a. 21 mg
   b. 30 mg
   c. 46 mg
   d. 101 mg

EXTENDED CASE STUDY

Psychotic Emergency

EMS responds to a local warehouse for a "man acting bizarre." While en route to the scene, it is requested that the police also respond.

On arrival, the warehouse foreman tells EMS that the patient is an excellent employee and has never before caused any problems. However, today he has been very loud, has broken several pieces of equipment, and has been rude to several of his fellow workers. He is now sitting quietly at a table in the corner. His wife is in the foreman's office, confused and scared.

Before making any attempt to approach the patient, try to obtain information about the patient from his wife. Family members can frequently provide some clues as to the nature of the patient's problem. The police can stand by (ideally out of sight) while EMS speaks with the patient's wife.

The patient's wife says that her husband has been under a lot of stress at work lately, because of increased project deadlines. He is 40, in good health, takes no medications, and has no history of psychiatric disorders.

It is very difficult for an out-of-hospital emergency care professional to eliminate probable causes of behavior emergencies in the out-of-hospital setting. It is not appropriate to draw any definite conclusions based solely on information gathered from history, which is often only suggestive at best.

Approach the patient with a suspected mental disorder in a slow, calm, deliberate manner. Calmly explain why you were called, and assure him or her that you are there to help in any way that you can.

It can be frustrating to try to communicate with this type of patient, who may not be dealing with reality. A common-sense approach to the patient, combining reinforcement of factual information and reassurance, is recommended.

So far, the patient has exhibited no aggressive behavior. He allowed his vital signs to be taken; they are:

Level of consciousness: Alert, disoriented.
Respirations: 16 breaths/min.
Pulse: 82 beats/min, regular.
Blood pressure: 156/96.

There are no other obvious signs of trauma or medical problems.

While helping the patient to the ambulance, he suddenly goes into a grand mal seizure. The immediate course of action should be to protect the patient from injuring himself and to protect the airway during the seizure. The seizure is clonic and subsides after approximately 2 min. The patient remains unconscious. At this point, place the patient in the ambulance and administer humidified oxygen.

While en route to the hospital, the patient goes into another seizure, which also lasts approximately 2 min. Medical control orders an IV of NS at a keep-open rate and 5 mg of diazepam by slow IV bolus. If necessary, another 5 mg can be given.

Patients with mental disorders are rarely sedated in the out-of-hospital setting. In this case, the diazepam is primarily to help control seizure activity. Diazepam depresses the CNS, causing seizure activity to subside.

During transport, monitor the patient closely, be alert for any changes. The patient is still unconscious. His reflexes are normal, his vital signs are stable, and his pupils are equal and reactive.

Patients with mental disorders are usually difficult to manage. The role of the out-of-hospital emergency care professional is primarily supportive. Occasionally these patients exhibit aggressive behavior and may perceive you as a threat to their safety or an ally of their enemies. A calm, nonthreatening approach can work toward patient confidence, regardless of whether the patient is behaving aggressively or passively. Expressing a desire to help frequently produces positive results.

Patients who experience severe psychotic episodes in the out-of-hospital setting may require antipsychotic drugs such as chlorpromazine or haloperidol. These drugs block dopamine receptors in the brain associated with behavior and mood. The adult dose of chlorpromazine is 25 mg IM, and the adult dose of haloperidol is 2–5 mg, also IM. Although it is rare for these drugs to be administered in the out-of-hospital setting, it is important for you to be familiar with them, because you may administer them while working in the hospital setting.

In most cases when a mental disorder is suspected, quiet transport to the emergency department is called for. The siren can be disturbing for the patient, and it should not be used unless a life-threatening emergency exists.

CHAPTER 17

PAIN MANAGEMENT

Therapeutic Classifications of Drugs for Pain Management

Anti-Inflammatory Agent
Ketorolac

Antipyretic Agent
Ketorolac

Benzodiazepine
Midazolam

Medicinal Gas
Nitrous oxide-oxygen mixture

Non-Opioid Analgesics
Ketorolac
Nitrous oxide-oxygen mixture

Opioid Analgesics (Agonist)
Fentanyl citrate

Meperidine
Morphine

Opioid Analgesics (Agonist/ Antagonist)
Butorphanol
Nalbuphine

OBJECTIVES

On completion of this chapter and study questions, you should be able to:

- Describe in detail the anti-inflammatory, non-opioid analgesic, ketorolac.
- Describe in detail the benzodiazepine drug, midazolam.
- Describe in detail the medicinal gas, nitrous oxide-oxygen mixture.
- Describe in detail the following opioid analgesic agonists: fentanyl citrate, meperidine, and morphine.
- Describe in detail the following opioid analgesic agonists/antagonists: butorphanol and nalbuphine.

KEY TERMS

Analgesic
Opioid

Pain

Physical dependence

CASE STUDIES

1. EMS responds to a motor vehicle accident. The driver, a 40-year-old female, is complaining of wrist pain with obvious deformity, and head pain. In assessing the scene it is noted that the windshield is cracked from the impact by the driver's head. The most appropriate analgesic to administer at this time to relieve the patient's pain is:
   a. Morphine
   b. Nitrous oxide-oxygen mixture
   c. Butorphanol
   d. None

2. EMS is transporting a 20-year-old male with a femur fracture to the hospital. Nitrous oxide has been ordered to relieve the patient's pain. The patient has been receiving the medication for approximately 10 minutes when he falls asleep and his hand falls, pulling the mask away from his face. The appropriate action to take at this time is to:
   a. Attach the mask to the patient's face to continue administering the medication
   b. Administer morphine 5 mg IM because the patient is no longer able to self-administer nitrous oxide
   c. Administer naloxone to reverse the effects of nitrous oxide
   d. Continue to monitor the patient's vital signs, level of consciousness, and respiratory status

INTRODUCTION

Pain is probably the most common patient complaint encountered by EMS providers. Although pain management is not the initial priority in out-of-hospital patient care, it is an important aspect of patient management. Pain is an unpleasant sensation that disturbs a patient's comfort, thought, sleep, or normal daily activity. Pain is caused by an underlying disorder. Pain is considered to be the fifth vital sign; however, it is the most difficult to assess because of its subjective nature. A patient's presentation of pain and the manner by which the pain is dealt with widely vary. Some patients may be in a great amount of pain but not exhibit significant symptoms; while other patients may be very anxious and emotional. Pain may greatly affect the anxiety level of the patient and result in physical symptoms such as: tachypnea, tachycardia, and hypertension. EMS providers must have an understanding of the importance of pain management and its effect on the overall condition of the patient.

Overview of Analgesics

The analgesics presented in this chapter include a medicinal gas, a non-opioid analgesic, and opioid analgesics, including those with agonist and antagonist properties. The inhalational analgesic, nitrous oxide, is administered with oxygen. It provides very effective analgesia, equivalent in most patients to that provided by morphine. Nitrous oxide is self-administered by the patient. This allows for very safe administration, as the patient must achieve a good seal with the mask in order to receive the drug. When the patient becomes drowsy the mask will fall away and the administration of nitrous oxide will be discontinued.

The non-opioid analgesic, ketorolac, is a non-steroidal anti-inflammatory drug. Ketorolac has analgesic, anti-inflammatory, and antipyretic properties. Non-steroidal anti-inflammatory drugs interfere with the pathway of prostaglandin synthesis. Prostaglandins are primary mediators of inflammation and pain. Ketorolac has fewer effects on respiratory function, mental status, and blood pressure than the opioid analgesics. In addition, ketorolac does not possess addictive properties. Ketorolac may be the analgesic of choice when there is doubt as to whether the patient is actually in pain or is displaying drug-seeking behavior.

The opioid analgesics bind to opiate receptors in the CNS and alter the perception of and response to painful stimuli. Opioid antagonists compete with opioid agonists for receptor sites and reverse the effects of the opioid agonist, including sedation, respiratory depression, and hypotension. Some opioids possess both agonist and antagonist properties. These agents act as agonist at some receptors and antagonist at other receptors. Opioid agonists/antagonists have less potential for overdose than do agonists, alone; however, they do have the potential to cause opioid withdrawal in patients physically dependent on opioids. The equi-analgesic dosages of opioid analgesics are compared in Table 17–1. Dosage requirements vary with the severity of pain, individual response to pain, age, weight, and the presence of concomitant diseases. Pain management must be individualized for each patient based on the patient's reporting of pain and the symptoms exhibited, as well as the occurrence of adverse effects. An opioid antagonist, naloxone or nalmefene, should be readily available for administration should symptoms of opioid overdose occur.

Table 17–1 Dosages of Opioid Analgesics. (© Delmar/Cengage Learning)

Drug	Route	Average Dose (mg)	Average Duration (hr)
Butorphanol	IM, SC	3	3
Fentanyl	IV, IM, SC	0.2	1
Meperidine	IM, SC	100	3
Morphine	IM, SC	10	4
Nalbuphine	IM, SC	20	4

Individual Drugs

BUTORPHANOL TARTRATE

(byou-TOR-fah-nohl)
Pregnancy Class: C
Stadol, Stadol NS (C-IV) (Rx)
Classification: Opioid analgesic (agonist/antagonist)

Mechanism of Action

Binds to opiate receptors in the CNS, altering the perception of and response to painful stimuli. Produces generalized CNS depression. Butorphanol has partial antagonist properties.

Indications

Management of moderate to severe pain. Analgesia during labor.

Contraindications

Hypersensitivity to butorphanol. Do not administer to patients physically dependent on opioids because it may precipitate withdrawal, because of its antagonistic properties.

Precautions

Use with caution in patients with: head trauma, increased intracranial pressure, renal or hepatic dysfunction, pulmonary disease, or undiagnosed abdominal pain. Elderly patients are at an increased risk of side effects and should receive half the usual initial dose at twice the usual interval. Safety has not been established in pregnancy, lactation, or children less than eighteen years of age.

Route and Dosage

Adults (IM): 2 mg every 3–4 hours as needed.
Adults (IV): 1 mg administered over 3–5 minutes every 3–4 hours as needed.
Geriatric (IM, IV): 1 mg every 4–6 hours, increased as needed.
Adults (Nasal): 1 mg (1 spray in 1 nostril) initially. An additional dose may be given 60–90 minutes later. This sequence may be repeated in 3–4 hours.
Geriatric (Nasal): 1 mg (1 spray in 1 nostril) initially. An additional dose may be given 90–120 minutes later. This sequence may be repeated in 3–4 hours.
Pediatrics: Not approved for use.

How Supplied

Injection: 1 mg/mL, 2 mg/mL.
Intranasal solution: 10 mg/mL in 2.5-mL metered-dose spray pump (14–15 doses; 1 mg/spray).

Adverse Reactions and Side Effects

CNS: Confusion, dysphoria, hallucinations, sedation, headache.
Respiratory: Respiratory depression.
CV: Hypertension or hypotension, palpitations.
GI: Nausea, vomiting, constipation.
GU: Urinary retention.
Dermatologic: Sweating.
HEENT: Blurred vision, double vision.

EMS Considerations

Monitor vital signs and CNS status closely. Naloxone should be available should respiratory depression or overdose occur.

Drug Interactions

May produce severe, potentially fatal reactions when administered to patients receiving monoamine oxidase inhibitors; the initial dose of butorphanol should be reduced to 25% of the usual dose. Additive CNS depression may occur with alcohol, antidepressants, antihistamines, and sedative/hypnotics. May precipitate withdrawal in patients who are physically dependent on opioid analgesics or sedative/hypnotics.

FENTANYL CITRATE

(FEN-tah-nil)
Pregnancy Class: C
Sublimaze (C-II) (Rx)
Classification: Opioid analgesic

Mechanism of Action

Binds to opiate receptors in the CNS, altering the response to and perception of painful stimuli. Produces CNS depression.

Indications

Treatment of severe pain. Analgesic supplement to general anesthesia.

Contraindications

Hypersensitivity to fentanyl.

Precautions

Use cautiously in patients with head trauma, increased intracranial pressure, undiagnosed abdominal pain, pulmonary or hepatic disease, or cardiac disease. Safety has not been established in pregnancy, lactation or children less than two years of age.

Route and Dosage

Adults (>12 years): Sedation for procedures/analgesia: (IM, IV): 0.5–1 mcg/kg/dose. May repeat every 30–60 minutes, as needed. Adjunct to general anesthesia: (IM, IV): 2–50 mcg/kg.

Pediatrics (1–12 years): Sedation for procedures/analgesia: (IM, IV): 1–2 mcg/kg/dose. May repeat every 30–60 minutes, as needed. Adjunct to general anesthesia: (IM, IV): 2–50 mcg/kg.

How Supplied

Injection: 0.05 mg/mL.

Adverse Reactions and Side Effects

CNS: Confusion, paradoxical excitation, delirium, drowsiness, mental depression.
Respiratory: Respiratory depression.
CV: Arrhythmias, bradycardia, hypotension.
GI: Nausea, vomiting.
Dermatologic: Itching.
HEENT: Blurred vision, double vision.

EMS Considerations

Monitor vital signs and ECG continuously. Have naloxone available in the event of respiratory depression or overdose.

Drug Interactions

Avoid use in patients who have received monoamine oxidase inhibitors within the previous 14 days; concurrent use may produce unpredictable, potentially fatal reactions. Additive CNS and respiratory depression may occur with other CNS depressants including: alcohol, antihistamines, antidepressants, sedative/hypnotics, and other opioids.

KETOROLAC

(kee-toh-ROH-lack)
Pregnancy Class: C
Toradol, Toradol IM (Rx)
Classifications: Anti-inflammatory, antipyretic, non-opioid analgesic

Mechanism of Action

Inhibits prostaglandin synthesis producing peripherally mediated analgesia. Provides anti-inflammatory and antipyretic effects.

Indications

Management of severe, acute pain.

Contraindications

Hypersensitivity to ketorolac or other non-steroidal anti-inflammatory drugs; intolerance to alcohol.

Precautions

Use cautiously in patients with a history of GI bleeding or cardiovascular disease. Patients with renal impairment require reduced dosages. Do not administer during the second half of pregnancy or to children.

Route and Dosage

Adults (IM-Single dose): <65 years: 60 mg IM; >65 years, renal impairment, or weight less than 50 kg: 30 mg IM.
Adults (IM-Multiple doses): <65 years: 30 mg IM every 6 hours. Not to exceed 120 mg/day; >65 years, renal impairment, or weight <50 kg: 15 mg IM every 6 hours. Not to exceed 60 mg/day.
Adults (IV-Single dose): <65 years: 30 mg IV; >65 years, renal impairment, or weight <50 kg: 15 mg IV.
Adults (IV-Multiple doses): <65 years: 30 mg IV every 6 hours. Not to exceed 120 mg/day; >65 years, renal impairment, or weight <50 kg: 15 mg IV every 6 hours. Not to exceed 60 mg/day.

How Supplied

Injection: 15 mg/mL, 30 mg/mL.

Adverse Reactions and Side Effects

CNS: Drowsiness, dizziness, headache.
Respiratory: Asthma, dyspnea.
CV: Edema, vasodilation.
GI: GI bleeding, diarrhea, dyspepsia, nausea.
GU: Renal toxicity.
Dermatologic: Pruritis, sweating, pallor.
Local: Pain at injection site.

EMS Considerations

IV doses should be given slowly over no less than 15 seconds. IM injections should be given slowly, deep into the muscle.

Drug Interactions

Additive GI effects may occur with concurrent use of aspirin, other non-steroidal anti-inflammatory drugs, potassium supplements, glucocorticoids, or alcohol.

MEPERIDINE

(meh-PER-ih-deen)
Pregnancy Class: C
Demerol, (C-II) (Rx)
Classification: Opioid analgesic

Mechanism of Action

Binds to opiate receptors in the CNS; which alters the perception of and response to painful stimuli. Produces generalized CNS depression.

Indications

Treatment of moderate to severe pain.

Contraindications

Hypersensitivity to meperidine or bisulfites. Avoid use in patients who have received monoamine oxidase inhibitors within the previous 14 to 21 days.

Precautions

Use cautiously in patients with head trauma, increased intracranial pressure, undiagnosed abdominal pain, severe renal or hepatic dysfunction, or pulmonary disease. Elderly patients are at increased risk of side effects, so dosage reductions are recommended. Use cautiously in children, because of an increased risk of seizures caused by an accumulation of the metabolite, normeperidine.

Route and Dosage

Adults (IM, SC): 50 mg every 3–4 hours, as needed.
Pediatrics (IM, SC): 1–1.5 mg/kg every 3–4 hours, as needed.

How Supplied

Injection: 25 mg/mL, 50 mg/mL, 75 mg/mL, 100 mg/mL.

Adverse Reactions and Side Effects

CNS: Seizures, confusion, sedation, dysphoria, hallucinations, headache.
Respiratory: Respiratory depression.
CV: Hypotension, bradycardia.
GI: Nausea, vomiting, constipation.
GU: Urinary retention.
Dermatologic: Flushing, sweating.

EMS Considerations

Monitor vital signs closely. Have naloxone available to reverse respiratory depression or overdose.

Drug Interactions

Avoid use in patients who have received monoamine oxidase inhibitors within the previous 14 to 21 days, because of the risk of potential fatal reactions. Additive CNS depression may occur with alcohol, antihistamines, sedative/hypnotics, or other opioid analgesics.

MIDAZOLAM

(mid-AY-zoe-lam)
Pregnancy Class: D
Versed (Rx)
Classification: benzodiazepine, antianxiety, sedative/hypnotic

Mechanism of Action

Produces generalized CNS depression, causing short-term sedation.

Indications

Provides sedation/anxiolysis/amnesia (conscious sedation) during therapeutic procedures.

Contraindications

Known hypersensitivity. Do not administer to patients with pre-existing CNS depression, uncontrolled severe pain, or acute-angle glaucoma.

Precautions

Use with caution in patients with pulmonary disease, CHF, renal impairment, severe hepatic impairment and in the obese patient (calculate dose at the ideal body weight).

Route and Dosage (Sedation in Critical Care Settings)

Adults: 0.01 to 0.05 mg/kg. May repeat q 10–15 minutes as necessary.

How Supplied

Injection: 1 mg/mL, 5 mg/mL.

Adverse Reactions and Side Effects

Resp.: apnea, respiratory depression, laryngospasm, coughing.
CV: arrhythmias, cardiac arrest.
CNS: headache, drowsiness, agitation.
GI: hiccups, nausea, vomiting.

EMS Considerations

Monitor BP closely. Administer the lowest possible dose, especially in the geriatric patient.

Drug Interactions

Increased CNS depression if used with antihistamines and other sedative/hypnotics. Increase risk of hypotension is used with antihypertensives, opioid analgesics, and nitrates.

MORPHINE

(MOR-feen)
Pregnancy Class: C
Astramorph, Avinza, DepoDur, Duramorph, Embeda (C-II) (Rx)
Classification: Opioid analgesic

Mechanism of Action

Binds to opiate receptors in the CNS, altering the perception of and response to painful stimuli. Produces generalized CNS depression.

Indications

Treatment of severe pain or pain associated with myocardial pain.

Contraindications

Hypersensitivity to morphine or bisulfites; intolerance to alcohol.

Precautions

Use cautiously in patients with head trauma, increased intracranial pressure, undiagnosed abdominal pain, severe renal or hepatic dysfunction, pulmonary disease, or a history of substance abuse. Elderly patients should receive reduced dosages, because of increased risk of side effects.

Route and Dosage

Adults >50 kg (IM, IV, SC): 4–10 mg every 3–4 hours.
Adults and Pediatrics <50 kg (IM, IV, SC): 0.05–0.2 mg/kg every 3–4 hours. Maximum dose = 15 mg.
For IV use, dilute 2–10 mg with at least 5 mL sterile water or NS and administer over 4–5 minutes.

How Supplied

Injection: 1 mg/mL, 2 mg/mL, 4 mg/mL, 5 mg/mL, 8 mg/mL, 10 mg/mL, 15 mg/mL, 25 mg/mL, 50 mg/mL.

Adverse Reactions and Side Effects

CNS: Confusion, sedation, dizziness, dysphoria, hallucinations, headache.
Respiratory: Respiratory depression.
CV: Hypotension, bradycardia.
GI: Nausea, vomiting, constipation.
GU: Urinary retention.
Dermatologic: Flushing, itching, sweating.
HEENT: Blurred vision, double vision, miosis.

EMS Considerations

Monitor vital signs continuously. Have naloxone available for administration to reverse respiratory depression and overdose.

Drug Interactions

The initial dose of morphine should be decreased to 25% of the usual dose in patients receiving monoamine oxidase inhibitors, because of the risk of unpredictable severe reactions. Additive CNS depression may occur with alcohol, sedative/hypnotics, antihistamines, and other opioid analgesics.

NALBUPHINE

(NAL-byou-feen)
Pregnancy Class: C
Nubain (Rx)
Classification: Opioid analgesic (agonist/antagonist)

Mechanism of Action

Binds to opiate receptors in the CNS, altering the perception of and response to painful stimuli. Has partial antagonist properties. Produces generalized CNS depression.

Indications

Moderate to severe pain.

Contraindications

Hypersensitivity to nalbuphine or bisulfites. Do not administer to patients physically dependent on opioids because it may precipitate withdrawal.

Precautions

Use cautiously in patients with head trauma, increased intracranial pressure, undiagnosed abdominal pain, severe renal or hepatic dysfunction, or pulmonary disease. Safety has not been established in pregnancy, lactation, or in children. Dosage reductions are recommended in elderly patients, because of an increased risk of side effects.

Route and Dosage

Adults (IM, SC, IV): 10 mg every 3–6 hours. A single dose should not exceed 20 mg. The total daily dose should not exceed 160 mg.
Pediatrics: Not recommended for use.

How Supplied

Injection: 10 mg/mL, 20 mg/mL.

Adverse Reactions and Side Effects

CNS: Dizziness, headache, sedation, confusion, hallucinations, dysphoria.
Respiratory: Respiratory depression.
CV: Hypertension or orthostatic hypotension, palpitations.
GI: Nausea, vomiting, constipation.
GU: Urinary urgency.
Dermatologic: Sweating.
HEENT: Blurred vision, double vision.

EMS Considerations

Monitor vital signs closely.

Drug Interactions

The dose of nalbuphine should be reduced to 25% of the usual dose in patients receiving monoamine oxidase inhibitors, because unpredictable, severe reactions may occur. Additive CNS depression may occur with concurrent use of alcohol, antihistamines, sedative/hypnotics, and other opioid analgesics.

NITROUS OXIDE-OXYGEN MIXTURE

(NYE-trus OX-ide)
Pregnancy Class: C
Nitronox, Entonox (Rx)
Classifications: Analgesic, medicinal gas

Mechanism of Action

Inhalation of a 50% mixture of nitrous oxide and oxygen produces CNS depression and rapid pain relief.

Indications

Treatment of moderate to severe pain.

Contraindications

Do not administer if any of the following exist: decreased level of consciousness, if the patient has taken a CNS depressant, thoracic trauma is present, respiratory compromise is present, cyanosis develops during administration, the patient is unable to follow simple instructions, the patient has sustained abdominal distention or trauma, or in pregnancy.

Precautions

Monitor the patient closely during administration. Some patients develop severe nausea and vomiting during administration.

Some patients experience syncope while receiving the medication.

Route and Dosage

Adult: Self-administration by the patient until pain is relieved.
Pediatric: Same.

How Supplied

A set containing an oxygen cylinder and a nitrous oxide cylinder joined by a valve that regulates flow to provide 20–50% of nitrous oxide concentration to oxygen. The mixture flows to a demand-valve apparatus.

Adverse Reactions and Side Effects

CNS: Lightheadedness, drowsiness.
Respiratory: Decreased respirations.
GI: Nausea, vomiting.

EMS Considerations

Patients with respiratory compromise should receive 100% oxygen to prevent nitrous oxide from collecting in dead air spaces and further aggravating chest injuries. Patients with myocardial pain should receive oxygen when the nitrous oxide-oxygen mixture is not being given. Do not administer a nitrous oxide-oxygen mixture to patients with abdominal pain unless it is certain that intestinal blockage is not present, because nitrous oxide may collect in the obstructed space, aggravating the obstruction.

Drug Interactions

Additive CNS depression may occur when other CNS depressants are administered.

CONCLUSION

The analgesics discussed in this chapter are very effective in alleviating pain. It is vital for EMS providers to understand when it is appropriate to administer analgesics. Analgesics should never be administered if they will preclude the correct diagnosis or assessment of the patient, such as head trauma or abdominal pain. Protocols for pain management vary widely among EMS systems. EMS providers should be aware of their local protocols.

STUDY QUESTIONS

1. Butorphanol and nalbuphine are opioid agonists/antagonists. They should not be administered to patients who are physically dependent on opioids because:
   a. Respiratory depression may occur
   b. Withdrawal may occur
   c. Hypotension may occur
   d. Loss of consciousness may occur

2. The appropriate initial dose of butorphanol for a 75-year-old female is:
   a. 2 mg IM every 3–4 hours as needed
   b. 1 mg IV every 3–4 hours as needed
   c. 0.5 mg IV every 4–6 hours as needed
   d. 1 mg IV every 4–6 hours as needed

3. Fentanyl is _____ times as potent as morphine.
   a. 50
   b. 1/5
   c. 5
   d. 2

4. The dose of ketorolac is dependent on all of the following *except*:
   a. Age
   b. Pain level
   c. Weight
   d. Renal function

5. Seizures may occur in children because of the accumulation of a metabolite of this drug:
   a. Morphine
   b. Fentanyl
   c. Ketorolac
   d. Meperidine

6. Adverse effects of morphine may include all of the following *except*:
   a. Diarrhea
   b. Respiratory depression
   c. Nausea
   d. Sedation

7. Patients receiving morphine while on monoamine oxidase inhibitors should:
   a. Receive a 25% increase in the usual dose of morphine
   b. Receive the usual dose of morphine
   c. Not receive morphine
   d. Receive a 25% decrease in the usual dose of morphine

8. The correct dosage of meperidine for a 5-year-old child is:
   a. 1–1.5 mg IM or SC every 3–4 hours
   b. 10 mg/kg IM or SC every 3–4 hours
   c. 1–1.5 mg/kg IM or SC every 3–4 hours
   d. 1–1.5 mg/kg IM or SC every 6–8 hours

9. Nitrous oxide-oxygen mixture is contraindicated in the following:
   a. Intestinal obstruction
   b. Myocardial infarction
   c. Pediatrics
   d. Chronic obstructive pulmonary disease

10. Which of the following analgesics has the potential adverse effect of GI bleeding?
    a. Morphine
    b. Ketorolac
    c. Nalbuphine
    d. Fentanyl

EXTENDED CASE STUDY

EMS receives a call to respond to a gym. A 60-year-old man has dropped a 50-pound weight on his foot and is complaining of severe pain. On examination, the foot has obvious deformity, swelling, and bruising.

Vital signs are as follows:
Respirations: 24/minute.
Pulse: 120/minute, regular.
BP: 180/92.

The patient weighs approximately 80 kg. After stabilizing the foot, an order is received to administer morphine. The appropriate dose for this patient is 4–8 mg IM or IV. This dose may be repeated every 3–4 hours. During transport the patient's vital signs, level of consciousness, and respiratory status should be continuously monitored. Nausea and vomiting are common with the administration of morphine. The EMS provider should be prepared should this occur. Keeping the patient still and lying down decreases the risk of nausea and vomiting. Antiemetics, such as promethazine or chlorpromazine, are frequently coadministered with morphine to prevent or treat nausea and vomiting. The EMS provider should have naloxone available to administer if signs or symptoms of opioid overdose occur. This may include loss of consciousness, respiratory depression, or hypotension. The appropriate dose of naloxone is 0.4–2 mg IV every 2–3 minutes as needed. The maximum total dose should not exceed 10 mg.

APPENDIX A

Drugs (Generic and Trade Names) and their Therapeutic Classifications*

Drug Name	Therapeutic Classification(s)	Drug Name	Therapeutic Classification(s)
A-Methapred (methylprednisolone)	Anti-inflammatory, immunosuppressant	alprazolam	Antianxiety agent—controlled substance, Schedule IV
Abeneton (biperiden)	Antiparkinsonian	Altace (ramipril)	Antihypertensive/ACE inhibitor
Accolate (zafirlukast)	Antiasthmatic	alteplase	Thrombolytic drug
acebutolol	Antihypertensive, antiarrhythmic	Alupent (metaproterenol)	Bronchodilator
Acephen (acetaminophen)	Non-narcotic analgesic, antipyretic	Alzapam (lorazepam)	Antianxiety agent, sedative/hypnotic—controlled substance, Schedule IV
acetaminophen	Non-narcotic analgesic, antipyretic	A-methapred (methylprednisolone)	Anti-inflammatory
acetazolamide	Anticonvulsant, diuretic	Aminophylline	Bronchodilator
acetohexamide	Antidiabetic	Amcill (ampicillin)	Antibiotic
acetophenazine	Antipsychotic	Aminophyllin (aminophylline)	Bronchodilator
Acetylcysteine	Antidote (acetaminophen)	aminophylline	Bronchodilator
Acetylsalicylic acid	Antiplatelet, analgesic	amiodarone	Ventricular and supraventricular antiarrhythmic
Activase (alteplase)	Thrombolytic drug		
Adalat (nifedipine)	Antianginal	amitriptyline	Antidepressant
Adapin (doxepin)	Antidepressant	amobarbital	Sedative/hypnotic, anticonvulsant—controlled substance, Schedule II
Adenosine	Antiarrhythmic		
Adrenalin Chloride (epinephrine	stimulant, local anesthetic adjunct, topical	Amodopa Tabs (methyldopa)	Antihypertensive
Bronchodilator, vasopressor, cardiac hydrochloride)	antihemorrhagic, antiglaucoma agent	Amoline (aminophylline)	Bronchodilator
Aerolate (theophylline)	Bronchodilator	amoxapine	Antidepressant
Akineton (biperiden)	Antiparkinsonian	amoxicillin	Antibiotic
Ak-Zol (acetazolamide)	Anticonvulsant, diuretic	Amoxil (amoxicillin)	Antibiotic
Alalat (nifedipine)	Antianginal	amphotericin B	Antifungal
Alazsine Tabs (hydralazine)	Antihypertensive	ampicillin	Antibiotic
albuterol	Bronchodilator	amrinone	Inotropic, vasodilator
albuterol/ipratropium	Combination bronchodilator	amyl nitrite	Cyanide poisoning adjunct
Aldactone (spironolactone)	Antihypertensive, diuretic	Amytal (amobarbital)	Sedative/hypnotic, anticonvulsant— controlled substance, Schedule II
Alphancaine (lidocaine)	Ventricular antiarrhythmic, local anesthetic		

*Drug names beginning with a capital letter are trade; drug names beginning with a lowercase letter are generic.

(continued)

Drug Name	Therapeutic Classification(s)
Anacin-3 (acetaminophen)	Non-narcotic analgesic, antipyretic
Anectine (succinylcholine chloride)	Depolarizing neuromuscular blocking drug
Anestucon (lidocaine)	Ventricular antiarrhythmic, local anesthetic
Ang-O-Span (nitroglycerin [oral])	Antianginal, vasodilator
anisoylated plasminogen strepto-kinase activator	thrombolytic
Anspor (cephradine)	Antibiotic
Antilirium (physostigmine)	Antimuscarinic
Apo-Amitriptyline (amitriptyline)	Antidepressant
Apresoline (hydralazine)	Antihypertensive
Aprozide (hydrochlorothiazide)	Diuretic, antihypertensive
Aquachloral (chloral hydrate)	Sedative/hypnotic—controlled substance, Schedule IV
Aquatensen (methyclothiazide)	Diuretic, antihypertensive
Arm-a-Med (isoetharine)	Bronchodilator
Asendin (amoxapine)	Antidepressant
Asthma Nefrin (epinephrine hydrochloride)	Bronchodilator, vasopressor, cardiac stimulant, local anesthetic adjunct, topical antihemorrhagic, antiglaucoma agent
AsthmaHaler (epinephrine bitartrate)	Bronchodilator, vasopressor, cardiac stimulant, local anesthetic adjunct, topical antihemorrhagic, antiglaucoma agent
Astromorph (morphine)	Analgesic—controlled substance, Schedule II
Atarax (hydroxyzine)	Antianxiety agent, sedative, anticholinergic, antiemetic, antihistamine
atenolol	Antihypertensive, antiarrhythmic
atracurium besylate	Nondepolarizing skeletal muscle relaxant
atropine	Antiarrhythmic, anticholinergic, antidote (cholinesterase inhibitors)
Atrovent (ipratropium)	Bronchodilator
Auto-Injector (lidocaine)	Ventricular antiarrhythmic, local anesthetic
Aventyl (nortriptyline)	Antidepressant
Azmacort (triamcinolone)	Corticosteroid
Bacampicillin	Antibiotic
Barbased (butabarbital)	Sedative/hypnotic—controlled substance, Schedule III
Barbita (phenobarbital)	Anticonvulsant, sedative/hypnotic— controlled substance, Schedule IV
beclomethasone	glucocorticoid

Drug Name	Therapeutic Classification(s)
Beclovent (beclomethasone)	Anti-inflammatory, antiasthmatic
Beconase (beclomethasone)	Anti-inflammatory, antiasthmatic
Beef Regular Iletin II	Antidiabetic agent (insulin [regular])
Beldin (diphenhydramine)	Antihistamine, antiemetic and antivertigo agent, antitussive, sedative/hypnotic, topical anesthetic
Benadryl (diphenhydramine)	Antihistamine, antiemetic and antivertigo agent, antitussive, sedative/hypnotic, topical anesthetic
Benadryl Children's Allergy (diphenhydramine)	Antihistamine, antiemetic and antivertigo agent, antitussive, sedative/hypnotic, topical anesthetic
Benadryl Complete Allergy (diphenhydramine)	Antihistamine, antiemetic and antivertigo agent, antitussive, sedative/hypnotic, topical anesthetic
Bendylate (diphenhydramine)	Antihistamine, antiemetic and antivertigo agent, antitussive, sedative/hypnotic, topical anesthetic
Benylin (diphenhydramine)	Antihistamine, antiemetic and antivertigo agent, antitussive, sedative/hypnotic, topical anesthetic
Benylin DM Cough (dextromethorphan)	Non-narcotic antitussive
benzphetamine	Anorexigenic agent
Beta$_2$ (isoetharine)	Bronchodilator
biperiden	Antiparkinsonian agent
Bisorine (isoetharine)	Bronchodilator
Bitolterol	Bronchodilator
Blocadren (timolol)	Antihypertensive, antiglaucoma agent
Brethine (terbutaline)	Bronchodilator
bretylium tosylate	Antiarrhythmic
Bretylol (bretylium)	Antiarrhythmic
Brevibloc (esmolol)	Antiarrhythmic (class II)/beta-blocker
Bricanyl (terbutaline)	Bronchodilator
Bromo-Seltzer (acetaminophen)	Non-narcotic analgesic, antipyretic
bromocriptine	Antiparkinsonian agent
Bronitin Mist (epinephrine bitartrate)	Bronchodilator, vasopressor, cardiac, stimulant, local anesthetic adjunct, topical antihemorrhagic, antiglaucoma agent
Bronkaid Mist (epinephrine)	Bronchodilator, vasopressor, cardiac stimulant, local anesthetic adjunct, topical antihemorrhagic, antiglaucoma agent
Bronkaid Mist Suspension (epinephrine bitartrate)	Bronchodilator, vasopressor, cardiac stimulant, local anesthetic adjunct, topical antihemorrhagic, antiglaucoma agent

Drug Name	Therapeutic Classification(s)
Bronkodyl (theophylline)	Bronchodilator
Bronkosol (isoetharine)	Bronchodilator
bumetanide	Antihypertensive, diuretic
Bumex	Antihypertensive, diuretic
butabarbital	Sedative/hypnotic—controlled substance, Schedule III
Butalan (butabarbital)	Sedative/hypnotic—controlled substance, Schedule III
Butatran (butabarbital)	Sedative/hypnotic—controlled substance, Schedule III
Buticaps (butabarbital)	Sedative/hypnotic—controlled substance, Schedule III
Butisol (butabarbital)	Sedative/hypnotic—controlled substance, Schedule III
butorphanol	Narcotic agonist-antagonist, opioid partial agonist analgesic
Calan (verapamil)	Antianginal, antiarrhythmic, antihypertensive
Capoten (captopril)	Antihypertensive
calcium chloride	Electrolyte modifier
calcium gluceptate	Electrolyte modifier
calcium gluconate	Electrolyte modifier
Capoten (captopril)	Antihypertensive/ACE inhibitor
captopril	Antihypertensive/ACE inhibitor
carbamazepine	Anticonvulsant, analgesic
carbenicillin	Antibiotic
Cardizem (diltiazem)	Antianginal
Catapres (clonidine)	Antihypertensive
Catapres-TTS (clonidine)	Antihypertensive
Ceclor (cefaclor)	Antibiotic
Cedilanid-D Injections (deslanoside)	Antiarrhythmic, inotropic
cefaclor	Antibiotic
Celontin Half Strength Kapseals (methsuximide)	Anticonvulsant
Celontin Kapseals (methsuximide)	Anticonvulsant
Centrax (prazepam)	Antianxiety agent—controlled substance, Schedule IV
cephradine	Antibiotic
chloral hydrate	Sedative/hypnotic—controlled substance, Schedule IV
Chlorpazine (prochlorpazine)	Antipsychotic, antiemetic, antianxiety agent
chlordiazepoxide	Antianxiety agent, anticonvulsant, sedative/hypnotic—controlled substance, Schedule IV
chlorothiazide	Diuretic, antihypertensive
chlorpromazine	Antipsychotic, antiemetic
chlorpropamide	Antidiabetic, antidiuretic agent
chlorprothixene	Antipsychotic
chlorthalidone	Diuretic, antihypertensive
Chlorzide (hydrochlorothiazide)	Diuretic, antihypertensive
Chlorzine (chlorpromazine)	Antipsychotic, antiemetic
Choledyl (oxtriphylline)	Bronchodilator
Cin-Quin (quinidine)	Ventricular and supraventricular antiarrhythmic, atrial antiarrhythmic
clemastine	Antihistamine
clonazepam	Anticonvulsant—controlled substance, Schedule IV
clonidine	Antihypertensive
clorazepate	Antianxiety agent, anticonvulsant, sedative/hypnotic—controlled substance, Schedule IV
codeine	Analgesic, antitussive—controlled substance, Schedule II
Combivent (albuterol/ipratropium)	Combination bronchodilator
Compazine (prochlorperazine)	Antipsychotic, antiemetic, antianxiety agent
Compazine Spansule (prochlorperazine)	Antipsychotic, antiemetic, antianxiety agent
Compoz (diphenhydramine)	Antihistamine, antiemetic and antivertigo agent, antitussive, sedative/hypnotic, topical anesthetic
Congesprin (dextromethorphan)	Non-narcotic antitussive
Constant-T (theophylline)	Bronchodilator
Cordarone (amiodarone)	Ventricular and supraventricular antiarrhythmic
Corgard (nadolol)	Antihypertensive, antianginal
Cortef (hydrocortisone)	Anti-inflammatory
Cortisol (hydrocortisone)	Anti-inflammatory
Coumadin (warfarin)	Anticoagulant
Covera HS (verapamil)	Antianginal, antiarrhythmic, antihypertensive
Cremacoat 1 (dextromethorphan)	Non-narcotic antitussive
Cromolyn sodium	Antiasthmatic, antiallergic
Crystodigin (digitoxin)	Antiarrhythmic agent, inotropic agent
Dalcaine (lidocaine)	Ventricular antiarrhythmic, local anesthetic
Dalmane (flurazepam)	Sedative/hypnotic—controlled substance, Schedule IV
Darvon (propoxyphene)	Analgesic—controlled substance, Schedule IV
Datril (acetaminophen)	Non-narcotic analgesic, antipyretic

(continued)

Drug Name	Therapeutic Classification(s)
Datril-500 (acetaminophen)	Non-narcotic analgesic, antipyretic
Decadron (dexamethasone)	Anti-inflammatory
Delsym (dextromethorphan)	Non-narcotic antitussive
Demerol (meperidine)	Analgesic—controlled substance, Schedule II
Depakene (valproic acid)	Anticonvulsant
desipramine	Antidepressant, antianxiety agent
deslanoside	Antiarrhythmic, inotropic
dexamethasone	glucocorticoid
dextromethorphan	Non-narcotic antitussive
dextrose 50% in water	Hyperglycemic antihypoglycemic
Dey-Dose (isoetharine)	Bronchodilator
Dey-Lute (isoetharine)	Bronchodilator
DiaBeta (glyburide)	Antidiabetic
Diabinese (chlorpropamide)	Antidiabetic, antidiuretic agent
Diachlor (chlorothiazide)	Diuretic, antihypertensive
Diahist (diphenhydramine)	Antihistamine, antiemetic, and antivertigo agent, antitussive, sedative/hypnotic, topical anesthetic
Diamox (acetazolamide)	Anticonvulsant, diuretic
Diamox Sequels (acetazolamide)	Anticonvulsant, diuretic
Diaqua (hydrochlorothiazide)	Diuretic, antihypertensive
diazepam	Antianxiety agent, skeletal muscle relaxant, amnesic agent, anticonvulsant, sedative/hypnotic
diazoxide	Antihypertensive, vasodilator
Didrex (benzphetamine)	Anorexigenic agent
digitoxin	Antiarrhythmic, inotropic
digoxin	Antiarrhythmic, inotropic
Dilantin (phenytoin)	Anticonvulsant, antiarrhythmic
Dilaudid (hydromorphone)	Analgesic, antitussive
Dilocaine (lidocaine)	Ventricular antiarrhythmic, local anesthetic
diltiazem	Antianginal, antiarrhythmic, antianginal, antihypertensive
Diphen (diphenhydramine)	Antihistamine, antiemetic, and antivertigo agent, antitussive, sedative/hypnotic
Diphen (diphenhydramine)	topical anesthetic
Diphenadril (diphenhydramine)	Antihistamine, antiemetic, antivertigo agent, antitussive, sedative/hypnotic, topical anesthetic

Drug Name	Therapeutic Classification(s)
diphenhydramine	Antihistamine, antiemetic, antivertigo agent, antitussive, anticholinergic sedative/hypnotic, topical anesthetic, anticholinergic
dipyridamole	Coronary vasodilator, platelet aggregation inhibitor
disopyramide	Ventricular/supraventricular antiarrhythmia, atrial antitachyarrhythmic
Dispos-a-Med (isoetharine)	Bronchodilator
Diuril (chlorothiazide)	Diuretic, antihypertensive
DM Cough (dextromethorphan)	Non-narcotic antitussive
dobutamine	Inotropic
Dobutrex (dobutamine)	Inotropic
Dolene (propoxyphene)	Analgesic—controlled substance, Schedule IV
Dolophine (methadone)	Analgesic, narcotic detoxification adjunct—controlled substance, Schedule II
dopamine	Inotropic, vasopressor
Dopastat (dopamine)	Inotropic, vasopressor
Doriden (glutethimide)	Sedative/hypnotic—controlled substance, Schedule III
Doriglute (glutethimide)	Sedative/hypnotic—controlled substance, Schedule III
Doxaphene (propoxyphene)	Analgesic—controlled substance, Schedule IV
doxepin	Antidepressant
droperidol	Antianxiety, antipsychotic sedative
Duramorph (morphine)	Analgesic—controlled substance, Schedule II
Durapam (flurazepam)	Sedative/hypnotic—controlled substance, Schedule IV
Dymelor (acetohexamide)	Antidiabetic
Edecrin (ethacrynic acid)	Diuretic
edrophonium	Antiarrhythmic, cholinergic agonist
Elavil (amitriptyline)	Antidepressant
Elixophyllin (theophylline)	Bronchodilator
Emitrip (amitriptyline)	Antidepressant
Enalapril	ACE inhibitor
Enalaprilat	vasodilator
Enalaprit	antihypertensive
Endep (amitriptyline)	Antidepressant
Enduron (methyclothiazide)	Diuretic, antihypertensive
Enovil (amitriptyline)	Antidepressant
Entonox (nitrous oxide-oxygen mixture)	Analgesic

Drug Name / Therapeutic Classification(s)

Drug Name	Therapeutic Classification(s)
Ephed II (ephedrine sulfate)	Adrenergic
ephedrine sulfate	Adrenergic
Epifrin (epinephrine hydrochloride)	Bronchodilator, vasopressor, cardiac stimulant, local anesthetic adjunct, topical antihemorrhagic, antiglaucoma agent adrenergic
epinephrine	Bronchodilator, vasopressor, cardiac stimulant, local anesthetic adjunct, topical antihemorrhagic, antiglaucoma agent
epinephrine bitartrate	Bronchodilator, vasopressor, cardiac stimulant, local anesthetic adjunct, topical antihemorrhagic, antiglaucoma agent
epinephrine hydrochloride	Bronchodilator, vasopressor, cardiac stimulant, local anesthetic adjunct, topical antihemorrhagic, antiglaucoma agent
EpiPen (epinephrine)	Bronchodilator, vasopressor, cardiac stimulant, local anesthetic adjunct, topical antihemorrhagic, antiglaucoma agent
EpiPen Jr. (epinephrine)	Bronchodilator, vasopressor, cardiac stimulant, local anesthetic adjunct, topical antihemorrhagic, antiglaucoma agent
Epitol (carbamazepine)	Anticonvulsant, analgesic
Epitrate (epinephrine bitartrate)	Bronchodilator, vasopressor, cardiac stimulant, local anesthetic adjunct, topical antihemorrhagic, antiglaucoma agent
Epsom Salts (magnesium sulfate)	Electrolyte
Equanil (meprobamate)	Antianxiety agent—controlled substance, Schedule IV
Esidrix (hydrochlorothiazide)	Diuretic, antihypertensive
Eskalith (lithium)	Antimanic, antipsychotic
Eskalith CR (lithium)	Antimanic, antipsychotic
esmolol	Antiarrhythmic (class II)/beta-blocker, beta adrenergic antagonist
ethacrynic acid	Diuretic
ethchlorvynol	Sedative/hypnotic—controlled substance, Schedule IV
ethosuximide	Anticonvulsant
Eutonil (pargyline)	Antihypertensive
Extentabs (quinidine)	Ventricular and supraventricular antiarrhythmic, atrial antiarrhythmic
fentanyl citrate	Opioid analgesic
Fenylhist (diphenhydramine)	Antihistamine, antiemetic, antivertigo agent, antitussive, sedative/hypnotic, topical anesthetic, anticholinergic
flecainide	Ventricular antiarrhythmic
Flovent (fluticasone propionate)	Corticosteroid
Flumazil	Benzodiazepine antagonist
Flumazenil	Benzodiazepine antagonist
fluphenazine	Antipsychotic
flurazepam	Sedative/hypnotic—controlled substance, Schedule IV
fluticasone propionate	Corticosteroid
Fortrol (pentazocine)	Analgesic—controlled substance, Schedule IV
Fosphenytoin	anticonvulsant
Fungizone (amphotericin B)	Antifungal
furosemide	Diuretic, antihypertensive
Fynex (diphenhydramine)	Antihistamine, antiemetic, antivertigo agent, antitussive, sedative/hypnotic, topical anesthetic, anticholinergic
Geopen (carbenicillin)	Antibiotic
Glaucon (epinephrine hydrochloride)	Bronchodilator, vasopressor, cardiac stimulant, local anesthetic adjunct, topical antihemorrhagic, antiglaucoma agent
glipizide	Glucotrol
Glucamide (chlorpropamide)	Antidiabetic, antidiuretic agent
glucagon	antihypoglycemic
Glucotrol (glipizide)	Antidiabetic agent
glutethimide	Sedative/hypnotic—controlled substance, Schedule III
glyburide	Antidiabetic
guanabenz	Antihypertensive
guanethidine	Antihypertensive
halazepam	Antianxiety agent—controlled substance, Schedule IV
Halcion (triazolam)	Sedative/hypnotic—controlled substance, Schedule III
Haldol (haloperidol)	Antipsychotic
haloperidol	Antipsychotic
heparin	anticoagulant
Hexadrol (dexamethasone)	Anti-inflammatory
Hold (dextromethorphan)	Non-narcotic antitussive
Humulin R (insulin [regular])	Antidiabetic agent
hydralazine	Antihypertensive
Hydramine (diphenhydramine)	Antihistamine, antiemetic, antivertigo agent, antitussive, sedative/hypnotic, topical anesthetic, anticholinergic
Hydril (diphenhydramine)	Antihistamine, antiemetic, antivertigo agent, antitussive, sedative/hypnotic, topical anesthetic

(continued)

Drug Name	Therapeutic Classification(s)
Hydro DIURIL (hydrochlorothiazide)	Diuretic, antihypertensive
Hydro-Z-50 (hydrochlorothiazide)	Diuretic, antihypertensive
hydrochlorothiazide	Diuretic, antihypertensive
hydrocortisone	corticosteroid
Hydrocortone (hydrocortisone)	Anti-inflammatory
Hydromal (hydrochlorothiazide)	Diuretic, antihypertensive
hydromorphone	Analgesic, antitussive
hydroxyzine	Antianxiety agent, sedative, anticholinergic, antiemetic, antihistamine
Hygroton (chlorthalidone)	Diuretic, antihypertensive
Hyperstat (diazoxide)	Antihypertensive
Hylidone (chlorthalidone)	Diuretic, antihypertensive
Ibutilide	antiarrhythmic
Inapsine (droperidol)	Antianxiety, antipsychotic
Inderal (propranolol)	Antihypertensive, antianginal, antiarrhythmic
Inderal LA (propranolol)	Antihypertensive, antianginal, antiarrhythmic
Inocor (amrinone)	Inotropic, vasodilator
insulin (regular)	Antidiabetic agent
Intal (cromolyn sodium)	Antiasthmatic, antiallergic
Intropin (dopamine)	Inotropic, vasopressor
ipratropium bromide	Bronchodilator
Ismelin (guanethidine)	Antihypertensive
Isomotic (isosorbide)	Antiglaucoma agent
isocarboxazid	Antidepressant
isoetharine	Bronchodilator
isoproterenol	Antiarrhythmic, bronchodilator, cardiac stimulant
Isoptin (verapamil)	Antianginal, antihypertensive, antiarrhythmic
isosorbide	Antiglaucoma agent
Ketorolac	Anti-inflammatory, antipyretic, non-opioid analgesic
Klavikordal (nitroglycerin [oral])	Antianginal, vasodilator
Klonopin (clonazepam)	Anticonvulsant—controlled substance, Schedule IV
L-caine (lidocaine)	Ventricular antiarrhythmic, local anesthetic
labetalol	Antihypertensive, antianginal, antiarrhythmic
Lanoxicaps (digoxin)	Antiarrhythmic agent, inotropic agent
Lanoxin (digoxin)	Antiarrhythmic, inotropic
Lasix (furosemide)	Diuretic, antihypertensive

Drug Name	Therapeutic Classification(s)
levalbuterol	Bronchodilator
Levoprome (methotrimeprazine)	Sedative, analgesic agent, antipruritic
Librium (chlordiazepoxide)	Antianxiety agent, anticonvulsant, sedative/hypnotic—controlled substance, Schedule IV
lidocaine	Ventricular antiarrhythmic, local anesthetic
Lidoject (lidocaine)	Ventricular antiarrhythmic, local anesthetic
LidoPen (lidocaine)	Ventricular antiarrhythmic, local anesthetic
Lipoxide (chlordiazepoxide)	Antianxiety agent, anticonvulsant, sedative/hypnotic—controlled substance, Schedule IV
lisinopril	Antihypertensive/ACE inhibitor
Lithane (lithium)	Antimanic, antipsychotic
lithium	Antimanic, antipsychotic
Lithobid (lithium)	Antimanic, antipsychotic
Lithonate (lithium)	Antimanic, antipsychotic
Lithotabs (lithium)	Antimanic, antipsychotic
Loniten (minoxidil)	Antihypertensive
lorazepam	Antianxiety agent, anticonvulsant sedative/hypnotic—controlled substance, Schedule IV
Lopressor (metoprolol)	Antihypertensive
Ludiomil (maprotiline)	Antidepressant
Luminal (phenobarbital)	Anticonvulsant, sedative/hypnotic—controlled substance, Schedule IV
magnesium sulfate	Electrolyte, antiarrhythmic, anticonvulsant
mannitol	Diuretic
maprotiline	Antidepressant
Marplan (isocarboxazid)	Antidepressant
Mazepine (carbamazepine)	Anticonvulsant, analgesic
Mebaral (mephobarbital)	Anticonvulsant—controlled substance, Schedule IV
Medihaler-Epi (epinephrine bitartrate)	Bronchodilator, vasopressor, cardiac stimulant, local anesthetic adjunct, topical antihemorrhagic, antiglaucoma agent
Mediquell (dextromethorphan)	Non-narcotic antitussive
Medrol (methylprednisolone)	Anti-inflammatory, immunosuppressant
Mellaril-S (thioridazine)	Antipsychotic
Mentaban (mephobarbital)	Anticonvulsant—controlled substance, Schedule IV
meperidine	Analgesic—controlled substance, Schedule II

Drug Name	Therapeutic Classification(s)
mephenytoin	Anticonvulsant
mephobarbital	Anticonvulsant—controlled substance, Schedule IV
meprobamate	Antianxiety agent—controlled substance, Schedule IV
Meprospan (meprobamate)	Antianxiety agent—controlled substance, Schedule IV
Mesantoin (mephenytoin)	Anticonvulsant
mesoridazine	Antipsychotic
Metaprel (metaproterenol)	Bronchodilator
metaprolol	Antihypertensive
metaproterenol	Bronchodilator
methadone	Analgesic, narcotic detoxification adjunct—controlled substance, Schedule II
Methadose (methadone)	Analgesic, narcotic detoxification adjunct—controlled substance, Schedule II
Methidate (methylphenidate)	CNS stimulant—controlled substance, Schedule II
methotrimeprazine	Sedative, analgesic agent, antipruritic
methyclothiazide	Diuretic, antihypertensive
methyldopa	Antihypertensive
methylphenidate	CNS stimulant—controlled substance, Schedule II
methylprednisolone	Anti-inflammatory, glucocorticoid
methyprylon	Sedative/hypnotic—controlled substance, Schedule III
metoprolol	Antihypertensive, antianginal, antiarrhythmic
mexiletine	Ventricular antiarrhythmic
Mexitil (mexiletine)	Ventricular antiarrhythmic
Micronase (glyburide)	Antidiabetic
MicroNefrin (epinephrine hydrochloride)	Bronchodilator, vasopressor, cardiac stimulant, local anesthetic adjunct, topical antihemorrhagic, anti-glaucoma agent
midazolam	Antianxiety/sedative/hypnotic
Milontin (phensuximide)	Anticonvulsant
milrinone	Inotropic
Miltown (meprobamate)	Antianxiety agent—controlled substance, Schedule IV
Minipress (prazosin)	Antihypertensive
minoxidil	Antihypertensive
morphine	Analgesic—controlled substance, Schedule II

Drug Name	Therapeutic Classification(s)
MS Contin (morphine)	Analgesic—controlled substance, Schedule II
Mucomyst (acetylcysteine)	Antidote (acetaminophen)
Murcil (chlordiazepoxide)	Antianxiety agent, anticonvulsant, sedative/hypnotic—controlled substance, Schedule IV
Myidone (primidone)	Anticonvulsant
Mysoline (primidone)	Anticonvulsant
N-G-C (nitroglycerin [oral])	Antianginal, vasodilator
nadolol	Antihypertensive, antianginal
nalbuphine	Analgesic
Nalicaine (lidocaine)	Ventricular antiarrhythmic, local anesthetic
nalmefene	Narcotic antagonist
naloxone	Narcotic antagonist
Napamide (disopyramide)	Ventricular/supraventricular antiarrhythmia, atrial antitachyarrhythmic
Narcan (naloxone)	Narcotic antagonist
nardil (phenelzine)	Antidepressant
Navane (thiothixene)	Antipsychotic
Nembutal (pentobarbital)	Anticonvulsant, sedative/hypnotic— controlled substance, Schedule II; suppositories under Schedule III
Nervine (diphenhydramine)	Antihistamine, antiemetic, antivertigo agent, antitussive, sedative/hypnotic, topical anesthetic
Nervocaine (lidocaine)	Ventricular antiarrhythmic, local anesthetic
Neuramate (meprobamate)	Antianxiety agent—controlled substance, Schedule IV
Neurate (meprobamate)	Antianxiety agent—controlled substance, Schedule IV
nifedipine	Antianginal, antihypertensive
Nighttime Sleep-Aid (diphenhydramine)	Antihistamine, antiemetic, antivertigo agent, antitussive, sedative/hypnotic, topical anesthetic
Niong (nitroglycerin [oral])	Antianginal, vasodilator
Nitro-bid (nitroglycerin [oral])	Antianginal, vasodilator
Nitrobid (nitroglycerin [topical])	Antianginal, vasodilator
Nitrocap (nitroglycerin [oral])	Antianginal, vasodilator
Nitrocap T.D. (nitroglycerin [oral])	Antianginal, vasodilator
nitroglycerin (oral)	Antianginal, vasodilator
nitroglycerin (sublingual)	Antianginal, vasodilator antihypertensive
nitroglycerin (topical)	Antianginal, vasodilator

(continued)

Drug Name / Therapeutic Classification(s)

Drug Name	Therapeutic Classification(s)
Nitroglyn (nitroglycerin [oral])	Antianginal, vasodilator
Nitrol (nitroglycerin [topical])	Antianginal, vasodilator
Nitrolin (nitroglycerin [oral])	Antianginal, vasodilator
Nitronet (nitroglycerin [oral])	Antianginal, vasodilator
Nitrong (nitroglycerin [oral])	Antianginal, vasodilator
Nitrong (nitroglycerin [topical])	Antianginal, vasodilator
Nitronox (nitrous oxide-oxygen mixture)	Analgesic
Nitropress (nitroprusside)	Antihypertensive
Nitroprusside	Antihypertensive vasodilator
Nitrospan (nitroglycerin [oral])	Antianginal, vasodilator
Nitrostat (nitroglycerin [sublingual])	Antianginal, vasodilator
Nitrostat (nitroglycerin [topical])	Antianginal, vasodilator
Nitrostat SR (nitroglycerin [oral])	Antianginal, vasodilator
nitrous oxide-oxygen mixture	non-opiod analgesic, medicinal gas
Noctec (chloral hydrate)	Sedative/hypnotic—controlled substance, Schedule IV
Noludar (methprylon)	Sedative/hypnotic—controlled substance, Schedule III
Norcuron (vecuronium bromide)	Nondepolarizing neuromuscular blocking drug
Nordryl (diphenhydramine)	Antihistamine, antiemetic, antivertigo agent, antitussive, sedative/hypnotic, topical anesthetic
Norepinephrine	vasocontrictor, vasopressor
Normodyne (labetalol)	Antihypertensive
Norpace (disopyramide)	Ventricular/supraventricular antiarrhythmic, atrial antitachyarrhythmic
Norpace CR (disopyramide)	Ventricular/supraventricular antiarrhythmic, atrial antitachyarrhythmic
Norpramin (desipramine)	Antidepressant, antianxiety agent
nortriptyline	Antidepressant
Novochlorhydrate (chloral hydrate)	Sedative/hypnotic—controlled substance, Schedule IV
Novolin (insulin [regular])	Antidiabetic agent
Nubain (nalbuphine)	Analgesic
Numorphan (oxymorphone)	Analgesic—controlled substance, Schedule II
Nytol with DPH (diphenhydramine)	Antihistamine, antiemetic, antivertigo agent, antitussive, sedative/hypnotic, topical anesthetic
Omnipen (ampicillin)	Antibiotic
Oramide (tolbutamide)	Antidiabetic agent
Oretic (hydrochlorothiazide)	Diuretic, antihypertensive
Orinase (tolbutamide)	Antidiabetic agent
Ormayine (chlorpromazine)	Antipsychotic, antiemetic
Osmitrol (mannitol)	Diuretic
oxazepam	Antianxiety, sedative/hypnotic—controlled substance, Schedule IV
oxtriphylline	Bronchodilator
Oxygen	medicinal gas
oxymorphone	Analgesic—controlled substance, Schedule II
oxytocin	Oxytocic
Pamelor (nortriptyline)	Antidepressant
pancuronium bromide	Neuromuscular blocking drug
Panwarfin (warfarin)	Anticoagulant
Parlodel (bromocriptine)	Antiparkinsonian agent
Parnate (tranylcypromine)	Antidepressant
Pavulon (pancuronium sulfate)	Neuromuscular blocking drug
Paxipam (halazepam)	Antianxiety agent—controlled substance, Schedule IV
Pedia Care (dextromethorphan)	Non-narcotic antitussive
pentazocine	Analgesic—controlled substance, Schedule IV
pentobarbital	Anticonvulsant, sedative/hypnotic— controlled substance, Schedule II; suppositories under Schedule III
perphenazine	Antipsychotic, antiemetic
Persantine (dipyridamole)	Coronary vasodilator, platelet aggregation inhibitor
Pertofrane (desipramine)	Antidepressant, antianxiety agent
Pertussin 8 Hour Cough Formula (dextromethorphan)	Non-narcotic antitussive
phenelzine	Antidepressant
Phenergan (promethazine)	Antihistamine
phenobarbital	Anticonvulsant, sedative/hypnotic— controlled substance, Schedule IV
phensuximide	Anticonvulsant
phentolamine	Agent for pheochromocytoma (alpha-adrenergic blocker) antihypertensive
phenytoin	Anticonvulsant, antiarrhythmic
Phyllocontin (aminophylline)	Bronchodilator
physostigmine	(Antimuscarinic)
pindolol	Antihypertensive

Drug Name	Therapeutic Classification(s)
Pitocin (oxytocin)	Oxytocic
Placidyl (ethchlorvynol)	Sedative/hypnotic—controlled substance, Schedule IV
Polycillin (ampicillin)	Antibiotic
Polymox (amoxicillin)	Antibiotic
Pork Regular Iletin II (insulin [regular])	Antidiabetic agent
pralidoxime	Antidote (nticholinesterase inhibitor)
prazepam	Antianxiety agent—controlled substance, Schedule IV
prazosin	Antihypertensive
Primacor (milrinone)	Inotropic
Primatene Mist Solution (epinephrine)	Bronchodilator, vasopressor, cardiac stimulant, local anesthetic adjunct, topical antihemorrhagic, antiglaucoma agent
Primatene Mist Suspension (epinephrine bitartrate)	Bronchodilator, vasopressor, cardiac stimulant, local anesthetic adjunct, topical antihemorrhagic, antiglaucoma agent
primidone	Anticonvulsant
Principen (ampicillin)	Antibiotic
Prinivil (lisinopril)	Antihypertensive/ACE inhibitor
procainamide	Ventricular and supraventricular antiarrhythmic, atrial antitachyarrhythmic
Procan SR (procainamide)	Ventricular and supraventricular antiarrhythmic, atrial antitachyarrhythmic
Procardia (nifedipine)	Antianginal
prochlorperazine	Antipsychotic, antiemetic, antianxiety agent
Profene (propoxyphene)	Analgesic—controlled substance, Schedule IV
Proglycem (diazoxide)	Antihypertensive
Prolixin (fluphenazine)	Antipsychotic
Promapar (chlorpromazine)	Antipsychotic, antiemetic
Promay (chlorpromazine)	Antipsychotic, antiemetic
promazine	Antipsychotic, antiemetic, analgesic— controlled substance, Schedule IV
promethazine	Antihistamine anticholinergic, antiemetic, antihistamine
Promine (procainamide)	Ventricular and supraventricular antiarrhythmic, atrial antitachyarrhythmic
Pronestyl (procainamide)	Ventricular and supraventricular antiarrhythmic, atrial antitachyarrhythmic
Pronestyl-SR (procainamide)	Ventricular and supraventricular antiarrhythmic, atrial antitachyarrhythmic

Drug Name	Therapeutic Classification(s)
propoxyphene	Analgesic—controlled substance, Schedule IV
propranolol	Antihypertensive, antianginal, antiarrhythmic
Protopam (pralidoxime)	Anticholinesterase inhibitor
protriptyline	Antidepressant
Proventil (albuterol)	Bronchodilator
Proventil Syrup (albuterol)	Bronchodilator
Prozine (promazine)	Antipsychotic, antiemetic, analgesic— controlled substance, Schedule IV
Purodigin (digitoxin)	Antiarrhythmic agent, inotropic agent
Pyopen (carbenicillin)	Antibiotic
Pyridamole (dipyridamole)	Coronary vasodilator, platelet aggregation inhibitor
Quinidex (quinidine)	Ventricular and supraventricular antiarrhythmic, atrial antiarrhythmic
quinidine	Ventricular and supraventricular antiarrhythmic, atrial antiarrhythmic
Quinora (quinidine)	Ventricular and supraventricular antiarrhythmic, atrial antiarrhythmic
Racemic epinephrine	adrenergic
ramipril	Antihypertensive/ACE inhibitor
Razepam (temazepam)	Sedative/hypnotic—controlled substance, Schedule IV
Regitine (phentolamine)	Agent for pheochromocytoma (alpha-adrenergic blocker)
Regular Iletin I (insulin [regular])	Antidiabetic agent
Regular Iletin II (insulin [regular])	Antidiabetic agent
Regular Pork Insulin (insulin [regular])	Antidiabetic agent
Reposans-10 (chlordiazepoxide)	Antianxiety agent, anticonvulsant, sedative/hypnotic—controlled substance, Schedule IV
reserpine	Antihypertensive, antipsychotic
Restoril (temazepam)	Sedative/hypnotic—controlled substance, Schedule IV
Reteplase	thrombolytic enzyme
Revex (nalmefene)	Narcotic antagonist
Rhythmin (procainamide)	Ventricular and supraventricular antiarrhythmic, atrial antitachyarrhythmic
Ritalin (methylphenidate)	CNS stimulant—controlled substance, Schedule II
Ritalin SR (methylphenidate)	CNS stimulant—controlled substance, Schedule II
Rivotril (clonazepam)	Anticonvulsant—controlled substance, Schedule IV

(continued)

Drug Name	Therapeutic Classification(s)	Drug Name	Therapeutic Classification(s)
RMS Uniserts (morphine)	Analgesic—controlled substance, Schedule II	SK-Bamate (meprobamate)	Antianxiety agent—controlled substance, Schedule IV
Ro-Chlorozide (chlorothiazide)	Diuretic, antihypertensive	SK-Chlorozide (chlorothiazide)	Diuretic, antihypertensive
Ro-Hydrazide (hydrochlorothiazide)	Diuretic, antihypertensive	SK-Hydrochlorothiazide (hydrochlorothiazide)	Diuretic, antihypertensive
Roampicillin (ampicillin)	Antibiotic	SK-Lasix (furosemide)	Diuretic, antihypertensive
Robalyn (diphenhydramine)	Antihistamine, antiemetic and antivertigo agent, antitussive, sedative/hypnotic, topical anesthetic	SK-Lygen (chlordiazepoxide)	Antianxiety agent, anticonvulsant, sedative/hypnotic—controlled substance, Schedule IV
rocuronium bromide	Neuromuscular blocking drug	SK-Quinidine Sulfate (quinidine)	Ventricular and supraventricular antiarrhythmic, atrial antiarrhythmic
Romazicon (flumazenil)	Benzodiazepine antagonist	SK-Tolbutamide (tolbutamide)	Antidiabetic agent
Ronase (tolazamide)	Antidiabetic agent	Sleep-Eye 3 (diphenhydramine)	Antihistamine, antiemetic and antivertigo agent, antitussive, sedative/hypnotic, topical anesthetic
Roxanol (morphine)	Analgesic—controlled substance, Schedule II	Slo-bid (theophylline)	Bronchodilator
S-2 Inhalant (epinephrine hydrochloride)	Bronchodilator, vasopressor, cardiac stimulant, local anesthetic adjunct, topical antihemorrhagic, antiglaucoma agent	Slo-Phyllin (theophylline)	Bronchodilator
Sandril (reserpine)	Antihypertensive, antipsychotic	Sodium bicarbonate	hydrogen ion buffer, urine alkalinizer
salmeterol xinafoate	Beta$_2$-adrenergic agonist	Sodium nitrite	cyanide poisoning agent
Sarisol No. 2 (butabarbital)	Sedative/hypnotic—controlled substance, Schedule III	sodium thiosulfate	Cyanide poisoning adjunct
Seconal (secobarbital)	Sedative/hypnotic, anticonvulsant— controlled substance, Schedule II; suppositories are under Schedule III	Sofarin (warfarin)	Anticoagulant
secobarbital	Sedative/hypnotic, anticonvulsant— controlled substance, Schedule II; suppositories are under Schedule III	Solfoton (phenobarbital)	Anticonvulsant, sedative/hypnotic— controlled substance, Schedule IV
Sectral (acebutolol)	Antihypertensive, antiarrhythmic	Solu-Medrol	Anti-inflammatory, immunosuppressant
Sedabamate (meprobamate)	Antianxiety agent—controlled substance, Schedule IV	Sominex Formula 2 (diphenhydramine)	Antihistamine, antiemetic and antivertigo agent, antitussive, sedative/hypnotic, topical anesthetic
Serax (oxazepam)	Antianxiety, sedative/hypnotic—controlled substance, Schedule IV	Somophyllin-T (theophylline)	Bronchodilator
Sereen (chlordiazepoxide)	Antianxiety agent, anticonvulsant, sedative/hypnotic—controlled substance, Schedule IV	Somophyllin (aminophylline)	Bronchodilator
Serentil (mesoridazine)	Antipsychotic	Sonayine (chlorpromazine)	Antipsychotic, antiemetic
Serevent (salmeterol xinafoate)	Beta$_2$-adrenergic agonist	Sparine (promazine)	Antipsychotic, antiemetic, analgesic—controlled substance, Schedule IV
Serpanray (reserpine)	Antihypertensive, antipsychotic	Spectrobid (bacampicillin)	Antibiotic
Serpasil (reserpine)	Antihypertensive, antipsychotic	spironolactone	Antihypertensive, diuretic
Serpate (reserpine)	Antihypertensive, antipsychotic	St. Joseph for Children	Non-narcotic antitussive (dextromethorphan)
Serpolan (reserpine)	Antihypertensive, antipsychotic	Stadol (butorphanol)	Narcotic agonist-antagonist, opioid partial agonist
Sertan (primidone)	Anticonvulsant	Stelazine (trifluoperazine)	Antipsychotic, antiemetic
Sinequan (doxepin)	Antidepressant	streptokinase	Thrombolytic
Sintocine (oxytocin)	Oxytocic	Sublimaze (fentanyl)	Opioid analgesic
SK-Amitriptyline (amitriptyline)	Antidepressant	Succinylcholine	Depolarizing neuromuscular blocking drug

Drug Name	Therapeutic Classification(s)
Sucrets Cough Control (dextromethorphan)	Non-narcotic antitussive
Super Totacillian (ampicillin)	Antibiotic
Suprazine (trifluoperazine)	Antipsychotic, antiemetic
Sus-Phrine (epinephrine)	Bronchodilator, vasopressor, cardiac stimulant, local anesthetic adjunct, topical antihemorrhagic, antiglaucoma agent
Sustaire (theophylline)	Bronchodilator
Syrup of ipecac	emetic
Talwin-NX (pentazocine)	Analgesic—controlled substance, Schedule IV
Tambocor (flecainide)	Ventricular antiarrhythmic
Taractan (chlorprothixene)	Antipsychotic
Tavist (clemastine)	Antihistamine
Tavist-1 (clemastine)	Antihistamine
Tegretol (carbamazepine)	Anticonvulsant, analgesic
temazepam	Sedative/hypnotic—controlled substance, Schedule IV
Tempay (temazepam)	Sedative/hypnotic—controlled substance, Schedule IV
Tempra (acetaminophen)	Non-narcotic analgesic, antipyretic
Tenormin (atenolol)	Antihypertensive, antianginal
Tensilon (edrophonium)	Antiarrhythmic, cholinergic agonist
terbutaline	Bronchodilator, tocolytic
Thalitone (chlorthalidone)	Diuretic, antihypertensive
Theo-24 (theophylline)	Bronchodilator
Theo-Dur (theophylline)	Bronchodilator
Theobid (theophylline)	Bronchodilator
Theoclear (theophylline)	Bronchodilator
Theophyl (theophylline)	Bronchodilator
theophylline	Bronchodilator
Theospan-SR (theophylline)	Bronchodilator
Theovent (theophylline)	Bronchodilator
thioridazine	Antipsychotic
thiothixene	Antipsychotic
Thor-Prom (chlorpromazine)	Antipsychotic, antiemetic
Thorayine (chlorpromazine)	Antipsychotic, antiemetic
timolol	Antihypertensive, antiglaucoma agent
Timoptic (timolol)	Antihypertensive, antiglaucoma agent

Drug Name	Therapeutic Classification(s)
Tindal (acetophenazine)	Antipsychotic
tocainide	Ventricular antiarrhythmic
tolazamide	Antidiabetic agent
tolbutamide	Antidiabetic agent
Tolinase (tolazamide)	Antidiabetic agent
Tonocard (tocainide)	Ventricular antiarrhythmic
Toradd (ketorolac)	Anti-inflammatory, non-opioid analgesic
Tornalate (bitolterol)	Bronchodilator
Tracrium (atracurium)	Nondepolarizing skeletal muscle relaxant
Trandate (labetalol)	Antihypertensive
Tranmep (meprobamate)	Antianxiety agent—controlled substance, Schedule IV
Tranxene-SD (clorazepate)	Antianxiety agent, anticonvulsant, sedative/hypnotic—controlled substance Schedule IV
Tranxene-SD Half Strength	Antianxiety agent, anticonvulsant, (clorazepate) sedative/hypnotic—controlled substance, Schedule IV
tranylcypromine	Antidepressant
triamcinolone	Corticosteroid
triazolam	Sedative/hypnotic—controlled substance, Schedule III
Tridione (trimethadione)	Anticonvulsant
trifluoperazine	Antipsychotic, antiemetic
Trilafon (perphenazine)	Antipsychotic, antiemetic
trimethadione	Anticonvulsant
Trimox (amoxicillin)	Antibiotic
Triptil (protriptyline)	Antidepressant
Truphylline (aminophylline)	Bronchodilator
Tubocurarine chloride	Nondepolarizing neuromuscular blocking drug
Tusstat (diphenhydramine)	Antihistamine, antiemetic and antivertigo agent, antitussive, sedative/hypnotic, topical anesthetic
Twilite (diphenhydramine)	Antihistamine, antiemetic and antivertigo agent, antitussive, sedative/hypnotic, topical anesthetic
Tylenol (acetaminophen)	Non-narcotic analgesic, antipyretic
Uniphyl (theophylline)	Bronchodilator
Utimox (amoxicillin)	Antibiotic
Valadol (acetaminophen)	Non-narcotic analgesic, antipyretic
Valdrene (diphenhydramine)	Antihistamine, antiemetic and antivertigo agent, antitussive, sedative/hypnotic, topical anesthetic

(continued)

Drug Name	Therapeutic Classification(s)	Drug Name	Therapeutic Classification(s)
Valium (diazepam)	Antianxiety agent, skeletal muscle relaxant, amnesic, anticonvulsant, sedative/ hypnotic—controlled substance, Schedule IV	Viscous (lidocaine)	Ventricular antiarrhythmic, local anesthetic
Valorin (acetaminophen)	Non-narcotic analgesic, antipyretic	Visken (pindolol)	Antihypertensive
valproic acid	Anticonvulsant	Vistaril (hydroxyzine)	Antianxiety agent, sedative, anticholinergic, antiemetic, antihistamine
Valrelease (diazepam)	Antianxiety agent, skeletal muscle relaxant, amnesic agent, anticonvulsant, sedative/hypnotic	Vivactil (protriptyline)	Antidepressant
Vancerase (beclomethasone)	Anti-inflammatory, antiasthmatic	Volmax (albuterol)	Bronchodilator
Vanceril (beclomethasone)	Anti-inflammatory, antiasthmatic	warfarin	Anticoagulant
Vaponefrin (epinephrine hydrochloride)	Bronchodilator, vasopressor, cardiac stimulant, local anesthetic adjunct, topical antihemorrhagic, antiglaucoma agent	Wymox (amoxicillin)	Antibiotic
		Wytensin (guanabenz)	Antihypertensive
vecuronium bromide	Nondepolarizing neuromuscular blocking drug	Xanax (alprazolam)	Antianxiety agent—controlled substance, Schedule IV
Velosef (cephradine)	Antibiotic	Xopenex (levalbuterol)	Bronchodilator
Velosulin (insulin [regular])	Antidiabetic agent	Xylocaine (lidocaine)	Ventricular antiarrhythmic, local anesthetic
Velosulin Human (insulin [regular])	Antidiabetic agent	zafirlukast	Antiasthmatic
Ventolin (albuterol)	Bronchodilator	Zarontin (ethosuximide)	Anticonvulsant
Ventolin Syrup (albuterol)	Bronchodilator	Zemuron (rocuronium bromide)	Neuromuscular blocking drug
verapamil	Antianginal, antihypertensive, antiarrhythmic	Zepine (reserpine)	Antihypertensive, antipsychotic
Versed (midazolam)	Antianxiety/sedative/hypnotic	Zestril (lisinopril)	Antihypertensive/ACE inhibitor
		zileuton	Antiasthmatic
		ZyFlo (zileuton)	Antiasthmatic

APPENDIX B

Pediatric Normal Values, Dosages, and Infusion Rates

Statistically Common Pediatric Normal Values

Age	Average Weight*	Respiratory Rate	Pulse Rate	Blood Pressure†
Birth–6 wk	4–5 kg (9–11 lb)	30–50 breaths/min	120–160 beats/min	74–100 mm Hg 50–68 mm Hg
7 wk–1 y	4–11 kg (9–24 lb)	20–30 breaths/min	80–140 beats/min	84–106 mm Hg 45–70 mm Hg
1–2 y	11–14 kg (24–31 lb)	20–30 breaths/min	80–130 beats/min	98–106 mm Hg 58–70 mm Hg
2–6 y	14–25 kg (31–55 lb)	20–30 breaths/min	80–120 beats/min	98–112 mm Hg 64–70 mm Hg
6–13 y	25–63 kg (55–139 lb)	12–20 breaths/min	60–100 beats/min	104–124 mm Hg 64–80 mm Hg
13–16 y	62–80 kg (136–176 lb)	12–20 breaths/min	60–100 beats/min	118–132 mm Hg 70–82 mm Hg

*Weight estimation: $8 + (12 \infty \text{age [y]}) = \text{weight in kg}$.
†Systolic blood pressure estimation: $80 + (2 \infty \text{age [y]}) = \text{approx systolic B/P}$.

Pediatric Drug Dosages

Drug	Body Weight (kg/lb)†				
	1 kg/2 lb	2 kg/4 lb	3 kg/7 lb	4 kg/9 lb	5 kg/11 lb
Adenosine	0.1 mg	0.2 mg	0.3 mg	0.4 mg	0.5 mg
Aminophylline*	6 mg	12 mg	18 mg	24 mg	30 mg
Amiodarone	5 mg	10 mg	15 mg	20 mg	25 mg
Atropine	0.02 mg	0.04 mg	0.06 mg	0.08 mg	0.10 mg
Calcium chloride	20 mg	40 mg	60 mg	80 mg	100 mg
Calcium gluconate	60–100 mg	120–200 mg	180–300 mg	240–400 mg	300–500 mg
Dextrose 50% in water	0.5–1 mg	1–2 mg	1.5–3 mg	2–4 mg	2.5–5 mg
Diazoxide	1–3 mg	2–6 mg	3–9 mg	4–12 mg	5–15 mg
Diphenhydramine	2–5 mg	4–10 mg	6–15 mg	8–20 mg	10–25 mg
Dopamine	2–20 *mcg*/min	4–40 *mcg*/min	6–60 *mcg*/min	8–80 *mcg*/min	10–100 *mcg*/min
Epinephrine (1:10,000)	0.01 mg	0.02 mg	0.03 mg	0.04 mg	0.05 mg

*Doses are the usual initial single dose.
†Pounds have been rounded to the nearest pound.

Pediatric Drug Dosages (*continued*)

Drug	Body Weight (kg/lb)[†]				
	1 kg/2 lb	**2 kg/4 lb**	**3 kg/7 lb**	**4 kg/9 lb**	**5 kg/11 lb**
Etomidate	0.2–0.4 mg	0.4–0.8 mg	0.6–1.2 mg	0.8–1.6 mg	1.0–2.0 mg
Furosemide	1 mg	2 mg	3 mg	4 mg	5 mg
Isoproterenol	0.1–0.2 *mcg*/min	0.2–0.4 *mcg*/min	0.3–0.6 *mcg*/min	0.4–0.8 *mcg*/min	0.5–1 *mcg*/min
Lidocaine	1 mg	2 mg	3 mg	4 mg	5 mg
Naloxone	0.1 mg	0.2 mg	0.3 mg	0.4 mg	0.5 mg
Propranolol	0.01 mg	0.02 mg	0.03 mg	0.04 mg	0.05 mg
Sodium bicarbonate	1 mEq	2 mEq	3 mEq	4 mEq	5 mEq
Verapamil	0.1–0.3 mg	0.2–0.6 mg	0.3–0.9 mg	0.4–1.2 mg	0.5–1.5 mg
	6 kg/13 lb	**7 kg/15 lb**	**8 kg/18 lb**	**9 kg/20 lb**	**10 kg/22 lb**
Adenosine	0.6 mg	0.7 mg	0.8 mg	0.9 mg	1.0 mg
Aminophylline	36 mg	42 mg	48 mg	54 mg	60 mg
Amiodarone	30 mg	35 mg	40 mg	45 mg	50 mg
Atropine	0.12 mg	0.14 mg	0.16 mg	0.18 mg	0.2 mg
Calcium chloride	120 mg	140 mg	160 mg	180 mg	200 mg
Calcium gluconate	360–600 mg	420–700 mg	480–800 mg	540–900 mg	600–1000 mg
Dextrose 50% in water	3–6 mg	3.5–7 mg	4–8 mg	4.6–9 mg	5–10 mg
Diazoxide	6–18 mg	7–21 mg	8–24 mg	9–27 mg	10–30 mg
Diphenhydramine	12–30 mg	14–35 mg	16–40 mg	18–45 mg	20–50 mg
Dopamine	12–120 *mcg*/min	14–140 *mcg*/min	16–160 *mcg*/min	18–180 *mcg*/min	20–200 *mcg*/min
Epinephrine (1:10,000)	0.06 mg	0.07 mg	0.08 mg	0.09 mg	0.1 mg
Etomidate	1.2–2.4 mg	1.4–2.8 mg	1.6–3.2 mg	1.8–3.6 mg	2.0–4.0 mg
Furosemide	6 mg	7 mg	8 mg	9 mg	10 mg
Isoproterenol	0.6–1.2 *mcg*/min	0.7–1.4 *mcg*/min	0.8–1.6 *mcg*/min	0.9–1.8 *mcg*/min	1.0–2 *mcg*/min
Lidocaine	6 mg	7 mg	8 mg	9 mg	10 mg
Naloxone	0.6 mg	0.7 mg	0.8 mg	0.9 mg	1.0 mg
Propranolol	0.06 mg	0.07 mg	0.08 mg	0.09 mg	0.1 mg
Sodium bicarbonate	6 mEq	7 mEq	8 mEq	9 mEq	10 mEq
Verapamil	0.6–1.8 mg	0.7–2.1 mg	0.8–2.4 mg	0.9–2.7 mg	1–3 mg
	12.5 kg/28 lb	**15 kg/33 lb**	**17.5 kg/39 lb**	**20 kg/44 lb**	**20.5 kg/50 lb**
Adenosine	1.25 mg	1.5 mg	1.75 mg	2.0 mg	2.05 mg
Aminophylline	75 mg	90 mg	105 mg	120 mg	135 mg
Amiodarone	62.5 mg	75 mg	87.5 mg	100 mg	102.5 mg
Atropine	0.25 mg	0.30 mg	0.35 mg	0.4 mg	0.45 mg
Calcium chloride	250 mg	300 mg	350 mg	400 mg	410 mg
Calcium gluconate	750–1250 mg	900–1500 mg	1.05–1.75 gm	1.2–2.0 gm	1.23–2.05 gm
Dextrose 50% in water	6.25–12.5 g	7.5–15 g	8.75–17.5 g	10–20 g	11.25–22.5 g
Diazoxide	12.5–37.5 mg	15–45 mg	17.5–52.5 mg	20–60 mg	22.5–67.5 mg
Diphenhydramine	25–62.5 mg	30–75 mg	35–87.5 mg	40–100 mg	45–112.5 mg
Dopamine	25–250 *mcg*/min	30–300 *mcg*/min	35–350 *mcg*/min	40–400 *mcg*/min	41–410 *mcg*/min

*Doses are the usual initial single dose.
[†]Pounds have been rounded to the nearest pound.

Pediatric Drug Dosages (*continued*)

	Body Weight (kg/lb)†				
	12.5 kg/28 lb	15 kg/33 lb	17.5 kg/39 lb	20 kg/44 lb	20.5 kg/50 lb
Epinephrine (1:10,000)	0.125 mg	0.15 mg	0.175 mg	0.2 mg	0.225 mg
Etomidate	2.5–5.0 mg	3.0–6.0 mg	3.5–7.0 mg	4.0–8.0 mg	4.1–8.2 mg
Furosemide	12.5 mg	15 mg	17.5 mg	20 mg	22.5 mg
Isoproterenol	1.25–2.5 *mcg*/min	1.5–3 *mcg*/min	1.75–3.5 *mcg*/min	2–4 *mcg*/min	2.25–4.5 *mcg*/min
Lidocaine	12.5 mg	15 mg	17.5 mg	20 mg	22.5 mg
Naloxone	1.25 mg	1.5 mg	2.0 mg	2.0 mg	2.0 mg
Propranolol	0.125 mg	0.15 mg	0.175 mg	0.2 mg	0.225 mg
Sodium bicarbonate	12.5 mEq	15 mEq	17.5 mEq	20 mEq	22.5 mEq
Verapamil	1.25–3.75 mg	1.5–4.5 mg	1.75–5 mg	2–5 mg	2–5 mg

	25 kg/55 lb	30 kg/66 lb	35 kg/77 lb	40 kg/88 lb	45 kg/99 lb
Adenosine	2.5 mg	3.0 mg	3.5 mg	4.0 mg	4.5 mg
Aminophylline	150 mg	180 mg	210 mg	240 mg	270 mg
Amiodarone	125 mg	150 mg	175 mg	200 mg	225 mg
Atropine	0.5 mg	0.5 mg	0.5 mg	0.5 mg	0.5 mg
Calcium chloride	500 mg	600 mg	700 mg	800 mg	900 mg
Calcium gluconate	1.5–2.5 gm	1.8–3.0 gm	2.1–3.5 gm	2.4–4.0 gm	2.7–4.5 gm
Dextrose 50% in water	12.5–25 g	15–30 g	17.5–35 g	20–40 g	22.5–45 g
Diazoxide	25–75 mg	30–90 mg	35–105 mg	40–120 mg	45–135 mg
Diphenhydramine	50–125 mg	60–150 mg	70–176 mg	80–200 mg	90–225 mg
Dopamine	50–500 *mcg*/min	60–600 *mcg*/min	70–700 *mcg*/min	80–800 *mcg*/min	90–900 *mcg*/min
Epinephrine (1:10,000)	0.25 mg	0.3 mg	0.35 mg	0.4 mg	0.45 mg
Etomidate	5.0–10.0 mg	6.0–12.0 mg	7.0–14.0 mg	8.0–16.0 mg	9.0–18.0 mg
Furosemide	25 mg	30 mg	35 mg	40 mg	45 mg
Isoproterenol	2.5–5 *mcg*/min	3–6 *mcg*/min	3.5–7 *mcg*/min	4–8 *mcg*/min	4.5–9 *mcg*/min
Lidocaine	25 mg	30 mg	35 mg	40 mg	45 mg
Naloxone	2.0 mg	2.0 mg	2.0 mg	2.0 mg	2.0 mg
Propranolol	0.25 mg	0.3 mg	0.35 mg	0.4 mg	0.45 mg
Sodium bicarbonate	25 mEq	30 mEq	35 mEq	40 mEq	45 mEq
Verapamil	2.5–7.5 mg	3–9 mg	3.5–10.5 mg	4–12 mg	4.5–13.5 mg

	50 kg/110 lb	55 kg/121 lb	60 kg/132 lb	65 kg/143 lb	70 kg/154 lb
Adenosine	5.0 mg	5.5 mg	6.0 mg	6.5 mg	7.0 mg
Aminophylline	300 mg	330 mg	360 mg	390 mg	420 mg
Amiodarone	250 mg	275 mg	300 mg	325 mg	350 mg
Atropine	0.5 mg	0.5 mg	0.5 mg	0.5 mg	0.5 mg
Calcium chloride	1 g	1.1 g	1.2 g	1.3 g	1.4 g
Calcium gluconate	3.0–5.0 gm	3.3–5.5 gm	3.6–6.0 gm	3.9–6.5 gm	4.2–7.0 mg
Dextrose 50% in water	25–50 g	27.5–55 g	30–60 g	32.5–65 g	35–70 g
Diazoxide	50–150 mg	55–150 mg	60–150 mg	65–150 mg	70–150 mg
Diphenhydramine	100–250 mg	110–275 mg	120–300 mg	130–325 mg	140–350 mg

*Doses are the usual initial single dose.
†Pounds have been rounded to the nearest pound.

Pediatric Drug Dosages (*continued*)

	Body Weight (kg/lb)[†]				
	50 kg/110 lb	55 kg/121 lb	60 kg/132 lb	65 kg/143 lb	70 kg/154 lb
Dopamine	100–1000 *mcg*/min	110–1100 *mcg*/min	120–1200 *mcg*/min	130–1300 *mcg*/min	140–1400 *mcg*/min
Epinephrine (1:10,000)	0.5 mg	0.55 mg	0.6 mg	0.65 mg	0.7 mg
Etomidate	10.0–20.0 mg	11.0–22.0 mg	12.0–24.0 mg	13–26 mg	14.0–28.0 mg
Furosemide	50 mg	55 mg	60 mg	65 mg	70 mg
Isoproterenol	5–10 *mcg*/min	5.5–11 *mcg*/min	6–12 *mcg*/min	6.5–13 *mcg*/min	7–14 *mcg*/min
Lidocaine	50 mg	55 mg	60 mg	65 mg	70 mg
Naloxone	2.0 mg	2.0 mg	2.0 mg	2.0 mg	2.0 mg
Propranolol	0.5 mg	0.55 mg	0.6 mg	0.65 mg	0.7 mg
Sodium bicarbonate	50 mEq	55 mEq	60 mEq	65 mEq	70 mEq
Verapamil	2–5 mg	2–5 mg	2–5 mg	2–5 mg	2–5 mg

*Doses are the usual initial single dose.
[†]Pounds have been rounded to the nearest pound.

Calculating Drug Concentrations and Infusion Rates for Common Pediatric Medications

Drug	Commonly Found Drug Concentration	Desired Rate of Administration	Amount of Drug Solution to Add to 100 mL of D$_5$W
Isoproterenol	0.2 mg/mL	0.1 *mcg*/kg/min	3 mL
Epinephrine	1:1000 (1 mg/mL)	0.1 *mcg*/kg/min	0.6 mL
Dopamine	40 mg/mL	10 *mcg*/kg/min	1.5 mL
Dobutamine	25 mg/mL	10 *mcg*/kg/min	2.4 mL
Lidocaine	1% (10 mg/mL)	20 *mcg*/kg/min	12 mL

Listed above are five out-of-hospital pediatric drugs. The chart shows, for each drug, the drug's concentration in its most common preparation and the rate of administration that medical control usually orders for the drug. The last column shows the amount of drug preparation to add to 100 mL of D$_5$W. By infusing the resulting solution at the rate of administration indicated on the body weight chart below, you will achieve the desired rate of drug administration.

Weight

kg	lb	Infusion Rate (mL/h)	kg	lb	Infusion Rate (mL/h)
3	6.6	3	30	66	30
7	15.4	7	35	77	35
10	22	10	40	88	40
12.5	27.5	12.5	45	99	45
15	33	15	55	110	50
17.5	38.5	17.5	55	121	55
20	44	20	60	132	60
22.5	49.5	22.5	65	143	65
25	55	25	70	154	70

Drugs Used in Pediatric Advanced Life Support*

Drugs Used in Pediatric Advanced Life Support*

Drug	Dose	Remarks
Adenosine	0.1 mg/kg Maximum 1st dose: 6 mg Maximum 2nd dose:12 mg Maximum single dose: 12 mg	Rapid IV push
Amiodarone	5 mg/kg (VF) 5 mg/kg (SVT)	Rapid IV/IO bolus IV/IO over 20–60 minutes
Amrinone	0.75–1.0 mg/kg	IV/IO over 5 minutes
Atropine sulfate	0.02 mg/kg per dose	Minimum dose: 0.1 mg Maximum single dose: 0.5 mg in child, 1.0 mg in adolescent
Calcium chloride 10%	20 mg/kg per dose	Give slowly
Calcium gluconate	60–100 mg/kg	Slow IV/IO push
Dobutamine hydrochloride	2–20 μg/kg/min	Titrate to desired effect
Dopamine hydrochloride	2–20 mcg/kg/min	α-Adrenergic action dominates at 15–20 mcg/kg/min
Epinephrine For bradycardia	IV/IO; 0.01 mg/kg (1:10,000) ET: 0.1 mg/kg (1:1000)	Be aware of effective dose of preservatives administered (if preservatives are present in epinephrine preparation) when high doses are used
For asystolic or pulseless arrest	First dose: IV/IO: 0.01 mg/kg (1: 10,000) ET: 0.1 mg/kg (1:1000) Doses as high as 0.2 mg/kg may be effective Subsequent doses: IV/IO/ET: 0.1 mg/kg (1:1000) Doses as high as 0.2 mg/kg may be effective	Be aware of effective dose of preservative administered (if preservatives present in epinephrine preparation) when high doses are used
Epinephrine infusion	Initial at 0.1 mcg/kg/min Higher infusion dose used if asystole present	Titrate to desired effect (0.1–1.0 mcg/kg/min)
Etomidate	0.2–0.4 mg/kg	Infused over 30–60 seconds
Glucose	0.5–1.0 g/kg	Maximum concentration: 25%, 2–4 mL/kg
Lidocaine	1 mg/kg per dose	
Lidocaine infusion	20–50 mcg/kg/min	
Magnesium sulfate	25–50 mg/kg	Maximum: 2 g over 10–20 minutes
Naloxone	0.1 mg/kg 2.0 mg	Up to 20 kg Over 20 kg
Nitroprusside	1 mcg/kg/min	Titrate up to 8 mcg/kg/min if needed
Norepinephrine	0.1–2.0 mcg/kg/min	Adjust infusion rate to achieve desired blood pressure
Procainamide	15 mg/kg	IV/IO over 30–60 minutes
Sodium bicarbonate	1 mEq/kg per dose or 0.3 × kg × base deficit	Infuse slowly and only if ventilation is adequate

*IV indicates intravenous route; IO, intraosseous route; and ET, endotracheal route.

Acute Pulmonary Edema

Confirm Acute Pulmonary Edema

Identify & Treat Possible Causes

Hypovolema
Hypoxia
Hydrogen ion
Hypoglycemia
Hypo-hyperkalemia
Hypothermia
Toxins
Tamponade
Tension pneumothorax
Thrombosis
Trauma

First-line Actions
(Per Protocol/Medical Control)

Oxygen & Advanced Airway as needed
Nitroglycerin 0.3–0.4 mg SL
Furosemide 0.5–1 mg/kg IV
Morphine 2–4 mg IV

Second-line Actions
(BP Dependent/Protocol/Medical Control)

Consider: Norepinephrine 0.5–30 mg/minute IV
Dopamine 2–20 mcg/kg/minute IV
Dobutamine 2–20 mcg/kg/minute IV
Nitroglycerin 10–20 mcg/minute

Expert Consultation

Stable Narrow-Complex Tachycardia

Primary/Secondary Survey (Supporting ABCs as needed)

Give Oxygen
Monitor ECG

Establish IV
Obtain 12-lead ECG

Regular/Irregular Rhythm ⟶ Transport for Consultation

Treat Possible Causes

Hypovolema
Hypoxia
Hydrogen ion
Hypoglycemia
Hypo-hyperkalemia
Hypothermia
Toxins
Tamponade
Tension pneumothorax
Thrombosis
Trauma

Attempt Vagal Maneuvers
Give adenosine, 6 mg (may
repeat at 12 mg x 2 if no conversion)

Transport

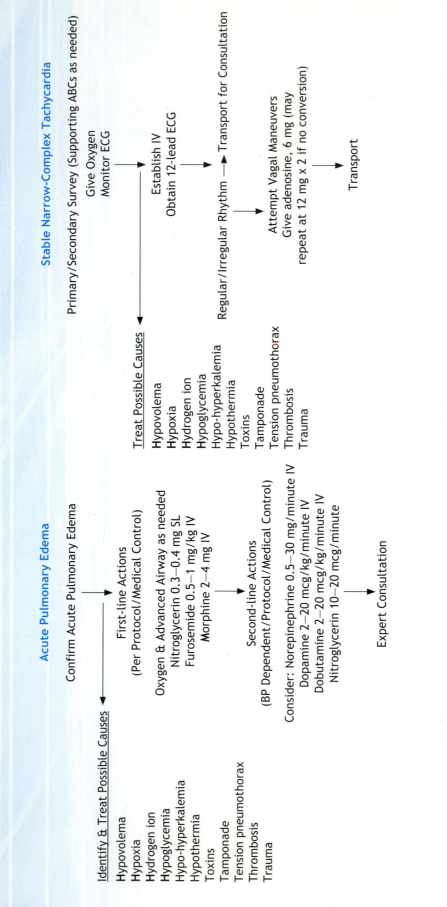

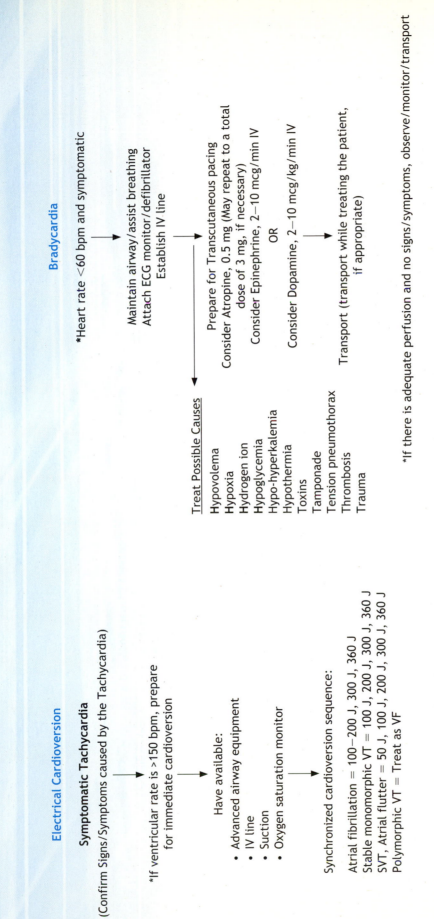

Bradycardia

*Heart rate <60 bpm and symptomatic

Maintain airway/assist breathing
Attach ECG monitor/defibrillator
Establish IV line

Treat Possible Causes

Hypovolema
Hypoxia
Hydrogen ion
Hypoglycemia
Hypo-hyperkalemia
Hypothermia
Toxins
Tamponade
Tension pneumothorax
Thrombosis
Trauma

Prepare for Transcutaneous pacing
Consider Atropine, 0.5 mg (May repeat to a total dose of 3 mg, if necessary)
Consider Epinephrine, 2–10 mcg/min IV

OR

Consider Dopamine, 2–10 mcg/kg/min IV

Transport (transport while treating the patient, if appropriate)

*If there is adequate perfusion and no signs/symptoms, observe/monitor/transport

Electrical Cardioversion

Symptomatic Tachycardia

(Confirm Signs/Symptoms caused by the Tachycardia)

*If ventricular rate is >150 bpm, prepare for immediate cardioversion

Have available:
• Advanced airway equipment
• IV line
• Suction
• Oxygen saturation monitor

Synchronized cardioversion sequence:

Atrial fibrillation = 100–200 J, 300 J, 360 J
Stable monomorphic VT = 100 J, 200 J, 300 J, 360 J
SVT, Atrial flutter = 50 J, 100 J, 200 J, 300 J, 360 J
Polymorphic VT = Treat as VF

*When preparing for synchronized cardioversion, premedicate the patient, when possible. Drug choices include:

• Diazepam
• Midozolam
• Etomidate
• Ketamine

These drugs can be used with or without fentanyl, norphase, or meperidine.

Pulseless Arrest
VF/VT

Primary & Secondary Survey
Give Oxygen when available
If no pulse, begin CPR
Attach AED/Monitor/Defibrillator

→

Confirm VF/VT

→

Give 1 Defibrillation
Resume CPR (5 cycles)

→

Check Rhythm
If VF/VT:
Give 1 Defibrillation
Resume CPR
When IV/IO available, give:
Epinephrine, 1 mg q 3-5 minutes

OR

May give 1, 40 unit dose of Vasopressin to replace 1st or 2nd dose of epinephrine

→

Check Rhythm
If VF/VT:
Give 1 Defibrillation
Resume CPR
Consider:

Amiodarone, 300 mg (may give additional 150 mg IV one time).

OR

Lidocaine, 1-1.5 mg/kg (may repeat at 0.5-0.75 mg/kg with a maximum dose of 3 doses or 3 mg/kg).

OR

Consider: Magnesium, 1-2 g if Torsades de pointes

After 5 cycles of CPR, repeat treatment from step 5, or follow protocols/medical control.

Asystole/PEA

Primary & Secondary Survey
Give Oxygen when available
If no pulse, begin CPR
Attach AED/Monitor/Defibrillator

→

Check Pulse

→

Asystole/PEA

→

Resume 5 Cycles of CPR

→

When IV/IO in place, give:
Epinephrine, 1 mg q 3-5 min

OR

May give 1 dose, 40 units of vasopression to replace 1st or 2nd dose of epinephrine

→

Check Pulse

→

If asystole or PEA continue, repeat treatment from step 4, or follow local protocol/medical control.

Treat Possible Causes

Hypovolema
Hypoxia
Hydrogen ion
Hypoglycemia
Hypo-hyperkalemia
Hypothermia
Toxins
Tamponade
Tension pneumothorax
Thrombosis
Trauma

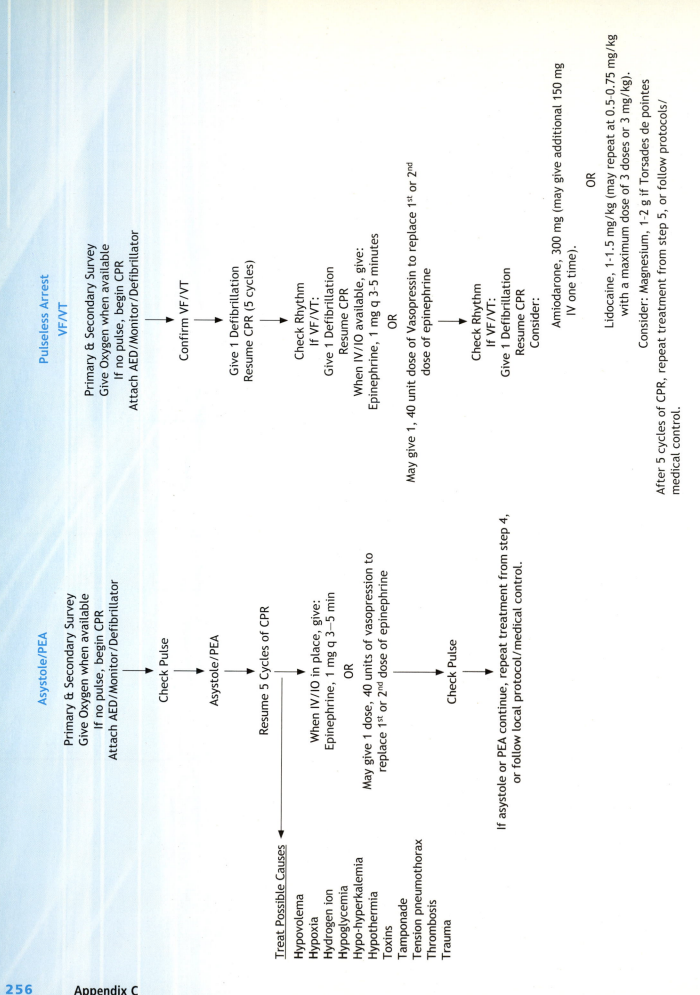

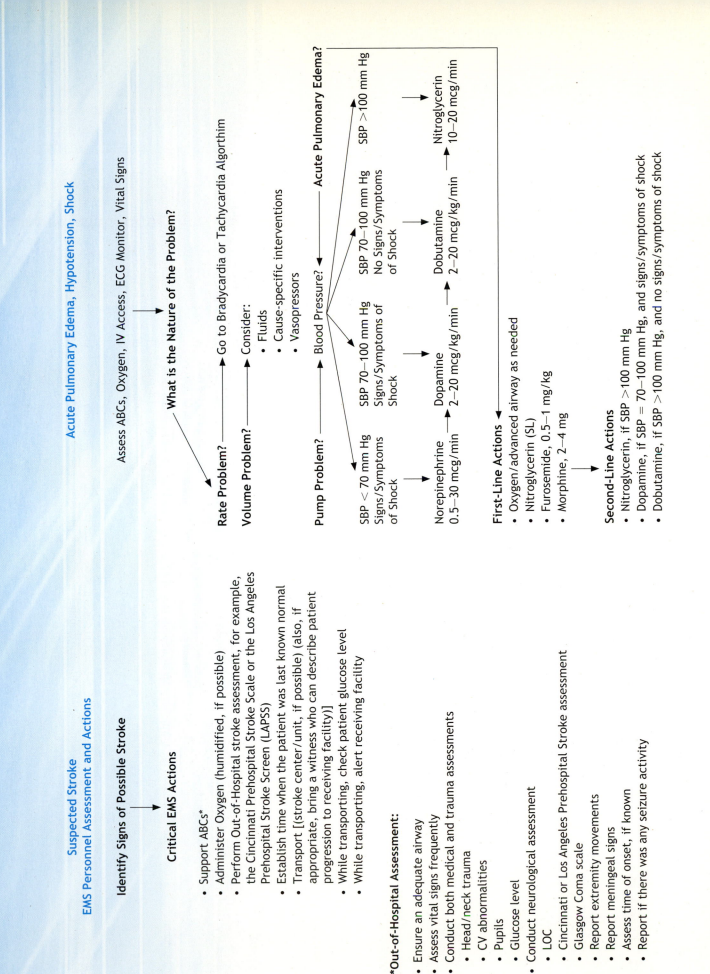

Suspected Stroke
EMS Personnel Assessment and Actions

Identify Signs of Possible Stroke →

Critical EMS Actions

- Support ABCs*
- Administer Oxygen (humidified, if possible)
- Perform Out-of-Hospital stroke assessment, for example, the Cincinnati Prehospital Stroke Scale or the Los Angeles Prehospital Stroke Screen (LAPSS)
- Establish time when the patient was last known normal
- Transport [(stroke center/unit, if possible) (also, if appropriate, bring a witness who can describe patient progression to receiving facility)]
- While transporting, check patient glucose level
- While transporting, alert receiving facility

*Out-of-Hospital Assessment:

- Ensure an adequate airway
- Assess vital signs frequently
- Conduct both medical and trauma assessments
  - Head/neck trauma
  - CV abnormalities
  - Pupils
  - Glucose level
- Conduct neurological assessment
  - LOC
  - Cincinnati or Los Angeles Prehospital Stroke assessment
  - Glasgow Coma scale
  - Report extremity movements
  - Report meningeal signs
  - Assess time of onset, if known
  - Report if there was any seizure activity

Acute Pulmonary Edema, Hypotension, Shock

Assess ABCs, Oxygen, IV Access, ECG Monitor, Vital Signs

What is the Nature of the Problem?

Rate Problem? → Go to Bradycardia or Tachycardia Algorthim

Volume Problem? → Consider:
- Fluids
- Cause-specific interventions
- Vasopressors

Pump Problem? → Blood Pressure?

Acute Pulmonary Edema?

- SBP <70 mm Hg Signs/Symptoms of Shock → Norepinephrine 0.5–30 mcg/min
- SBP 70–100 mm Hg Signs/Symptoms of Shock → Dopamine 2–20 mcg/kg/min
- SBP 70–100 mm Hg No Signs/Symptoms of Shock → Dobutamine 2–20 mcg/kg/min
- SBP >100 mm Hg → Nitroglycerin 10–20 mcg/min

First-Line Actions
- Oxygen/advanced airway as needed
- Nitroglycerin (SL)
- Furosemide, 0.5–1 mg/kg
- Morphine, 2–4 mg

Second-Line Actions
- Nitroglycerin, if SBP >100 mm Hg
- Dopamine, if SBP = 70–100 mm Hg, and signs/symptoms of shock
- Dobutamine, if SBP >100 mm Hg, and no signs/symptoms of shock

APPENDIX D

Herbal Remedies

Herb	Possible Uses	Possible Side Effects	Cautions	Drug Interactions
Alfalfa	Reduce LDL cholesterol levels. May reduce blood sugar levels in diabetic patients.	Stomach discomfort, diarrhea, and dermatitis.	Caution is advised in patients with hypoglycemia due to a possible reduction in blood sugar levels.	May reduce the blood-thinning effects of warfarin. May add to the effects of atrovastatin or simvastatin.
Aloe	Used topically to assist in healing of minor wounds, burns, and other skin irritations. Used orally as a laxative and to treat colic.	Cramps, diarrhea, allergic reactions	Some wound healing may be delayed when using topical gel. Patients with allergies to plants should use caution.	With oral use: digoxin, diuretics, corticosteroids, antiarrhythmics, AZT
Arginine (L-arginine)	May improve exercise tolerance and blood flow in arteries of the heart. Adding arginine to ibuprofen may decrease migraine headache pain. May decrease the severity of diabetes.	Nausea, stomach cramps.	May increase blood sugar levels.	May reduce the effectiveness of ranitidine or esomeprazole. May increase the risk of bleeding when used with anticoagulants.
Ashwagandha	Enhances mental and physical performance. Improves learning, ability. Decreases stress and fatigue. Provides chemotherapy and radiation protection.	Nausea, vomiting, GI distress	Do not use in pregnancy or lactation. Use with caution in patients receiving narcotic analgesics.	CNS depressants
Astragalus (Milk Vetch)	Increases stamina and energy. Support for chemotherapy and radiation. Improves immune function. Improves tissue oxygenation.	Nausea, vomiting, GI distress	Use with caution in acute infections, especially when accompanied by fever	Immunosuppressants
Bacopa	Enhances memory. Improves cognitive function.	CNS depression, seizures	Not for chronic use. Do not use in patients with seizure disorders.	CNS depressants, tricyclic antidepressants, antipsychotics
Bearberry	Diuretic. Short-term use for kidney stones and cystitis.	CNS depression, hypotension	Do not use in kidney disease or digestive disorders. Long-term use not recommended—may lead to GI distress.	Antihypertensives
Belladonna	Can cause relaxation of the airway and reduce the amount of mucus produced. Used for the treatment of irritable bowel.	Small amounts may cause death in children. Dry mouth, rapid heartbeat, nervousness. Large amounts may cause death in adults.	Older adults and children should avoid belladonna. Not recommended during pregnancy or during breastfeeding.	May interact with alkaloids, atropine, ergot derivatives, hormonal drugs, drugs that increase sun sensitivity, and drug cleared by the kidneys.
Bilberry	Treatment of eye disorders: myopia, decreased visual acuity, macular degeneration, night blindness, diabetic retinopathy, and cataracts. Treatment of vascular disorders: varicose veins, capillary permeability/stability, phlebitis.	Bleeding, impaired glucose control in diabetics	Use with caution in pregnancy and lactation. Diabetics should use cautiously because of potential to alter glucose regulation. Discontinue use at least 14 days prior to dental or surgical procedures.	Insulin, oral hypoglycemics, hormone replacement therapy

Herb	Possible Uses	Possible Side Effects	Cautions	Drug Interactions
Black Alder	Used as a cathartic	Diarrhea, vomiting, hypokalemia, abdominal cramping	Do not use in intestinal obstruction, inflammatory bowel disease, or children. Do not use for >8–10 days.	Antiarrhythmics, digoxin, corticosteroids, diuretics. May alter absorption of oral medications.
Black Cohosh	Treatment of menopausal disorders, PMS, mild depression, and arthritis	Nausea, vomiting, headache, hypotension, vertigo, impaired vision	Do not use in pregnancy or lactation. Do not use for >6 months. Use with caution with history of breast or endometrial cancer, thromboembolic disease, or CVA. Use with caution in patients with allergy to salicylates.	Oral contraceptives, hormone replacement therapy
Blessed thistle	May have activity against several types of bacteria.	Stomach irritation and vomiting.	May increase the risk of bleeding. Therefore, caution advised in patients with bleeding disorders or taking drugs that may increase the risk of bleeding.	
Bromelain	Treatment of inflammation and sports injuries. Use as a digestive aid. Treatment of respiratory tract infections. Aid in vision and circulation.	Nausea, vomiting, diarrhea, menstrual irregularities, hypotension	Use with caution in peptic ulcer disease, hypertension, and cardiovascular active bleeding. Stop use at least 14 days prior to dental or surgical procedures.	Anticoagulants, antiplatelet agents, aspirin, NSAIDs
Buckthorn	Used as a cathartic	Diarrhea, vomiting, hypokalemia, abdominal cramping	Should not be used for >8–10 days. Do not use in intestinal obstruction, inflammatory bowel disease, or children.	Antiarrhythmics, digoxin, diuretics, corticosteroids. May alter absorption of oral medications.
Burdock	Treatment of diabetes due to the possible blood sugar lowering effects.	Dry mouth and bradycardia.	Use with caution during pregnancy due to uterine stimulation.	May increase the risk of bleeding when taking with drugs that increase the risk of bleeding. Patients taking drug for diabetes should be monitored closely.
Bupleurum	Treatment of chronic inflammatory disease. Hepatoprotective against liver toxins.	Hypertension, tachycardia, sweating, hyperglycemia, edema	Use with caution in patients with diabetes, hypertension, or edema	Corticosteroids, diuretics, antihypertensives
Calendula	Used topically to treat minor wounds and burns	Contact dermatitis	Use caution in patients with allergies to plants	None
Cascara	Used as a laxative	Hypokalemia, diarrhea, abdominal cramping	Avoid use in children less than 12 years of age. Do not use in bowel obstruction, diarrhea, or dehydration. Use with caution in bowel disorders, inflammatory bowel disease, or appendicitis. Use with caution in cardiovascular disease.	Antiarrhythmics, digoxin, phenytoin, laxatives, lithium, theophylline, diuretics. May alter the absorption of oral medications.
Cat's Claw	Stimulates the immune system. Used as an adjunct therapy for AIDS and cancer therapy and post-radiation therapy. Anti-inflammatory activity in the treatment of allergies and arthritis. Used to treat bacterial, fungal, and viral infections.	Bleeding, diarrhea, or changes in bowel movements	Do not take in pregnancy or lactation. Use with caution in transplant patients, patients on immunosuppressants, or IV immunoglobulin.	IV immunoglobulin, immunosuppressants, anticoagulants, aspirin, NSAIDs, antiplatelet agents

(continued)

Herb	Possible Uses	Possible Side Effects	Cautions	Drug Interactions
Cayenne	Used topically to relieve pain associated with arthritis, rheumatism, and cold injuries. Taken orally to increase peripheral circulation and improve digestion.	Burning sensation when used topically. Oral use may cause GI distress, nausea, and vomiting.	Use with caution in patients with peptic ulcer disease	Monoamine oxidase inhibitors, aspirin, antihypertensives
Chamomile	Treatment of anxiety and insomnia. Treatment of GI disturbances: indigestion, heartburn, and flatulence. Used as a mouthwash for the treatment of gingivitis and pharyngitis. Used topically for the treatment of acne, superficial infections, minor wounds, and burns.	Allergic reactions, vomiting. Large doses may cause depression and drowsiness.	Avoid use in patients with allergies to plants in the chrysanthemum or daisy family, or to ragweed pollens. Do not use in pregnancy or lactation. Large doses may cause drowsiness—use caution when driving or operating machinery. Not for chronic use.	CNS depressants
Chasteberry	Progesterone-like action that is used to treat PMS, menopausal symptoms, endometriosis, menstrual cycle irregularities, corpus luteum insufficieny, insufficient lactation, hyperprolactinemia, and acne vulgaris	Heavy menstrual flow	Do not use in pregnancy	Hormone replacement therapy, oral contraceptives, metoclopramide, levodopa, bromocriptine, pramipexole, antipsychotics
Clove	Used topically to relieve toothache and teething problems	Use for >48 hours may cause gingival damage	Not for internal use. Use cautiously in patients allergic to plants.	None
Coleus	Treatment for allergies, asthma, hypertension, congestive heart failure, eczema, and psoriasis	Hypotension, bleeding	Use with caution in patients at risk of hypotension, who are elderly, or those who would not tolerate hypotension. Do not use in patients with active bleeding. Use with caution in patients with history of bleeding or hematologic disorders. Discontinue use at least 14 days prior to dental or surgical procedures.	Anticoagulants, antiplatelet agents, aspirin, NSAIDs, antihistamines, decongestants, antihypertensives
Cordyceps	Enhances endurance and stamina. Improves energy in patients with fatigue. Adjunctive treatment for chemotherapy and radiation. Protects liver from toxins. Enhances sexual vitality. Treatment of lung and kidney disorders.	Bleeding, hypertension	Use with caution in patients allergic to molds or fungi. Do not use in patients taking monoamine oxidase inhibitors. Do not use in patients with active bleeding. Use with caution in patients with history of bleeding or hematologic disorders. Discontinue use at least 14 days prior to dental or surgical procedures.	Monoamine oxidase inhibitors, anticoagulants, antiplatelet agents
Cranberry	Prevention of kidney stones. Treatment of urinary tract infections.	Large doses may cause GI symptoms	None	Drugs that increase uric acid levels
Creatine	May increase muscle mass. May also improve heart muscle strength. Potential benefit in the treatment of depression. May improve cognition.	Stomach discomfort, diarrhea, or nausea. May cause muscle cramps. Patients with kidney disease should avoid creatine.	Long-term use of large amounts of creating may increase the production of formaldehyde, which may cause serious side effects. Not recommended during pregnancy.	May interact with stimulants such as caffeine. May alter the effectiveness of insulin.
Dandelion	Use in digestive disorders to increase bile secretion, increase appetite, and to treat dyspepsia. Diuretic.	Electrolyte disturbances, allergic reactions	Avoid use in biliary obstruction or if gallstones are present	Diuretics, lithium, digoxin

Herb	Possible Uses	Possible Side Effects	Cautions	Drug Interactions
Devil's Claw	Used as an analgesic in the treatment of arthritis, tendonitis, gout, myalgia, and other inflammatory conditions	Bleeding, GI distress	Do not use in pregnancy or lactation. Use with caution in patients with GI disorders. Do not use in patients with active bleeding. Use with caution in patients with history of bleeding or hematologic disorders. Discontinue use at least 14 days prior to dental or surgical procedures.	Antiarrhythmics, digoxin, aspirin, NSAIDs, anticoagulants, antiplatelet agents
DHEA	May improve the quality of life in patients with Addison's disease. May be beneficial as a supplement in lowering cholesterol levels.	Fatigue, nasal congestion, headache and irregular heartbeats.	There is a risk of developing prostate, breast or ovarian cancer. Not recommended during pregnancy or during breastfeeding.	Should be used with caution with medications that affect heart rhythm. Alcohol may increase the effects of DHEA.
Dong Quai	Used to improve energy, especially in women. Used to treat anemia, menopausal symptoms, dysmenorrheal, PMS, and amenorrhea. Used to treat hypertension.	Hypotension, bleeding, photosensitivity	Do not use during the 1st trimester of pregnancy, in patients with excessive menses, hematologic disorders, or severe flu. Use caution in patients with GI distress, patients at risk of hypotension, or those who would not tolerate a hypotensive episode. May cause photosensitivity, so prolonged exposure to sunlight or UV radiation should be avoided. Use with caution in patients with a histor of breast or endometrial cancer, thromboembolism or CVA.	Antihypertensives, hormonal replacement therapy, oral contraceptives, tamoxifen, anticoagulants, antiplatelet agents
Echinacea	Used to stimulate the immune system. Prevention and treatment of colds, flus, allergies, and other upper respiratory infections. Used topically to treat boils, abscesses, tonsillitis, eczema, mild burns, canker sores, herpes, and minor wounds.	Immunosuppression with prolonged use. Allergic reactions.	Should not take for >8 weeks because of potential immunosuppressive effects. Should not be used for >10 days in patients with acute infection, or immunosuppression. Use with caution in patients allergic to ragweed, daisies, asters, chrysanthemums, and other pollens	Immunosuppressants, corticosteroids
Elder	Used to prevent or treat colds, flu, or other respiratory infections. Diuretic. Promotes sweating.	Hypokalemia with prolonged use or high doses	Use caution with drugs that cause hypokalemia or drugs whose toxicity is increased by hypokalemia	Diuretics, digoxin, lithium
Ephedra (Ma Huang)	Used as a bronchodilator in the treatment of asthma. Used as a decongestant in allergies, colds, sinusitis, and hay fever. Used to suppress appetite for weight loss.	CNS stimulation, nervousness, insomnia, headache, dizziness, skin flushing, palpitations, MI, hypertension, CVA	Should only be used under medical supervision. Do not use in pregnancy, lactation, or patients taking monoamine oxidase inhibitors. Use with extreme caution in patients with renal impairment, hypertension, cardiovascular disease, thyroid disease, diabetes, prostate disorder glaucoma, and seizure disorders. Ephedra has been used as a drug of abuse.	Caffeine, oxytocin, decongestants, methyldopa, beta-blockers, calcium channel blockers, thyroid medications, antiarrhythmias, digoxin, halothane, theophyllines,

Herb	Possible Uses	Possible Side Effects	Cautions	Drug Interactions
Evening Primrose	Used as a digestive aid in irritable bowel syndrome. Used in the treatment of eczema, dermatitis, and psoriasis. Used in the treatment of endometriosis, PMS, and menopausal symptoms. Also used for the treatment of diabetic neuropathy, rheumatoid arthritis, and multiple sclerosis. A source of omega-6 fatty acids.	Seizures, bleeding	Do not use in patients with seizure disorders, schizophrenia, and active bleeding. Use with caution in patients with a history of bleeding or hematologic disorders. Discontinue use at least 14 days prior to dental or surgical procedures.	Anticoagulants, anticonvulsants, antiplatelet agents, phenothiazines, antipsychotics
Fenugreek	Blood glucose regulation	Hypoglycemia	Blood glucose levels should be monitored closely. May alter insulin and/or oral hypoglycemic requirements in diabetics.	Insulin, oral hypoglycemic agents
Feverfew	Prevention of migraine headaches. Treatment of rheumatoid arthritis.	Mouth ulcers, unpleasant taste, abdominal pain, indigestion, tachycardia, bleeding. Post-feverfew syndrome may occur with abrupt discontinuation: nervousness, insomnia, joint stiffness and pain. Abrupt discontinuation may increase migraine frequency.	Do not use in pregnancy, lactation, children <2 years, or patients with allergies to chrysanthemums or daisies. The onset of effect may take weeks; patients should be advised to take for 1 month before deciding it is not effective. Do not take in active bleeding. Use with caution in patients with a history of bleeding or hematologic disorders. Discontinue use at least 14 days prior to dental procedures.	Anticoagulants, antiplatelet agents, aspirin, NSAIDs
Flaxseed Oil	Omega-3 fatty acid supplement	None	Must be refrigerated	May delay absorption of oral medications. Do not take within 2 hours of medications.
Garcinia	Glucose regulation in diabetes. Weight loss.	Hypoglycemia	Blood glucose should be closely monitored if taking insulin or oral hypoglycemics. Dosages of these drugs may need to be adjusted. Use with caution in diabetes or patients predisposed to hypoglycemia.	Insulin, oral hypoglycemics, hypolipidemic agents
Garlic	Digestive aid. Lowers cholesterol and blood pressure. Protects against heart disease by antiplatelet activity. Stimulates immune system. Prevents infection, including bacterial and fungal. Protection from cancer and liver toxicity.	GI distress at beginning of therapy, bleeding, sweating, hypoglycemia, hypotension	Do not use in patients with active bleeding. Use with caution in patients with history of bleeding or hematologic disorders. Discontinue use at least 14 days prior to dental or surgical procedures. Use caution in patients at risk of hypotension, who are elderly, or patients who would not tolerate hypotensive episodes. May alter glucose regulation. Use with caution in diabetes or patients predisposed to hypoglycemia. Monitor blood glucose closely.	Anticoagulants, aspirin, antiplatelet agents, NSAIDs, antihypertensives, insulin, oral hypoglycemics
Ginger	Treatment for motion sickness, dyspepsia, and nausea. Anticoagulant activity. Treatment of arthritis. Treatment of cough, colds, and flu.	High doses (>6 g) may cause a burning sensation and nausea. Bleeding.	Do not use in active bleeding or hematologic disorders. Discontinue use at least 14 days prior to dental or surgical procedures.	Anticoagulants, antiplatelet agents, aspirin, NSAIDs

Herb	Possible Uses	Possible Side Effects	Cautions	Drug Interactions
Ginkgo	Improves cerebral vascular and peripheral blood flow and oxygen delivery. Improves cognitive function in Alzheimer's disease. Treatment of peripheral vascular disease, Raynaud's disease, and coronary artery disease. Treatment of impotence, tinnitus, depression, macular degeneration, and asthma.	GI distress, headache, dizziness, bleeding (including hypema and subdural hematoma), palpitations dermatitis	Do not use in patients with active bleeding or hematologic disorders . Discontinue use at least 14 days prior to dental or surgical procedures.	Monoamine oxidase inhibitors, acetylcholinesterase inhibitors, aspirin, NSAIDs, antiplatelet agents, anticoagulants
Ginseng	Enhances mental and physical performance. Increases energy. Decreases stress. Improves immune function. Adjunct support for chemotherapy and radiation.	Nervousness, depression, insomnia, hypertension at low doses, tachycardia and hypotension at high doses, dermatitis, fever, bleeding, diarrhea, and gynecomastia with prolonged use or high doses	Do not use in renal failure, acute infection, pregnancy, lactation, or active bleeding. Use with caution in patients with hypertension and those at risk of hypotension, who are elderly, those who would not tolerate hypotensive episodes or patients with hematologic disorders.	Anticoagulants, antiplatelet agents, aspirin, NSAIDs, antihypertensives, monoamine oxidase inhibitors, CNS stimulants, caffeine, decongestants, hormonal , therapies, and drugs that cause gynecomastia: calcium channel blockers, digoxin, methyldopa, phenothiazines, and spironolactone
Glucosamine	Possible benefits in the treatment of general osteoarthritis of various joints of the body. May also benefit patients with rheumatoid arthritis.	Stomach upset, drowsiness, insomnia, headache, sun sensitivity.	Use cautiously in patients with bleeding disorders or taking drugs that may increase the risk of bleeding	May decrease the effectiveness of insulin. Used in combination with diuretics may cause an increased risk of side effects.
Golden Seal	Treats inflamed mucous membranes, gastritis, bronchitis, cystitis, and infectious diarrhea	Doses of 2–3 g may decrease heart rate, cause GI distress, and hypotension. High doses of 18 g may cause CNS depression, hypertension, paralysis, and seizures. Extended use of high doses may cause CNS stimulation, hallucinations, delirium, and GI disorders.	Do not use in pregnancy or lactation. Use with caution in patients with cardiovascular disease or hypertension. Should not be taken for an extended period of time.	Antihypertensives, anticoagulants
Gotu Kola	Used topically to promote healing of wounds from trauma, inflammation, or infection. Also used topically to treat hemorrhoids. Used orally to treat scleroderma.	Topical use may cause contact dermatitis. Large oral doses may cause sedation, and elevated cholesterol levels.	Do not use in pregnancy. May cause drowsiness—use caution when driving or operating machinery.	CNS depressants
Grape Seed	Treatment of allergies and asthma. Improves circulation by antiplatelet activity, and improvement of capillary fragility. Used to treat intermittent claudication, varicose veins, and rterial/venous insufficiency.	Bleeding	Do not use in patients with active bleeding. Use with caution in patients with hematologic disorders. Discontinue use at least 14 days prior to dental or surgical procedures.	Anticoagulants, aspirin, NSAIDs, antiplatelet agents, xanthine oxidase inhibitors, methotrexate
Green Tea	Preventative for cancer and cardiovascular disease. Adjunctive treatment for chemotherapy and radiation. Lowers cholesterol and inhibits platelet aggregation.	Contains caffeine: may cause GI irritation, decreased appetite, insomnia, tachycardia, palpitations and nervousness. Bleeding.	Use with caution in patients with peptic ulcer disease, cardiovascular disease, and patients with hematologic disorders. Do not use in patients with active bleeding. Discontinue use at least 14 days prior to dental or surgical procedures.	Monoamine oxidase inhibitors, CNS stimulants, caffeine, decongestants, aspirin, NSAIDs, antihypertensives, anticoagulants, antiplatelet agents, theophylline

(continued)

Herb	Possible Uses	Possible Side Effects	Cautions	Drug Interactions
Gymnema	Used in diabetes to regulate blood glucose levels	Hypoglycemia	Monitor blood glucose closely. Dosage of insulin or oral hypoglycemics may require adjustments. Patients should take only under medical supervision.	Insulin, oral hypoglycemics
Hawthorn	Treatment of angina, arrhythmias, tachycardia, hypotension or hypertension, peripheral vascular disease, and mild congestive heart failure	Hypotension, dizziness, headache	Do not use in pregnancy. Use with caution in patients at risk of hypotension, who are elderly, or those who would not tolerate hypotensive episodes.	Antihypertensives, digoxin, antiarrhythmics
Horse Chestnut	Used orally and topically for the treatment of varicose veins, hemorrhoids, deep venous thrombosis, lower extremity edema, and other venous insufficiencies	Gastroenteritis, bleeding	Use with caution in hepatic or renal impairment, or hematologic disorders. Do not use in patients with digestive disorders, or with active bleeding. Discontinue use at least 14 days prior to dental or surgical procedures.	Anticoagulants, aspirin, NSAIDs, antiplatelet agents
Horsetail	Used as a diuretic. Used in osteoporosis to strengthen bone and connective tissue	Electrolyte disorders, thiamine. (vitamin B_1) deficiency	Do not use in patients with hypotension or hypokalemia	Antiarrhythmics, digoxin, phenytoin, diuretics, lithium, theophylline
Isoflavones (Soy)	Prevention of cancer. Adjunctive treatment for chemotherapy. Decreases bone loss. Treatment of hypercholesterolemia. Treatment of menopausal symptoms.	None	Use with caution in patients with history of breast or endometrial cancer	Oral contraceptives, hormone replacement therapy
Kava Kava	Relieves anxiety and treats insomnia. Protects against CNS ischemia. Provides skeletal muscle relaxation. Used in children to treat ADD/ADHD.	Long-term use may cause rash, drowsiness, or hallucinations	Do not use in pregnancy, lactation, or Parkinson's disease. May cause drowsiness—use with caution when driving or operating machinery.	CNS depression, antipsychotics, levodopa
Lavender	Used topically as a wound-healing agent and on minor burns	None	For topical use only	None
Lemon Balm	Used topically for cold sores and fever blisters. Used orally in pediatrics for teething.	None	None	None
Licorice	Treatment of gastric and duodenal ulcers, adrenal insufficiency, and cough	Pseudohyperaldosteronism: hypokalemia, sodium retention, edema, and hypertension. Hepatotoxicity.	Do not use in pregnancy, diabetes, severe renal insufficiency, hypertension, cardiac disease, hypokalemia, or liver disease. Prolonged use (>4–6 weeks) not recommended.	Laxatives, diuretics, corticosteroids, nitrofurantoin
Marshmallow	Treatment of peptic ulcers. Cough suppressant and expectorant.	Hypoglycemia	Blood glucose should be monitored closely in patients receiving insulin or oral hypoglycemics	Insulin, oral hypoglycemics
Milk Thistle	Antidote in Death Cup mushroom poisoning. Promotes bile flow. Protects the liver when damaged by chronic drug abuse or drugs that are hepatotoxic. Relieves symptoms of jaundice and hepatiti	Diarrhea, gastroenteritis, thrombocytopenia	Do not use in hematologic or digestive disorders	None

Herb	Possible Uses	Possible Side Effects	Cautions	Drug Interactions
Passion Flower (Maypop)	Used to treat anxiety and insomnia	Drowsiness, vasculitis	May cause drowsiness—use caution when driving or operating machinery. Not for chronic use.	CNS depressants
Peppermint	Used as a digestive aid to treat abdominal cramps, nausea, flatulence, heartburn, and irritable bowel syndrome	None	Do not use in biliary tract obstruction, cholecystitis, gallstones, hiatal hernia, or severe liver damage	Calcium channel blockers
Propolis	Treatment of minor burns. Also has anti-viral and anti-inflammatory effects.	Generalized allergic reactions.	Contains high levels of alcohol and should be avoided during pregnancy and during breastfeeding.	May interact with anticoagulants, antibiotics, antineoplastics, antifungals and immunosuppressants.
Pycnogenol	Treatment of asthma. Also used in the treatment of Attention Deficit Hyperactivity Disorder (ADHD) to improve cognition. May decrease systolic blood pressure and reduce LDL cholesterol.	Minor stomach discomfort.	Used with caution in patients with diabetes or hypoglycemia.	May interact with angiotensin converting enzyme (ACE) inhibitors.
Psyllium	Used as a bulk-forming laxative	Abdominal cramps, diarrhea, or constipation	Avoid use in bowel obstruction	May decrease absorption of oral medications. Do not take within 2 hours of medications.
Pygeum	Improve urinary symptoms associated with benign prostatic hypertrophy (BPH)	Stomach pain, diarrhea, nausea, constipation.	Use beyond one year has not been studied.	None
Saw Palmetto	Treatment of benign prostatic hypertrophy	Rarely—headache, nausea Hypokalemia and other electrolyte disorders.	Prostatic cancer should be ruled out by prostatic exam and PSA prior to taking Saw Palmetto	Finasteride, alpha-adrenergic blockers
Senna	Used as a laxative	Overuse may cause bowel atony.	Avoid use in children less than 12 years of age, in bowel obstruction, diarrhea, or dehydration. Use with caution in bowel disorders, inflammatory bowel disease, and appendicitis. Use with caution in cardiovascular disease.	Antiarrhythmics, diuretics, digoxin, phenytoin, laxatives, lithium, theophylline. May decrease absorption of oral medications.
St. John's Wort	Used in the treatment of depression and anxiety. Used topically for minor wounds, burns, and infections, neuralgia, bruises, muscle soreness, and sprains.	Drowsiness, GI distress, fatigue, restlessness, photosensitivity, hypertension, hypomania, serotonin syndrome	Do not use in pregnancy, hypertension, patients who are bipolar, suicidal, psychotic, or severely depressed. May cause drowsiness—use caution when driving or operating machinery. May cause photosensitivity; avoid prolonged exposure to sunlight or UV radiation.	Pseudoephedrine, CNS depressants, meperidine, dextromethorphan, lithium, selegiline, monoamine oxidase inhibitors, antidepressants, yohimbine, serotonergic drugs, cyclosporin, digoxin, oral contraceptives, theophylline, anticoagulants
Schisandra	Hepatic protection and detoxification. Adjunct support for chemotherapy and radiation. Increases endurance, stamina, and work performance.	None	Do not use in pregnancy. Use caution in patients with liver damage, acute infections, and fever.	Calcium channel blockers, warfarin, phenytoin, cimetidine, theophylline
Soy	Adding soy to a diet can moderately decrease total cholesterol. Soy can treat diarrhea in infants and young children (2-38 months old).	GI blotting, nausea, constipation.	Use of soy is safe during pregnancy and during breastfeeding. High doses of soy at any age is not recommended.	Soy may interact with warfarin.

(continued)

Herb	Possible Uses	Possible Side Effects	Cautions	Drug Interactions
Spirulina	Used to treat nasal allergies due to anti-inflammatory properties. May lower cholesterol and triglyceride levels.	Headache, muscle pain, flushing of the face.	Not recommended during pregnancy or during breastfeeding.	May react with ACE inhibitors.
Tea Tree	Used as a mouthwash for dental and oral health. Used topically for burns, cuts, scrapes, and insect bites.	Allergic dermatitis	For external use only	None
Valerian	Used as a sedative/hypnotic to treat anxiety and insomnia. Treatment of nervous tension during PMS and menopause. Used in restless motor syndromes and muscle spasms.	Drowsiness, increased muscle relaxation, ataxia, hallucinations, headache, hepatotoxicity	May cause drowsiness—use caution when driving or operating machinery. Use with caution in pregnancy. Do not use in children less than 3 years of age.	CNS depressants
White Oak	Used as a mouthwash in the treatment of mild inflammation of the throat and mouth	None	Should not be swallowed	None
White Willow	Used to reduce fever and treat arthritis	GI distress or ulceration	Do not use in children or patients allergic to salicylates. Use with caution in patients with renal or hepatic dysfunction. Do not use in pregnancy, hypertension, or cardiovascular disease	Aspirin, NSAIDs, methotrexate, warfarin, metoclopramide, phenytoin, probenecid, spironolactone, valproic acid Monoamine oxidase inhibitors, antihypertensives, naloxone, tricyclic antidepressants, alpha$_2$-adrenergic blockers, caffeine, sympathomimetics
Yohimbe	Increases sexual vitality in men and women. Used to treat male erectile dysfunction.	Hypertension, tachycardia, palpitations, anxiety, insomnia		

APPENDIX E

Street Drugs

Cannabinoids:

Hashish:

Broom

Chronic

Gangster

Hash

Hash oil

Hemp

Marijuana:

A-bomb (with heroin or opium)

Acapulco gold

Acapulco red

Ace (with PCP)

African

Angola

Ashes

Assassin of Youth

Astro turf

Atshitshi

Aunt Mary

Baby bhang

Blunt

Dope

Ganja

Grass

Happy sticks (with PCP)

Herb

Joints

Kif

Love boat (with PCP)

Mary Jane

Maui Wowie

Pot

Primos (with Crack)

Reefer

Sinsemilla

Skunk

Texas tea

Tical (with PCP)

Weed

Woolies (with Crack)

Effects of Cannabinoids:

Euphoria

Slowed thinking and reaction time

Confusion

Impaired balance and coordination

Cough

Frequent respiratory infections

Impaired memory and learning

Tachycardia

Anxiety

Panic attacks

Hypertension

Increased thirst and appetite

Tolerance

Addiction

Club Drugs:

Flunitrazepam (Rohypnol):

Circles

Forget-me-drug

Forget-pill

La Roche

Mexican valium

Pappas

Pastas

Peanuts

R-2

Reynol

Rib

Roaches

Robinol

Roches

Rohibinol

Roofenol

Roofies

Roopies

Ropanyl

Rope

Rophies

Ro-shays

Rubies

Ruffiew

Whiteys

Used for:

Incapacitation of women/ sexual assault

Clinical Effects:

Sedation (onset within 15-20 minutes)

CNS depressant

Disinhibitory

Dizziness

Disorientation

Slurred speech

Loss of muscle control/coordination

Unconsciousness

Amnesia

Respiratory depression

Hot and cold flashes in rapid alteration

Nausea

Effects last 4-6 hrs/up to 12 hrs

Gamma-hydroxybutyrate (GHB):

Easy lay

Georgia homeboy

Great hormones at bedtime

Grievous bodily harm

G-riffic k

Jolt

Liquid

Liquid E

Liquid X

Max

Natural sleep-500

Organic quaalude

Salty water

Scoop

Soap

Somatomax

Used for:

Incapacitation of women/ sexual assault

Anabolic effects/increased muscle mass

Clinical Effects (onset 15-30 minutes):

CNS depressant

Drowsiness

Dizziness

Euphoria

Asymptomatic bradycardia

Nausea/vomiting

Unconsciousness

Hallucinations

Seizures

Respiratory depression

Respiratory acidosis

Delirium

Amnesia

Hypotonia

Mild hypothermia

Coma

Ketamine hydrochloride:

Bump

Cat Valium

Green

Honey oil

Jet

K

Kay

Keets

Kit-kat

Mauve

Purple

Special "K"

Special LA coke

Super acid

Super C

Vitamin K

Clinical Effects
(onset of effects 15-30 minutes):

Sedation

Hallucinations (duration ≤ 1 hour)

Impaired judgment

Impaired coordination

Hypertension

Vomiting

Hypersalivation

Rapid movements

Dizziness

Disorientation

Vivid dreams

Delirium

Nystagmus

Blurred or temporary loss of vision

Duration of effects 18-24 hours

Methylenedioxymetham-phetamine (MDMA):

Adam

B-bombs

Bens

Blue kisses

Blue lips

Cristal

Disco Biscuit

Ecstasy

Go

Hug Drug

XTC

Clinical Effects:

Confusion

Depression

Anxiety

Paranoia

Nausea

Syncope

Hypertension

Tachycardia

Rhabdomyolysis

Renal failure

Cardiovascular failure

Desired Effect:

CNS stimulant

Psychedelic

CNS Depressants:
Barbiturates (Amytal, Nembutal, Phenobarbital, Seconal):

Barb

Barbies

Barbs

Phennies

Red birds

Reds

Seccy

Tooies

Yellow Jackets

Yellows

Benzodiazepines (Ativan, Halcion, Librium, Valium, Xanax):

Candy

Downers

Green and whites

Sleeping pills

Tranks

Clinical Effects:

Sedation/drowsiness

Reduced pain

Reduced anxiety

Feeling of well-being

Dizziness

Disinhibition

Bradycardia

Respiratory depression

Poor concentration

Confusion

Impaired coordination

Impaired memory

Impaired judgment

Depression

Paradoxic excitation

Fever

Irritability

Slurred speech

Addiction

CNS Stimulants:
Amphetamine:

A

Aimies

Amp

B-bombs

Back dex

Bam

Bambita

Beans

Bennie

Bens

Benz

Benzedrine

Candy

Chalk

Christina

Christmas tree

Coasts to coasts

Crisscross

Crystal methadrine

Dex

Dexedrine

Dexies

Diet pills

Drivers

Eye opener

Fastin

Glass

Go

Head drugs

Hearts

Iboga

Jolly bean

L.A.

Lid poppers

Lid proppers

Marathons

Methedrine

Mini beans

Minibennie

Oranges

Peaches

Pep pills

Pink hearts

Pixies

Powder

Purple hearts

Red phosphorus

Snow

Speed

Speedball

Tens

Truck drivers

Uppers

Uppies

Alpha-ethyltryptamine:

Alpha-ET

ET

Love pearls

Love pills

Trip

Cocaine:

All-American Drug

Angie

Aunt Nora

Bazooka

Beam-me-up Scottie (w/PCP)

Belushi (with heroin)

Bernie

Big C

Big flake

Big rush

Blanco

Blast

Blow

C

C&M (with morphine)

C-dust

Cadillac

Caine

California cornflakes

Came

Candy

Candy C

Candy flipping on a string (with LSD/MDMA)

Caviar (with marijuana)

Champagne (with marijuana)

Charlie

Coca

Coke

Cola

Crystal

Dust

El diablito (with marijuana/ heroin/PCP)

El diablo (with marijuana/ heroin)

Flake

Florida snow

Freebase

Girlfriend

Glad stuff

Gold dust

Half piece (1/2 ounce)

Happy dust
Happy powder
Ice
Love affair
Marching dust
Movie star drug
Murder one (with heroin)
Nose
Nose candy
Nose powder
Nose stuff
Paradise white
Peruvian flake
Powder
Rock(s)
Rush
Snow
Snowball (with heroin)
Speed ball (with heroin)
Stardust
Sugar
Toot
White dragon
White horse
White mosquito
White powder

2-(4-Bromo-2,5 diethoxyphenyethylamine:

2-CB
Nexus
Spectrum
Toonies
Venus

Crack:

24-7
Apple Jacks
B.J.'s
Baby T
Bad
Badrock
Ball
Base
Baseball
Basing
Beamers
Beans
Beautiful boulders
Bill Blass
Biscuit (50 rocks)

Blanca
Blowcaine (with procaine)
Blowout
Bollo
Bomb
Boulder
Brick
Bubble gum
Butter
Caine
Cakes
Candy
Casper
Chalk
Chasing the dragon (with heroin)
Cheap basing
Climax
Cloud nine
Coke
Cookies
Crank
Crib
Crumbs
Crunch and Munch
Cubes
Devil drug
Hard ball
Hard rock
Hot cakes
Ice
Ice cube
Kryptonite
Liprimo (with marijuana)
Moonrock (with heroin)
Nuggets
One tissue box (1 ounce)
Outerlimits (with LSD)
Pebbles
Pee Wee ($5 worth)
Piles
Pony
Primo
Rock(s)
Smoke
Snow coke
Space base (with PCP)
Space cadet (with PCP)
Space dust (with PCP)
Spaceball (with PCP)

Stones
Sugarblock
White ghost

Dimethyltryptamine:

45-Minute Psychosis
AMT
Businessman's LSD
Businessman's special
Businessman's trip
DET
DMT
Fantasia

Methamphetamine:

Bathtub crank
Batu
Blue meth
Crink
Cris
Cristina
Cristy
Croak (with crack)
Crypto
Crystal
Crystal meth
Fire (with crack)
Hanyak
Hironpon
Hot ice
Ice
L.A. glass
L.A. ice
Meth
Meth speedball (with heroin)
Methlies Quik
Mexican crack
Mexican speedballs (with crack)
Quartz
Redneck cocaine
Super ice
Trash
White cross
Working man's cocaine
Yellow powder

Methcathinone:

Bathtub speed
Cadillac express
Cat

Ephedrone
Gaggers
Go-fast
Khat
Qat
Slick superspeed
Somali tea
Stat
Wild cat (with cocaine)
Wonder star

Methylphenidate (Ritalin[R]):

Crackers (with Talwin)
One and ones (with Talwin)
Poor man's heroin (with Talwin)
Ritz and T's (with Talwin)
Speedball (with heroin)
Ts and Rits (with Talwin)
Ts and Rs (with Talwin)
West Coast

4-Methylthioamphetamine:

Flatliners
Golden eagle

Clinical Effects of CNS Stimulants:

Hypertension
Decreased appetite
Tremors
Hyperreflexia
Irritability
Insomnia
Diaphoresis
Aggressive behavior
Anxiety
Delirium
Suicidal/homicidal tendencies
Violent behavior
Palpitations
Arrhythmias
Nausea
Abdominal cramps
Agitation
Temporary illusion of enhanced power and energy
Myocardial infarction
CVAs
Seizures
Paranoia

Cocaine: necrosis of the septum of the nose

Withdrawal: severe depression

Hallucinogens:

Lysergic acid diethylamide (LSD):

Acid

Acid cube

Back breakers (with strychnine)

Beavis & Butthead

Big D

Blotter

Blotter acid

Blue dots

Boomers

D

Dots

Microdot

Owsleys

Pane

Paper acid

Sugar

Sugar cubes

Window glass

Window pane

Yellow sunshines

Mescaline:

Beans

Buttons

Cactus

Mesc

Morning glory seeds:

Pearly gates

Psilocybin:

Magic mushroom

Mexico mushroom

Purple passion

Shrooms

Clinical Effects of Hallucinogens:

Hallucinations

Hyperthermia

Tachycardia

Dilated pupils

"Bad trip": 24 hr period of pain or loss of control

Hypertension

Decreased perception of pain

Insomnia

Alternating agitation and depression

Tremors

Numbness/weakness

Persisting perception disorder (flashbacks)

Cardiovascular collapse

Death

Inhalants:

Air blast

Aimes (amyl nitrate)

Aimies (amyl nitrate)

Ames (amyl nitrate)

Aroma of men (isobutyl nitrate)

Bagging (using inhalants)

Bolt (isobutyl nitrate)

Boppers (amyl nitrate)

Bullet (isobutyl nitrate)

Buzz bomb (nitrous oxide)

Climax (isobutyl nitrate)

Gluey (one who sniffs or inhales glue)

Huffing (sniffing an inhalant)

Laughing gas (nitrous oxide)

Locker room (isobutyl nitrate)

Pearls (amyl nitrate)

Poppers (isobutyl nitrate, amyl nitrate)

Quicksilver (isobutyl nitrate)

Rush (isobutyl nitrate)

Rush snappers (isobutyl nitrate)

Shoot the breeze (nitrous oxide)

Snappers (isobutyl nitrate)

Snorting (using inhalants)

Snotballs (rubber cement)

Thrust (isobutyl nitrate)

toncho (octane booster)

Whippets (nitrous oxide)

Whiteout

Commercial Products:

Adhesives

Aerosols

Anesthetics

Cleaning agents

Food products (vegetable cooking spray, dessert spray)

Gases

Solvents

Indicators of Inhalant Abuse:

Paint or stains on the body or clothing

Spots or sores around the mouth

Red or runny eyes and nose

Chemical odor on the breath

Intoxicated, dazed, or dizzy appearance

Loss of appetite

Excitability or irritability

Clinical Effects of Inhalants:

Initially:

CNS stimulation

Disinhibition

Distorted perception

Followed by:

CNS depression

Lethargy

Headache

Nausea/vomiting

Slurred speech

Loss of motor coordination

Wheezing

Acoustic nerve damage may cause deafness

Inhibition of oxygen-carrying capacity of the blood

Benzene may cause leukemias

Damage to the cerebral cortex and cerebellum:

Personality changes

Memory impairment

Hallucinations

Loss of coordination

Slurred speech

Sudden sniffing death syndrome (SSD):

Fatal cardiac arrhythmias

Kidney stones

Metabolic acidosis

Hepatotoxicity

Muscle wasting

Peripheral nerve damage:

Numbness

Tingling

Paralysis

"Glue sniffers rash": aroun nose and mouth

Withdrawal symptoms:

Diaphoresis

Tachycardia

Hand tremors

Insomnia

Nausea/vomiting

Agitation

Anxiety

Hallucinations

Generalized motor seizures

Opium Derivatives:

Codeine:

AC/DC

Captain Cody

Cody

Doors & fours (with glutethimide)

Lean

Loads (with glutethimide)

Nods

Pancakes & syrup (with glutethimide)

Schoolboy

Terp (with terpin hydrate)

Dextromethorphan:

DXM

Robo

Fentanyl:

Apache

China girl

China white

Dance fever

Friend

Goodfella

Jackpot

King ivory

Murder 8

TNT

Tango and Cash

Heroin:

AIP
Al Capone
Antifreeze
Aunt Hazel
Bart Simpson
Black tar
Brown sugar
Chinese white
Dope
H
H and stuff
Horse
Junk
Mexican mud
Scat
Skag
Skunk
Smack
Snow
White horse

Hydromorphone (Dilaudid^R):

Hospital heroin

Methadone:

Amidone
Dollies

Morphine:

M
Microdots
Miss Emma
Mister blue
Monkey
Morf
M.S.
White stuff

Opium:

Ah-pen-yen
Auntie
Aunti Emma
Big O
Black stuff
Block
Gum
Hop
Pingon
Pin yen
Poppy
Tar

Oxycontin:

Hillbillie heroin
OC
Oxi cotton
Oxy 80's
Oxy
Oxycet
Oxycotton

Paregoric:

Blue velvet (with amphetamine)
PG or PO
Propoxyphene hydrochloride
Pinks and grays

Clinical Effects of Opium Derivatives:

Pain relief
Euphoria
Respiratory depression/arrest
Nausea/vomiting
Confusion
Constipation
Sedation
Unconsciousness
Coma
Tolerance
Addiction
Withdrawal symptoms:
    Chills
    Diaphoresis
    Rhinitis
    Tearing
    Abdominal cramps
Muscle pain
Insomnia
Nausea/vomiting/diarrhea
Dextromethorphan (effects similar to PCP and ketamine)

Phencyclidine (PCP):

Ace
Amoeba
Angel
Angel dust
Angel hair
Angel mist
Animal trank
Animal tranquilizer
Aurora borealis
Black acid (with LSD)
Boat
Bush
Cheap cocaine
Cosmos
Devil's dust
DOA
Domex (with MDMA)
Dummy dust
Dummy mist
Hog
Jet
K
Kools (with marijuana)
Lemon 714
Love boat
Magic dust
Mauve
Monkey tranquilizer
Octane (with gasoline)
Ozone
Peace
Rocket fuel
Special LA coke
Superacid
Supercoke
Supergrass
Superjoint
Superweed
Trangs
Wack
Zombie
Clinical Effects
Acute onset of unusual behavior:
    Agitation
    Excitement
    Euphoria
    Hallucinations
    Incoordination
    Slurred speech
Catatonic rigidity
Hostility
Apathy
Amnesia
Nystagmus
Constricted pupils
Decreased pain perception
Seizures
Tremors
Weakness
Coma
Death
Involuntary muscle contractions
Hypertension
Arrhythmias
Flushing
Nausea/vomiting
Hypersalivation
Fever/hyperthermia
Diaphoresis
Psychosis
Violent or suicidal behavior
Rhadomyolysis/renal failure

Steroids:
Oral:

Anadrol (oxymetholone)
Oxandrin (Oxandrolone)
Dianobol (methandrostenolone)
Winstrol (stanozolol)

Injectable:

Deca-Durabolin (nandrolone decanoate)
Durabolin (nandrolone phenpropionate)
Depo-Testosterone (testosterone cypionate)
Equipoise (boldenone undecylenate)

Desired Effect:

Growth of skeletal muscle

Adverse Side Effects:

Acne
Tendon rupture
Irritability
Delusions
Mania
Aggression/homicidal rage
Liver cancer
MIs
CVAs

Left ventricular
   hypertrophy
Hypercholesterolemia
Adolescent use:
   stunted growth

Men:
   gynecomastia
   Infertility
   Testicular atrophy

Women:
   masculinization
   Decreased breast size
   Decreased body fat
   Coarsening of skin

Deepening of voice
Excessive growth of body
hair
   Menstral irregularities
Both sexes:

NOTE: Slang terminology for street drugs change regularly. Appendix F covers some of the more common street drug names. Included here are two websites that are comprehensive for slang terminology world-wide. 1. http://www.swapotraining.com/street_names.htm (Drug & Awareness & Specialist Training) 2. http://www.spraakservice.net/slangportal/drug.htm (Street Drug Names Around the World)

Commonly Used Abbreviations and Symbols

a	before	AST	aspartate aminotransferase
aa,A	of each	ATC	around the clock
abd	abdominal/abdomen	ATP	adenosine triphosphate
ABG	arterial blood gas	ATS/CDC	American Thoracic Society/Centers for
a.c.	before meals		Disease Control and Prevention
ACE	angiotensin-converting enzyme	ATU	antithrombin unit
ACH	acetylcholine	ATX	antibiotics
ACLS	advanced cardiac life support	a.u.	each ear, both ears
ACS	acute coronary syndrome	AV	atrioventricular
ACTH	adrenocorticotropic hormone	BCLS	basic cardiac life support
ad	to, up to	b.i.d.	two times per day
a.d.	right ear	b.i.n.	two times per night
add.	add	BMR	basal metabolic rate
ADD	attention deficit disorder	BP	blood pressure
ad lib	as desired, at pleasure	BPD	bronchopulmonary dysplasia
ADP	adenosine diphosphate	BPH	benign prostatic hypertrophy
ADA	adenosine deaminase	bpm	beats per minute
ADH	antidiuretic hormone	BS	blood sugar, bowel sounds
ADL	activities of daily living	BSA	body surface area
AFB	acid fast bacillus	BSE	breast self-exam
AHF	antihemophilic factor	BSP	Bromsulphalein
AIDS	acquired immune deficiency syndrome	BTLS	basic trauma life support
a.l.	left ear	BUN	blood urea nitrogen
ALT	alanine aminotransferase	C	Celsius/Centigrade
a.m., A.M.	morning	c	with
AMI	acute myocardial infarction	CABG	coronary artery bypass graft
AML	acute myeloid leukemia	C&DB	cough and deep breathe
AMP	adenosine monophosphate	CAD	coronary artery disease
ANA	antinuclear antibody	caps, Caps	capsule(s)
ANC	active neutrophil count	CBC	complete blood count
ANS	autonomic nervous system	CCB	calcium channel blocker
APLS	advanced pediatric life support	C_{CR}	creatinine clearance
APTT	activated partial thromboplastin time	CD_4	helper T_4 lymphocyte cells
aq	water	CDC	Centers for Disease Control and
aq dist.	distilled water		Prevention
ARC	AIDS-related complex	CF	cystic fibrosis
ARDS	adult respiratory distress syndrome	CHD	Congenital heart disease; coronary heart
ASA	aspirin		disease
ASAP	as soon as possible	CHF	congestive heart failure
ASCVD	atherosclerotic cardiovascular disease	CHO	carbohydrate
ASD	artial septic defect	CLL	chronic lymphocytic leukemia
ASHD	arteriosclerotic heart disease	cm	centimeter

CML	chronic myelocytic leukemia	e.g.	for example
CMV	cytomegalovirus	elix	elixir
CN	cranial nerve	EMS	emergency medical services
c.n.	tomorrow night	emuls.	emulsion
CNS	central nervous system	ENL	erythema nodosum leprosum
CO	cardiac output	ENT	ear, nose, throat
COMT	catechol-o-methyltransferase	EPS	electrophysiologic studies, extrapyramidal
COPD	chronic obstructive pulmonary disease		symptoms
CP	cardiopulmonary	ER	extended release/emergency room
CPAP	continuous positive airway pressure	ESR	erythrocyte sedimentation rate
CPB	cardiopulmonary bypass	ESRD	end-stage renal disease
CPK	creatine phosphokinase	ET	endotracheal
CPR	cardiopulmonary resuscitation	ETOH	alcohol
CRF	chronic renal failure	ext.	extract
C&S	culture and sensitivity	F	Fahrenheit, fluoride
CSF	cerebrospinal fluid	f	female
CSID	congenital sucrase-isomaltase deficiency	FBS	fasting blood sugar
CT	computerized tomography	FD	fatal dose
CTS	carpal tunnel syndrome	FDA	Food and Drug Administration
CTZ	chemoreceptor trigger zone	FEV	forced expiratory volume
CV	cardiovascular	FFP	fresh frozen plasma
CVA	cerebrovascular accident	FOB	fecal occult blood
CVP	central venous pressure	FS	finger stick
CXR	chest X-ray	FSH	follicle-stimulating hormone
/d	per day	F/U	follow-up
dATP	deoxy ATP	FUO	fever of unknown origin
DBP	diastolic BP	FVC	forced vital capacity
dc	discontinue	g, gm	gram (1,000 mg)
DEA	Drug Enforcement Agency	GABA	gamma-aminobutyric acid
DI	diabetes insipidus	GERD	gastroesophageal reflux disease
DIC	disseminated intravascular coagulation	GFR	glomerular filtration rate
dil.	dilute	GGT	gamma-glutamyl transferase:
dL	deciliter (one-tenth of a liter)		*syn.* gamma-glutamyl transpeptidase
DM	diabetes mellitus	gi, GI	gastrointestinal
DNA	deoxyribonucleic acid	GnRH	gonadotropin-releasing hormone
DNR	do not resuscitate	GP	glycoprotein
DOA	dead on arrival	G6PD	glucose-6-phosphate dehydrogenase
DOB	date of birth	gr	grain
DOE	dyspnea on exertion	Gtt/gtt	a drop, drops
dr.	dram (0.0625 ounce)	GU	genitourinary
DTR	deep tendon reflex	GYN	gynecology
DVT	deep vein thrombosis	H+	hydrogen ion
EC	enteric-coated	h, hr	hour
ECB	extracorporeal cardiopulmonary bypass	HA, HAL	hyperalimentation
ECG, EKG	electrocardiogram, electrocardiograph	HCG	human chorionic gonadotropin
ED	emergency department/effective dose	HCP	health-care provider
EDTA	ethylenediaminetetraacetic acid	HCV	hepatitis C virus
EEG	electroencephalogram	HDL	high-density lipoprotein
EENT	eye, ear, nose, and throat	HFN	high flow nebulizer
EF	ejection fraction	H&H	hematocrit and hemoglobin

HIT	heparin-induced thrombocytopenia	m^2, M^2	square meter
HIV	human immunodeficiency virus	m	meter/male
HMG-CoA	3-hydroxy-3methyl-glutaryl-coenzyme A	MAC	*Mycobacterium avium* complex
h/o	history of	MAO	monoamine oxidase
HOB	head of bed	MAP	mean arterial pressure
HR	heart rate	max	maximum
h.s.	at bedtime	mcg	microgram
HSE	herpes simplex encephalitis	mCi	millicurie
HSV	herpes simplex virus	MDI	metered-dose inhaler
5-HT	5-hydroxytryptamine	MED	minimum effective dose
HTN	hypertension	mEq	milliequivalent
Hx, hx	history	mg	milligram
IA	intra-arterial	MI	myocardial infarction
IBD	inflammatory bowel disease	MIC	minimum inhibitory concentration
ICP	intracranial pressure	min	minute, minim
ICU	intensive care unit	mist, mixt	mixture
IDDM	insulin-dependent diabetes mellitus	mL	milliliter
Ig	immunoglobulin	MLD	minimum lethal dose
im, IM	intramuscular	mm	millimeter
IMV	intermittent mandatory ventilation	MRI	magnetic resonance imaging
in d.	daily	MS	multiple sclerosis/mitral stenosis
inj.	injection	mg	microgram
INR	international normalized ratio	NaCl	sodium chloride
I&O	intake and output	ng	nanogram
IOP	intraocular pressure	NG	nasogastric
IPPB	intermittent positive pressure breathing	NGT	nasogastric tube
ITP	idiopathic thrombocytopenia purpura	NICU	neonatal intensive care unit
IU	international units	NIDDM	non-insulin dependent diabetes mellitus
iv, IV	intravenous	NKA	no known allergies
IVPB	IV piggyback, a secondary IV line	NKDA	no known drug allergies
J	joule	noct	at night, during the night
JVD	jugular venous distention	non rep	do not repeat
kg	kilogram (2.2 lb)	NPN	nonprotein nitrogen
KVO	keep vein open	NPO	nothing by mouth
L	liter (1,000 mL)	NR	do not refill (e.g., a prescription)
L	left	NS	normal saline
L&D	labor and delivery	NSAID	non-steroidal anti-inflammatory drug
LDH	lactic dehydrogenase	NSR	normal sinus rhythm
LDL	low density lipoprotein	NSS	normal saline solution
LFTs	liver function tests	N&V, N/V	nausea and vomiting
LH	luteinizing hormone	O_2	oxygen
LHRH	luteinizing hormone-releasing hormone	OB	obstetrics
LLL	left lower lobe	o.d.	once a day
LLQ	left lower quadrant	O.D.	right eye
LOC	level of consciousness	OH	orthostatic hypotension
LR	lactated ringers	OOB	out of bed
LTD	lowest tolerated dose	OR	operating room
LV	left ventricular	os	mouth
LVFP	left ventricular function pressure	O.S.	left eye
M	mix	O_2 sat	oxygen saturation

OTC	over the counter	q8hr	every eight hours
OU	each eye, both eyes	qhs	every night
oz	ounce	q.i.d.	four times a day
PA	pulmonary artery	qmo	every month
PABA	para-aminobenzoic acid	q.o.d.	every other day
PALS	pediatric advanced life support	q.s.	as much as needed, quantity sufficient
PAWP	pulmonary artery wedge pressure	RA	right atrium; rheumatoid arthritis
PBI	protein-bound iodine	RBC	red blood cell
p.c.	after meals	RDA	recommended daily allowance
PCA	patient-controlled analgesia	REM	rapid eye movement
PCI	percutaneous coronary intervention	Rept.	let it be repeated
PCN	penicillin	RNA	ribonucleic acid
PCP	*Pneumocystis carinii* pneumonia	ROM	range of motion
PCWP	pulmonary capillary wedge pressure	ROS	review of systems
PDR	*Physician's Desk Reference*	RRMS	relapsing-remitting multiple sclerosis
PE	pulmonary embolus	R/T	related to
PEEP	positive end expiratory pressure	RV	right ventricular
per	by, through	RUQ	right upper quadrant
PFTs	pulmonary function tests	Rx	symbol for a prescription
pH	hydrogen ion concentration	s	without
Pharm.	pharmacy	SA	sinoatrial or sustained-action
PHTLS	prehospital trauma life support	SAH	subarachnoid hemorrhage
PID	pelvic inflammatory disease	SBE	subacute bacterial endocarditis
PMH	past medical history	SBP	systolic BP
PMI	point of maximal intensity	sc, SC, SQ	subcutaneous
PMS	premenstrual syndrome	SCID	severe combined immunodeficiency disease
PND	paroxysmal nocturnal dyspnea		
po, p.o., PO	by mouth	S.D.	standard deviation
PPD	purified protein derivative	SGOT	serum glutamic-oxaloacetic transaminase
PR	by rectum	SGPT	serum glutamic-pyruvic transaminase
p.r.n., PRN	when needed or necessary	S., Sig.	mark on the label
PSA	prostatic specific antigen	SI	sacroiliac
PSP	phenolsulfonphthalein	SIADH	syndrome inappropriate antidiuretic hormone
PT	prothrombin time		
PTCA	percutaneous transluminal coronary angioplasty	SIMV	synchronized intermittent mandatory ventilation
PTH	parathyroid hormone	SL	sublingual
PTSD	post-traumatic stress disorder	SLE	systemic lupus erythematosus
PTT	partial thromboplastin time	SOB	shortness of breath
PUD	peptic ulcer disease	sol	solution
PVC	premature ventricular contraction; polyvinyl chloride	sp	spirits
		S/P	no change after
PVD	peripheral vascular disease	SR	sustained-release
q.	every	ss	one-half
q.d.	every day	S&S	signs and symptoms
q.h.	every hour	SSS	sick sinus syndrome
q2hr	every two hours	stat	immediately, first dose
q3hr	every three hours	STD	sexually transmitted disease
q4hr	every four hours	SV	stroke volume
q6hr	every six hours	SVT	supraventricular tachycardia

syr	syrup	ut dict	as directed
tab	tablet	UTI	urinary tract infection
TB	tuberculosis	UV	ultraviolet
TCA	tricyclic antidepressant	v	vein
TENS	transcutaneous electric nerve stimulation	VAD	venous access device
TIA	transient ischemic attack	VF	ventricular fibrillation
TIBC	total iron binding capacity	vin	wine
t.i.d.	three times per day	vit	vitamin
t.i.n.	three times per night	VLDL	very low density lipoprotein
TKR	total knee replacement	VMA	vanillylmandelic acid
TNF	tumor necrosis factor	vol.	volume
T.O.	telephone order	V.O.	verbal order
TPN	total parenteral nutrition	VS	vital signs/volumetric solution
TSH	thyroid stimulating hormone	VT	ventricular tachycardia
U	unit	WBC	white blood cell
m	micron	XRT	radiation therapy
mCi	microcurie	&	and
mg	microgram	>	greater than
mm	micrometer	<	less than
UGI	upper gastrointestinal	↑	increased, higher
ULN	upper limit of normal	↓	decreased, lower
ung	ointment	−	negative
UO	urine output	/	per
URI, URTI	upper respiratory infection	%	percent
US	ultrasound	+	positive
USP	U.S. Pharmacopeia	X	times, frequency

GLOSSARY

Absorption: passage of a substance through a body surface into body fluids and tissues.

ACE Inhibitors: angiotensin-converting enzyme inhibitors are a classification of drugs used to treat hypertension and congestive heart failure (CHF).

Acetylcholine: naturally occurring body substance necessary for the functioning of the parasympathetic nervous system.

Acidosis: condition resulting from an excess of acid or deficit of alkalines (bicarbonate) in body fluid.

Active transport: mechanism for moving substances across cell membranes from a dilute solution to a concentrated solution.

Adams-Stokes syndrome: also referred to as Stokes-Adams syndrome, a loss of consciousness caused by decreased flow of blood to the brain.

Adrenergic: term for (sympathetic) nerve fibers that, when stimulated, release epinephrine; also, a class of drugs that produces the effect of epinephrine.

Affinity: in pharmacology, the attraction between a receptor and a drug.

Afterload: arterial pressure that the heart must push against to eject blood; tension in the ventricular wall during systole.

Agglutination: a type of antigen-antibody reaction.

Agglutinin: an antibody present in the blood that causes antigens to bind together.

Agglutinogen: a specific antigen that stimulates the recognition of an antibody.

Agonist: substance that activates a receptor.

Alimentary route: route of drug administration via the alimentary canal.

Alkalosis: condition resulting from an excess of alkalines or a deficit of acid in the body fluid.

Alpha$_1$-adrenergic receptor: a site on the post-synaptic adrenergic nerve pathway that responds when norepinephrine is released.

Alpha$_2$-adrenergic receptor: a site on the pre-synaptic adrenergic nerve pathway that responds when norepinephrine is released.

Analgesic: drug that relieves pain.

Angina pectoris: chest pain possibly spreading to the jaws and arms. Anginal attacks occur when the demand for blood by the heart exceeds the supply of the coronary arteries.

Angiotensin converting enzyme (ACE) inhibitor: a drug that prevents the conversion of angiotension I to angiotensin II. This action results in a decrease in peripheral resistance and decreased aldosterone secretion (leading to fluid loss) and, therefore, a decrease in blood pressure.

Anion: see *ion*.

Antagonist: drug that interferes with the action of an agonist.

Antianginal: drug that relieves the pain of angina pectoris.

Antianxiety agent: a drug that is used to treat anxiety.

Antiarrhythmic: drug that controls or prevents cardiac arrhythmias.

Antiasthmatic: drug that is used to treat asthma.

Antibody: a substance produced by the body in response to an *antigen*; each antibody reacts only with its specific antigen.

Anticholinergic: a drug that inhibits the action of acetylcholine.

Anticholinesterase agent: a drug that opposes the action of cholinesterase.

Anticoagulant: drug that prevents or dissolves blood clots.

Anticonvulsant: a drug that prevents, terminates, or reduces seizures.

Antidote: substance that neutralizes a poison or the toxic effects of a drug.

Antiemetic: to prevent or relieve nausea and vomiting.

Antigen: foreign particle or substance whose presence in the body causes *antibody* production.

Antihistamine: drug that blocks the effects of histamine.

Antihypertensive: drug that lowers blood pressure.

Anti-inflammatory agent: a drug that reduces inflammation.

Antimuscarinic agent: a drug that opposes the action of muscarine.

Antiplatelet: a drug used to prevent platelet aggregation. Used in the treatment of angina and the prophylaxis of myocardial infarction.

Antipsychotic: a drug used to treat psychosis.

Antitussive: drug used to prevent or relieve coughing.

Anxiety: a vague feeling of discomfort accompanied by an autonomic response.

Apothecaries' system: a system of weight and measure used mostly by pharmacists.

Asepsis: a condition free from any form of life.

Assay: chemical processing that determines the ingredients present in a drug and their amounts.

Asthma: a disease caused by a narrowing and inflammation of the tracheobronchial tree by various stimuli.

Autonomic nervous system: the component of the peripheral nervous system that controls automatic functions.

Beta₁-adrenergic receptor: a site within the autonomic nervous system that, when stimulated, causes an excitatory response to the heart.

Beta₂-adrenergic receptor: a site located within the autonomic nervous system that, when stimulated, produces bronchial dilation.

Beta-blocker: a beta-adrenergic blocking agent. A substance that blocks the inhibitory effects of sympathetic nervous system agents, such as epinephrine.

Bioassay: biological method that determines the amount of preparation to produce a predetermined effect on a laboratory animal.

Bioavailability: the rate at which a drug enters the general circulation, permitting access to the site of action.

Biotransformation: changes in chemical makeup resulting from metabolism.

Blood-brain barrier (also called the blood-cerebro spinal fluid barrier): membrane that separates the brain and spinal fluid from circulating blood and prevents certain substances in blood (such as drugs) from reaching brain tissue or spinal fluid.

Blood typing: test run to determine the patient's blood type.

Body substance isolation: see *Standard Precautions*.

Bolus: a concentrated mass of a substance; pharmacologically, a rounded preparation for oral ingestion or a single dose, injected all at once.

Bound drug: portion of a drug dose that chemically binds with blood proteins or becomes stored in fatty tissue and is unavailable for therapeutic action; see *free drug*.

Bronchodilator: drug used to relieve airway obstruction caused by constriction of the bronchi.

Calcium channel blocker: a drug that inhibits the influx of calcium through the cell membrane, resulting in depression of automaticity and conduction velocity in smooth and cardiac muscle.

Capnography: the continuous monitoring of CO_2 levels in expired air of mechanically ventilated patients.

Cardiogenic shock: a state of shock caused from failure of the heart to pump an adequate amount of blood to body tissues.

Cation: see *ion*.

Celsius: system of temperature measurement; the freezing and boiling points of water are 0 and 100 degrees, respectively.

Central nervous system (CNS): the brain and spinal cord.

Cerebrovascular accident (CVA): the sudden cessation of blood flow to a region of the brain, caused by a thrombus, embolus, or hemorrhage.

Chemical name: description, in the specialized language of chemistry, of the structure of a drug; see *generic name, official name, trade name*.

Chemoreceptor: a nerve ending that is stimulated by certain chemical stimuli and located outside the central nervous system (CNS).

Cholinergic: term for (parasympathetic) nerve fibers that, when stimulated, release acetylcholine; class of drugs that mimic the action of acetylcholine.

Chronotropic: having an influence on the rate of occurrence of an event, such as a heartbeat.

Colloid: substance that forms a suspension instead of a true solution; the molecules of a colloid do not cross body membranes.

Concentration: the amount of an ingredient relative to the whole compound; in pharmacology, the *strength* of a drug.

Congestive heart failure (CHF): a condition that reflects abnormal cardiac pumping, including alterations in rate, rhythm, and electrical conduction.

Contraindication: symptom or circumstance that makes an otherwise desirable action or treatment unadvisable.

Corticosteroids: any of several steroid hormones secreted by the adrenal gland.

Crossmatching: process that determines the compatibility between blood donor and patient (recipient).

Crystalloid: crystal-forming substance that can dissolve and cross body membranes in solution.

Cumulative drug effects: effects of repeated doses of a drug that the body does not completely or immediately eliminate; such drugs accumulate in the system, and their effects can be greater than the sum of the effects of individual doses.

Diabetes mellitus: a chronic metabolic disorder marked by hyperglycemia.

Diabetic ketoacidosis: acidosis caused by an accumulation of ketone bodies, in advanced stages of uncontrolled diabetes mellitus.

Depressant: agent that depresses a body function.

Diffusion: the tendency of particles of substances in solution to move about until the concentration of the substance is the same throughout the solution.

Distribution: the dividing and spreading. The presence of entities throughout the body.

Diuretic: a drug that increases the volume of urine produced by increasing the excretion of sodium and water from the kidney.

Dopaminergic: receptors that are stimulated by dopamine. Stimulation results in renal and mesenteric vasodilation to improve blood flow to these regions.

Dose-dependent: drug effects that vary with changes in the amount administered.

Drug: substance that, when introduced into the body, causes a change in the way the body functions.

Eclampsia: coma and convulsive seizures between the 20th week of pregnancy and the 1st week after delivery, occurring in 1 out of 200 patients with *preeclampsia*.

Effector organ: muscle or gland that, when stimulated by the nervous system, produces an effect.

Efficacy: power to produce a therapeutic effect.

Electrolyte: a substance that, in solution, separates into *ions* and, thus, becomes capable of conduction electricity. In the body fluid, the electrolytes (sodium, potassium, calcium, magnesium, and chloride) are necessary for cell function and *acid-base balance*.

End-tidal carbon dioxide (ETCO$_2$) detector: device used in capnography.

Endotracheal (ET): through the throat; also called transtracheal; a method of introducing medication into the airway through a tube down the throat (endotracheal tube).

Epitope: portion of the antigen an antibody combines with.

Excretion: elimination of waste products, including drug metabolites, from the body.

Facilitated diffusion: when active transport is required for diffusion to take place.

Fahrenheit: system of temperature measurement; the freezing and boiling points of water are 32 and 212 degrees, respectively.

Filtration: the movement of fluid through a membrane, caused by differences in hydrostatic pressure.

Fluid, body: the nonsolid, liquid portion of the body, consisting of:

> *Intracellular fluid*—the liquid content of body cells.
> *Extracellular fluid*—all other body fluid, consisting of:
>> *Interstitial fluid*—the liquid in the spaces between cells, and
>> Intravascular fluid—the nonsolid portion of the blood, or *plasma*.

Food and Drug Administration (FDA): the official United States regulatory agency for food, drugs, cosmetics, and medical devices. The FDA is part of the Department of Health and Human Services.

Free drug: portion of a drug dose not bound to blood protein or stored in fatty tissue and thereby available for therapeutic action; see *bound drug*.

Ganglia: nervous tissue composed mainly of neuron cell bodies outside the brain and spinal cord.

Generalized motor seizure: a type of seizure that has no definable focus in the brain. This class includes petit mal and grand mal seizures.

Generic name (nonproprietary name): name, usually the shortened form of the chemical name, by which a drug is identified; see *chemical name, official name, trade name*.

Genotype: special combination of genes unique to each person.

Glucocorticoid: a steroid hormone produced by the adrenal gland with very potent anti-inflammatory effects.

Glycogen: starch, the form in which carbohydrates are stored in the body; when needed for metabolism, it is converted to glucose.

Gram: basic unit of mass (weight) in the metric system.

Homeostasis: state of equilibrium the internal environment of the body is kept within.

Hydrogen ion buffer: a substance in a fluid that minimizes changes in the hydrogen ion concentration (pH) in the body fluids that would otherwise result from the addition of acid or base to the fluid.

Hydrostatic pressure: the force exerted by the weight of a solution.

Hypersensitivity: above-normal susceptibility to a foreign substance, such as pollen.

Hypertensive crisis: any severe elevation in blood pressure (generally greater than 130 mm Hg diastolic).

Hypertonic: having higher osmotic pressure than another solution.

Hypnotic: drug that induces sleep.

Hypotonic: having lower osmotic pressure than another solution.

Hypoxic drive: stimulus for respiration triggered by a deficiency of oxygen.

Immune response: ability of the immune system to recognize and respond to foreign invaders.

Immunity: condition in which a person is protected from disease.

Inhalation: act of drawing in air or gas into the lungs; a route of drug administration.

Inhaler: small hand-held device, usually an aerosol unit, containing a microcrystalline suspension of a drug.

Innervate: to stimulate.

Inotropic: influencing the force of muscle contraction.

Intradermal: into the upper layers of the skin; route of drug administration.

Intramuscular (IM): into the muscle; route of drug administration.

Intraosseous (IO): into the bone; route of drug administration.

Intravenous (IV): into the vein; route of drug administration.

Intravenous infusion (IV infusion): controlled introduction of a drug into the bloodstream over a period of time.

Ion: an atom with an excess or shortage of electrons, which gives it a charge of negative *(anion)* or positive *(cation)* electrical energy. See *electrolyte.*

Isoantigen: substance that can stimulate production of antibodies when introduced into the body.

Isotonic: having the same osmotic pressure.

Ketone: compound produced during the oxidation of fatty acids.

Korsakoff's syndrome: a neurological disorder caused by the lack of thiamine (vitamin B_1 in the brain.

Kussmaul's respirations: very deep, gasping breaths associated with diabetic acidosis and coma.

Length: the distance between two points.

Leukotriene: substance that induces smooth muscle contraction.

Liter: basic unit of volume in the metric system.

Local: limited area of effect; topical, not systemic.

Mass: weight; how much matter is in an object or substance.

Mechanism of action: explanation of what a drug does to achieve its therapeutic effect.

Metabolism: all the physical and chemical changes within an organism resulting in the transformation of ingested substances (food, oxygen, etc.) into cell material of energy.

Metabolite: any substance that results from metabolism.

Meter: basic unit of length in the metric system.

Metered-dose inhaler: an inhaler designed to administer a specific amount (dose) of a drug.

Metric system: decimal system for weights and measures used in all scientific disciplines.

Minimum therapeutic concentration: minimum concentration necessary for a drug to produce the desired therapeutic response.

Motoneuron: a neuron that stimulates a muscle or gland.

Myocardial infarction (MI): death of heart muscle caused by blockage or blood flow through a coronary artery.

Narcotic: a drug that depresses the central nervous system.

Narrow-angle glaucoma: disease in which the pressure inside the eye is higher than normal because of structural abnormality.

Neurogenic shock: shock caused by vasodilation and pooling of the blood in the peripheral vessels so that adequate perfusion of tissues cannot be maintained.

Neuromuscular blocking agents: compete with acetylcholine for receptor sites in muscle cells and cause paralysis.

Neurotransmitter: substance (e.g., acetylcholine, norepinephrine) that allows the transmission of impulses between synapses in a neural pathway.

Nitrates: a classification of drugs that cause arteriovenous dilation and used to treat angina pectoris, hypertension, and congestive heart failure (CHF).

Nonelectrolytes: compounds with no electrical charges.

Norepinephrine: a hormone produced by the adrenal medulla that chiefly caused vasoconstriction.

Official name: the name of a drug given to it by the U.S. Pharmacopeial Convention; usually it is the generic name, followed by the letters USP. See *chemical name, generic name, trade name.*

Onset of drug action: the time required for a drug preparation to reach an effective concentration at the desired site.

Opioid: a synthetic narcotic that is not derived from opium.

Organophosphate: chemical compound, common in pesticides, that inhibits *cholinesterase.*

Osmosis: the movement of a solvent through a semipermeable membrane (such as a cell wall) into a solution with a higher solute concentration, so as to equalize the concentration of solute on both sides of the membrane.

Osmotic diuretic: drug or agent that causes increased excretion of water and electrolytes (diuresis) by increasing the osmotic pressure of the glomerular filtrate.

Osmotic pressure: the pressure produced by the difference in solute concentration between two solutions separated by a semipermeable membrane.

Overdose: dose of a drug sufficient to cause an acute reaction.

Oxytocic: an agent that stimulates uterine contractions.

Pain: an unpleasant sensory and emotional experience that occurs from actual or potential tissue damage.

Parasympathetic nervous system: a division of the autonomic nervous system.

Parasympatholytic: having the ability to block parasympathetic nerves.

Parasympathomimetic: having the ability to produce effects similar to those resulting from stimulation of the parasympathetic nervous system.

Parenteral: describing any route of administration other than the alimentary canal, including intravenous and intramuscular.

Passive transport: the mechanisms for moving substances across cell membranes from a solution with a higher concentration of the substance to a solution with a lower concentration.

Peripheral nervous system (PNS): all nervous tissue found outside the central nervous system.

pH (potential of hydrogen): a number on a scale of 0 to 14 that expresses the acidity or alkalinity of a substance. A substance with a pH of 7 is neutral, one with a pH of <7 is acidic, and one with a pH of >7 is alkaline.

Pharmacodynamics: the study of the actions of drugs on the body.

Pharmacogenetics: study of the influence of hereditary factors on the response to drugs.

Pharmacokinetics: the study of the movement of drugs through the systems of the body.

Pharmacology: the study of drugs, their sources, characteristics, and effects.

Pharmacotherapy: the use of drugs in the treatment of disease.

Physical dependence: a physiological state that occurs after prolonged use of drugs.

Physicians' Desk Reference (PDR): a book, published annually, that describes all currently used drugs.

Piggyback: attaching an additional IV bag (different medication) to an already established IV infusion.

Plasma: the liquid part of blood and lymph that forms 52-62% of the total blood volume.

Poison: any substance taken into the body that interferes with normal physiologic function.

Postpartum hemorrhage: in a woman who has given birth, the loss of more than 500 mL of blood within 24 hours of delivery.

Preeclampsia: hypertension and other abnormalities resulting from toxemia of pregnancy and, in some cases, leading to eclampsia.

Preload: the degree of stretch of the heart muscle fibers at the beginning of a contraction; the volume or pressure within the ventricle at the end of diastole.

Preterm labor: occurs between the beginning of the 21st and end of the 37th week of pregnancy.

Prodrug: drug that becomes therapeutically active as a result of biotransformation.

Prophylactic: an agent, device, or process designed to prevent an unhealthy outcome.

Proportion: formed by using two ratios that are equal.

Proprietary name: trade name.

Psychosis: mental disorder characterized by loss of contact with reality.

Pulmonary embolus: see *embolus*.

Pulse oximetry: tool used to determine the oxygenation status of patients.

Ratio: the relationship of two quantities.

Receptor: in pharmacology, a part of a cell that combines with a drug or body substance to alter the cell's function.

Rectal: into the rectum; route of drug administration.

Reflex arc: the neural pathway of a reflex action.

Sedative: a drug that has a soothing or tranquilizing effect.

Seizure: a sudden attack of pain or other symptoms. Seizures associated with epilepsy include tonic-clonic (grand-mal) and partial or absence (petit mal).

Seizure threshold: level of stimulus intensity sufficient to set off a seizure.

Semipermeable membrane: see *membrane*.

Sick sinus syndrome: an abnormality caused by a malfunction of the sinoatrial (SA) node of the heart.

Skeletal muscle relaxant: a drug that causes relaxation of voluntary muscles.

Small-volume nebulizer: device that allows both a drug and oxygen to be inhaled simultaneously.

Solubility: the ability to dissolve in a substance.

Solute: see *solution*.

Solution: a mixture of a liquid (solvent) and a solid (solute) in which the particles of the solid are so well mixed that they cannot be distinguished from the resulting fluid; see *suspension*.

Solvent: see *solution*.

Somatic nervous system: that part of the nervous system that controls the skeletal muscles of the body.

Standard Precautions (body substance isolation precautions): uniform procedures of infection control through the use of barrier precautions; determined by the degree of risk of exposure to body substance and not by the diagnosis of infectious disease.

Status asthmaticus: continuous asthma attacks; may be fatal.

Status epilepticus: the occurrence of two or more seizures without a period of consciousness between them.

Steroid: any of a class of complex compounds important in body chemistry, including sex and other hormones and vitamins.

Stevens-Johnson syndrome: a rare but serious adverse effect of phenytoin that is characterized by inflammation of the mucous membranes and skin. Blistering occurs. Skin sloughing, high fever, and possibly infection occur as the disorder progresses.

Subcutaneous (SC or SQ): under the skin; a route of drug administration.

Sublingual (SL): under the tongue; a route of drug administration.

Suppository: a semisolid drug preparation in the form of a cone or cylinder that is inserted into the rectum, vagina, or urethra.

Suspension: a mixture of a solid and a fluid in which the particles of the solid are mixed with, but not dissolved in, the fluid; see *solution*.

Sympathetic nervous system: division of the autonomic nervous system.

Sympatholytic: drug or agent that produces effects like those produced by inhibiting the sympathetic nervous system.

Sympathomimetic: drug or agent that produces effects like those produced by stimulating the sympathetic nervous system.

Synapse: the connecting space between two neurons in a neural pathway.

Synergism: the acting together of two substances (drugs, hormones, or other body chemicals) whose combined effect is different from, and perhaps greater than, the individual effect of each substance.

Systemic: effective throughout the body via the circulation.

Therapeutic index: a number representing the ratio of the lethal or toxic dose of a drug to its therapeutic dose; an expression of the relative safety of a drug—the higher the number, the wider the margin of safety.

Therapeutics: the study of the effects of remedies, such as drugs, and the treatment of disease.

Tocolytic: drug used to decrease or inhibit uterine contraction.

Toxemia of pregnancy: pathologic condition resulting from metabolic disturbances in pregnant women, manifested in preeclampsia and, less often, in eclampsia.

Toxicity: the quality of being poisonous.

Toxicology: the study of poisons.

Trade name: the name of a drug given to it by a manufacturer and registered as a trademark; see *chemical name, generic name, official name*.

Unit: one of anything.

United States Pharmacopeia (USP): a book, published every 5 years by the U.S. Pharmacopeial Convention, that sets forth the official formulas for all drugs used in the United States and the specifications and standards for preparing and administering them. Since 1975, a similar publication, the *National Formulary*, has been included in the *Pharmacopeia*.

Universal donor: a person who has type O blood.

Universal recipient: a person who has type AB blood.

U.S.P. unit: a standard of measurement determined by the *United States Pharmacopeia* for a "biologic" (derived from living substance) drug, such as a vaccine, penicillin, and so forth; the amount of such a drug that produces a determined therapeutic effect under controlled conditions.

U.S. system: system for weights and measures in use in the United States.

Vagus nerve: one of a pair of cranial nerves, the major sensory and motor nerve of the parasympathetic nervous system.

Vasoconstrictor: a drug used to decrease the diameter of blood vessels.

Vasodilator: a drug used to increase the diameter of blood vessels.

Vasopressor: a drug that causes the muscles of the arteries and capillaries to contract.

Volatile: easily evaporated.

Volume: amount of space occupied by an object or substance.

Volume of distribution: the amount of fluid (body water or plasma) necessary to achieve the desired concentration of a drug in the body.

Wernicke's encephalopathy a neurological disorder caused by the lack of thiamine (vitamin B_1 in the brain.

Withdrawal syndrome: partial collapse resulting from withdrawal of alcohol, stimulants, or some opiates.

Wolff-Parkinson-White syndrome: abnormality of cardiac rhythm characterized by an initial slurring of the R wave (called the delta wave), a shortened P-R interval, and a widened QRS complex.

BIBLIOGRAPHY

American Heart Association. *Textbook of Advanced Cardiac Life Support*. Dallas, TX: Author; 2008.

American Heart Association. *Textbook of Pediatric Advanced Life Support*. Dallas, TX: Author; 2008.

Audet PR. *Davis's Physician's Drug Guide*. Philadelphia, PA: FA Davis; 1989.

Beck RK. *Drug Reference for EMS Providers*. Albany, NY: Delmar, a division of Thomson Learning, Inc. 2002.

Bledsoe BE, Bosker G, Papa FJ. *Prehospital Emergency Pharmacology*, 2nd ed. Englewood Cliffs, NJ: Prentice-Hall; 1988.

Caroline, NC. *Emergency Care in the Streets*. Boston, MA: Little, Brown & Co; 1987.

Chameides L, ed. *Textbook of Pediatric Advanced Life Support*. Dallas, TX: American Heart Association; 1988.

Clark JB, Queener SF, Karb VB. *Pharmacological Basis of Nursing Practice*. St. Louis, MO: CV Mosby; 1982.

Conn PM, Gebhart GF. *Essentials of Pharmacology*. Philadelphia, PA: FA Davis; 1989.

Deglin JH, Vallerand AH. *Davis's Drug Guide for Nurses*, 12th ed. Philadelphia, PA: FA Davis; 2011.

Eichelberger MR, et al. *Pediatric Emergencies*. Englewood Cliffs, NJ: Brady (Prentice-Hall Division); 1992.

Emergency Cardiac Care Committee and Subcommittees, American Heart Association: Guidelines for Cardiopulmonary Resuscitation and Emergency Cardiac Care, I: Introduction. *JAMA*, 1992 268:2172-2183.

Finucane BT, Santora AH. *Principles of Airway Management*. Philadelphia, PA: FA Davis; 1988.

Fujisawa Pharmaceutical Company: *Adenocard Monograph*. Deerfield, IL: Author.

Guy JS. *Pharmacology for the Prehospital Professional*. St. Louis, MO: Mosby, Inc., an affiliate of Elsevier, Inc. 2010.

Hahn AB, Oestreich SJK, Barkin RL. *Mosby's Pharmacology in Nursing*. St. Louis, MO: CV Mosby; 1986.

Jones SA, et al. *Advanced Emergency Care for Paramedic Practice*. Philadelphia, PA: JB Lippincott Company; 1992.

Springhouse Drug Reference. Springhouse, PA: Springhouse Corporation; 1988.

Thomas CL, ed. *Taber's Cyclopedic Medical Dictionary*, 21st ed. Philadelphia, PA: FA Davis; 2005.

Vallerand AH, Deglin JH. *Drug Guide for Critical Care and Emergency Nursing*, 2nd ed. Philadelphia, PA: FA Davis; 1991.

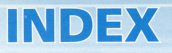

INDEX

DRUG INDEX

Amyl nitrite (Amyl Nitrite Aspirols; Amyl Nitrite Vaporole), 210, 237

Amyl Nitrite Aspirols. *See* Amyl nitrite

Amyl Nitrite Vaporole. *See* Amyl nitrite

Amytal. *See* Amobarbital

Anadrol. *See* Oxymetholone

Analgesics, 11, 73
narcotic, 12

Anecin-3. *See* Acetaminophen

Anectine. *See* Succinylcholine chloride

Anergan 50. *See* Promethazine hydrochloride

Anestacon. *See* Lidocaine hydrochloride

Ang-O-Span. *See* Nitroglycerine

Anisoylate plasminogen streptokinase activator (Eminase), 135

Anspor. *See* Cephradine

Antilirium. *See* Physostigmine

Apo-Amitriptyline. *See* Amitriptyline

Apresoline. *See* Hydralazine

Aprozide. *See* Hydrochlorothiazide

Aquachloral. *See* Chloral hydrate

Aquatensen. *See* Methyclothiazide

Arginine (L-arginine), 258

Arm-a-Med. *See* Isoetharine

ASA. *See* Acetylsalicylic acid

Ascriptin. *See* Acetylsalicylic acid

Asendin. *See* Amoxapine

Ashwagandha, 258

Aspergum. *See* Acetylsalicylic acid

Aspirin, 9t

Aspirtab. *See* Acetylsalicylic acid

Asthma Nefrin. *See* Epinephrine hydrochloride

AsthmaHaler. *See* Epinephrine bitartrate

Astragalus (Milk Vetch), 258

Astramorph. *See* Morphine sulfate

Atarax. *See* Hydroxyzine

Atenolol (Tenormin), 7, 11, 136, 238, 247

Ativan. *See* Lorazepam

Atorvastatin calcium (Lipitor), 54

Atracurium besylate (Tracrium), 107–108, 238, 247
rapid-sequence intubation and, 123

Atro-Pen. *See* Atropine sulfate

Atropine sulfate (Atro-Pen), 32, 75, 108, 238
cardiovascular use of, 136–137
in pediatric advanced life support, 253
pediatric dosage of, 249, 250, 251
for toxicologic emergencies, 210–211

Atrovent. *See* Ipratropium bromide

Auranofin, 10f

Auto-Injector. *See* Lidocaine hydrochloride

Aventyl. *See* Nortriptyline

Azmacort. *See* Triamcinolone

B

Bacampicillin (Spectrobid), 238, 246

Bacopa, 258

Banophen Caplets. *See* Diphenhydramine hydrochloride

Barbased. *See* Butabarbital

Barbita. *See* Phenobarbital

Baycol. *See* Cervistatin sodium

Bayer Aspirin. *See* Acetylsalicylic acid

Bearberry, 258

Beclomethasone dipropionate (Beconase; Beclovent; Vancenase; Vanceril), 108–109, 238, 248

Beclovent. *See* Beclomethasone dipropionate

Beconase. *See* Beclomethasone dipropionate

Beef Regular Iletin II, 238

Beldin. *See* Diphenhydramine hydrochloride

Belladonna, 258

Benadryl. *See* Diphenhydramine hydrochloride

Benylin. *See* Diphenhydramine hydrochloride

Benylin DM Cough. *See* Dextromethorphan

Benzphetamine (Didrex), 238, 240

Beta₂. *See* Isoetharine

Betalin S. *See* Vitamin B-1

Biamine. *See* Vitamin B-1

Bilberry, 258

Biperiden (Abeneton; Akineton), 237, 238

Bisorine. *See* Isoetharine

Bitolterol mesylate (Tornalate Aerosol), 109, 238, 247

Black Alder, 258

Black Cohosh, 259

Blessed thistle, 259

Blocadren. *See* Ttimolol

Boldenone undecylenate (Equipoise), 271

Brethaire. *See* Terbutaline sulfate

Brethine. *See* Terbutaline sulfate

Bricanyl. *See* Terbutaline sulfate

Bromelain, 259

Bromocriptine (Parlodel), 238, 244

Bromo-Seltzer. *See* Acetaminophen

Bronitin Mist. *See* Epinephrine bitartrate

Bronkaid Mist. *See* Epinephrine hydrochloride

Bronkaid Mist Suspension. *See* Epinephrine bitartrate

Bronkodyl. *See* Theophylline

Bronkosol. *See* Isoetharine

Buckthorn, 259

Bufferin. *See* Acetylsalicylic acid

Bumetanide (Bumex), 137, 238

Bumex. *See* Bumetanide

Bupleurum, 259

Burdock, 259

Butabarbital (Barbased; Butalan; Butatran; Buticaps; Butisol; Sarisol No. 2), 16t, 238, 246

Butalan. *See* Butabarbital

Butatran. *See* Butabarbital

Buticaps. *See* Butabarbital

Butisol. *See* Butabarbital

Butorphanol tartrate (Stadol; Stadol NS), 137–138, 230, 238, 246

C

Calan. *See* Verapamil

Calcium chloride, 9, 239
  pediatric dosage of, 249, 250, 251

Calcium chloride 10%, in pediatric advanced life support, 253

Calcium gluceptate, 239

Calcium gluconate (Kalcinate), 138–139, 239
  in pediatric advanced life support, 253
  pediatric dosage of, 249, 250, 251

Calendula, 259

Capoten. *See* Captopril

Captopril (Capoten), 139, 238, 239

Carbamazepine (Epitol; Mazepine; Tegretol), 239, 241, 242, 247

Carbenicillin (Geopen; Pyopen), 239, 241, 245

Cardizem Injectable. *See* Diltiazem

Cardizem Lyo-Ject. *See* Diltiazem

Cascara, 259

Catapres. *See* Clonidine

Catapres-TTS. *See* Clonidine

Cat's Claw, 259

Cayenne, 259

Ceclor. *See* Cefaclor

Cedilanid-D Injections. *See* Deslanoside

Cefaclor (Ceclor), 239

Celontin Half Strength Kapseals. *See* Methsuximide

Celontin Kapseals. *See* Methsuximide

Centrax. *See* Prazepam

Cephradine (Anspor), 239

Cephradine (Anspor; Velosef), 237, 248

Cerebyx. *See* Fosphenytoin

Cervistatin sodium (Baycol), 54

Chamomile, 260

Charcoaid. *See* Activated charcoal

Charcocaps. *See* Activated charcoal

Chasteberry, 260

Chloral hydrate (Aquachloral; Noctec; Novochlorhydrate), 237, 239, 244

Chlordiazepoxide (Librium; Lipoxide; Murcil; Reposans-10; Sereen; SK-Lygen), 16t, 239, 242, 243, 245, 246
  as street drug, 268

Chloroform, 7

Chlorothiazide (Diachlor; Diuril; Ro-Chlorozide; SK-Chlorozide), 239, 240, 245, 246

Chlorpazine. *See* Prochlorpazine

Chlorpromazine (Chlorzine; Ormazine; Promapar; Promay; Sonayine; Thorazine; Thor-Prom), 221–222, 239, 244, 245, 246, 247

Chlorpropamide (Diabinese; Glucamide), 240

Chlorprothixene (Taractan), 239, 247

Chlorthalidone, 239

Chlorthalidone (Hygroton; Hylidone; Thalitone), 241, 242, 247

Chlorzide. *See* Hydrochlorothiazide

Chlorzine. *See* Chlorpromazine

Choledyl. *See* Oxtriphylline

Cin-Quin. *See* Quinidine

Clemastine (Tavist; Tavist-1), 239, 247

Clonazepam (Klonopin; Rivotril), 239, 242, 245

Clonidine (Catapres; Catapres-TTS), 239

Clopidogrel (Plavix), 139

Clorazepate (Tranxene-SD), 239, 247

Clove, 260

Coca, 7

Cocaine, 16t, 268

Codeine, 16t, 239, 270

Combivent. *See* Albuterol/Ipratropium

Compazine. *See* Prochlorperazine

Compazine Spansule, 239

Compoz. *See* Diphenhydramine hydrochloride

Congesprin. *See* Dextromethorphan

Constant-T. *See* Theophylline

Cordarone. *See* Amiodarone

Cordyceps, 260

Corgard. *See* Nadolol

Cortef. *See* Hydrocortisone

Cortisol. *See* Hydrocortisone

Corvert. *See* Ibutilide

Coumadin. *See* Warfarin

Covera HS. *See* Verapamil

Crack, 269

Cranberry, 260

Creatine, 260

Cremacoat 1. *See* Dextromethorphan

Cromolyn sodium, 239

Cromolyn sodium (Intal), 109–110, 242

Crystodigin. *See* Digitoxin

D

Dalcaine. *See* Lidocaine hydrochloride

Dalmane. *See* Flurazepam

Dandelion, 260

Darvon. *See* Propoxyphene hydrochloride

Datril. *See* Acetaminophen

Decadron. *See* Dexamethasone

Deca-Durabolin. *See* Nandrolone decanoate

Delsym. *See* Dextromethorphan

Demerol. *See* Meperidine

Depakene. *See* Valproic acid

Deponit. *See* Nitroglycerine

Depo-Testosterone. *See* Testosterone cypionate

Desipramine (Desipramine; Pertofrane), 239, 244

Deslanoside (Cedilanid-D Injections), 239

Devil's Claw, 261

Dexamethasone (Decadron; Hexadrol; Solurex), 110, 181–182, 239, 241

Dextran, 52

Dextromethorphan (Benylin DM Cough; Congesprin; Cremacoat 1; Delsym; DM Cough; Hold; Mediquell; Pedia Care; Pertussin 8 Hour Cough Formula; Pertussin 8 Hour Cough Formula; St. Joseph for Children; Sucrets Cough Control), 238, 239, 240, 241, 242, 244, 246
   as street drug, 270

Dextromethorphan (Congesprin), 239

Dextrose 5% in 0.45% Sodium chloride ($D_5 1/2NS$), 53

Dextrose 5% in 0.9% Sodium chloride (D_5NS), 53

Dextrose 5% in lactated Ringer's solution (D_5LR), 54

Dextrose 5% in water (D_5W), 53

Dextrose 50% in water ($D_{50}W$), 59, 168–169, 182, 240
   pediatric dosage of, 249, 250, 251

Dey-Dose. *See* Isoetharine

Dey-Lute. *See* Isoetharine

DHEA, 261

Diabeta. *See* Glyburide

Diabinese, 240

Diachlor. *See* Chlorothiazide

Diahist. *See* Diphenhydramine hydrochloride

Diamox. *See* Acetazolamide

Diamox Sequels. *See* Acetazolamide

Dianobol. *See* Methandrostenolone

Diaqua. *See* Hydrochlorothiazide

Diazepam (Valium; Valrelease), 16t, 182–183, 201, 211–212, 222–223, 240, 248
   as street drug, 268

Diazoxide (Hyperstat IV; Proglycem), 139–140, 240, 242, 245
   pediatric dosage of, 249, 250, 251

Didrex. *See* Benzphetamine

Digitalis, 7, 10f

Digitoxin (Crystodigin; Purodigin), 239, 240, 245

Digoxin (Lanoxicaps; Lanoxin), 6, 9t, 11, 140–141, 240, 242

Dilantin. *See* Phenytoin

Dilaudid. *See* Hydromorphone

Dilocain. *See* Lidocaine hydrochloride

Diltiazem (Cardizem Injectable; Cardizem Lyo-Ject), 6, 141, 239, 240

Dimethyltryptamine, 269

Diphen. *See* Diphenhydramine hydrochloride

Diphenadril. *See* Diphenhydramine hydrochloride

Diphenhist. *See* Diphenhydramine hydrochloride

Diphenhydramine hydrochloride (AllerMax; Allermed; Banophen Caplets; Beldin; Benadryl; Benylin; Compoz; Diahist; Diphen; Diphenhist; Diphenadril; Fenylhist; Fynex; Genahist; Hydramine; Hydril; Hyrexin-50; Nervine; Nighttime Sleep-Aid; Nordryl; Nytol with DPH; Robalyn; Siladryl; Sleep-Eye 3; Sominex Formula 2; Tusstat; Twilite; Valdrene), 9t, 110, 238, 239, 240, 241, 243, 244, 246, 247
   for gastrointestinal emergencies, 194–195
   pediatric dosage of, 249, 250, 251

Diphenoxylate (Lomotil), 10f, 16t

Dipyridamole (Persantine; Pyridamole), 240, 244, 245

Disopyramide (Napamide; Norpace; Norpace CR), 11, 240, 243, 244

Dispos-a-Med. *See* Isoetharine

Diuretic, antihypertensive. *See* Hydrochlorothiazide

Diuril. *See* Chlorothiazide

DM cough. *See* Dextromethorphan

Dobutamine hydrochloride (Dobutrex), 8, 142, 240
   concentrations and infusion rates for pediatric use, 252
   in pediatric advanced life support, 253

Dobutrex. *See* Dobutamine hydrochloride (Dobutrex)

Dolene. *See* Propoxyphene hydrochloride

Dolophine. *See* Methadone

Dong Quai, 261

Donnagel-PG, 16t

Dopamine hydrochloride (Dopastat; Intropin), 9t, 60, 142–143, 240, 242
   concentrations and infusion rates for pediatric use, 252
   in pediatric advanced life support, 253
   pediatric dosage of, 249, 250, 251, 252

Dopastat. *See* Dopamine hydrochloride

Doriden. *See* Glutethimide

Doriglute. *See* Glutethimide

Doxaphene. *See* Propoxyphene hydrochloride

Doxepin (Adapin; Sinequan), 237, 240, 246

Droperidol (Inapsine), 223, 240, 242

DuoNeb,(Rx). *See* Albuterol/Ipratropium

Durabolin. *See* Nandrolone phenpropionate

Duramorph. *See* Morphine sulfate

Durapam. *See* Flurazepam

Pitocin. *See* Oxytocin
Pitressin. *See* Vasopressin
Placidyl. *See* Ethchlorvynol
Plasma protein (Albumin), 52
Polio vaccine, 8
Polycillin. *See* Ampicillin
Polymox. *See* Amoxicillin
Pralidoxime (Protopam),
    214–215, 245
Pravacol. *See* Pravastatin sodium
Pravastatin sodium (Pravacol), 55
Prazepam (Centrax), 239, 245
Prazosin (Minipress), 243, 245
Primacor. *See* Milrinone
Primatene. *See* Epinephrine
    hydrochloride
Primatene Mist Suspension. *See*
    Epinephrine bitartrate
Primidone (Myidone; Mysoline;
    Sertan), 243, 245, 246
Principen. *See* Ampicillin
Prinivil. *See* Lisinopril
Procainamide (Procan SR;
    Promine; Pronestyl;
    Pronestyl-SR; Rhythmin),
    11, 158, 245
Procainamide (Procan SR; Promine;
    Pronestyl; Rhythmin)
    in pediatric advanced life
    support, 253
Procan SR. *See* Procainamide
Procardia. *See* Nifedipine
Prochlorpazine (Chlorpazine), 239
Prochlorperazine (Compazine),
    239, 245
Profene. *See* Propoxyphene
    hydrochloride
Proglycem. *See* Diazoxide
Prolixin Decanoate. *See*
    Fluphenazine
Promapar. *See* Chlorpromazine
Promay. *See* Chlorpromazine
Promazine (Prozine; Sparine),
    245, 246
Promethacon. *See* Promethazine
    hydrochloride
Promethazine hydrochloride
    (Anergan 50; Phenergan,
    Promethacon), 73, 117,
    196, 245

Promine. *See* Procainamide
Pronestyl. *See* Procainamide
Propolis, 265
Propoxyphene hydrochloride
    (Darvon; Dolene;
    Doxaphene; Profene), 16t,
    239, 240, 245
Propranolol (Inderal; Inderal LA),
    11, 158–159, 242, 245
    pediatric dosage of, 250,
    251, 252
Protopam. *See* Pralidoxime
Protriptyline (Triptil; Vivactil),
    245, 247, 248
Proventil. *See* Albuterol
Prozine. *See* Promazine
Psyllium, 265
Purodigin. *See* Digitoxin
Pycnogenol, 265
Pygeum, 265
Pyopen. *See* Carbenicillin
Pyridamole. *See* Dipyridamole

Q

Quinidex. *See* Quinidine
Quinidine (Cin-Quin; Extentabs;
    Quinidex; Quinora; SK-
    Quinidine Sulfate), 10f, 239,
    241, 245, 246

R

Racemic epinephrine, 117–118
Ramipril (Altace), 159, 237, 245
Razepam. *See* Temazepam
Regitine. *See* Phentolamine
Reposans-10. *See*
    Chlordiazepoxide
Reserpine. *See* Reserpine
Reserpine (Sandril; Serpanray;
    Serpasil; Serpolan; Zepine),
    245, 246, 248
Restoril. *See* Temazepam
Retavase. *See* Reteplase
Reteplase (Retavase), 159–160
Revex. *See* Nalmefene
Rhythmin. *See* Procainamide
Ritalin. *See* Methylphenidate
Ritalin SR. *See* Methylphenidate
Rivotril. *See* Clonazepam
RMS inserts. *See* Morphine sulfate

Roampicillin. *See* Ampicillin
Robalyn. *See* Diphenhydramine
    hydrochloride
Robitussin A-C, 16t
Ro-Chlorozide. *See*
    Chlorothiazide
Rocuronium bromide (Zemuron),
    118, 246, 248
Ro-Hydrazide. *See*
    Hydrochlorothiazide
Romazicon. *See* Flumazenil
Ronase. *See* Tolazamide
Roxanol. *See* Morphine sulfate

S

S-2 Inhalant. *See* Epinephrine
    hydrochloride
Salmeterol xinafoate (Serevent),
    118–119, 246
Sandril. *See* Reserpine
Sarisol No. 2. *See* Butabarbital
Saw Palmetto, 265
Schisandra, 265
Secobarbital (Seconal), 246
Seconal. *See* Secobarbital
Sectral. *See* Acebutolol
Sedabamate. *See* Meprobamate
Senna, 265
Serax. *See* Oxazepam
Sereen. *See* Chlordiazepoxide
Serentil. *See* Mesoridazine
Serevent. *See* Salmeterol
    xinafoate
Serpasil. *See* Reserpine
Serpolan. *See* Reserpine
Sertan. *See* Primidone
Siladryl. *See* Diphenhydramine
    hydrochloride
Simvastatin (Zocor), 55
Sinequan. *See* Doxepin
Sintocine. *See* Oxytocin
SK-Amitriptyline. *See*
    Amitriptyline
SK-Bamate. *See* Meprobamate
SK-Chlorozide. *See*
    Chlorothiazide
SK-Hydrochlorothiazide. *See*
    Hydrochlorothiazide
SK-Lasix. *See* Furosemide
SK-Lygen. *See* Chlordiazepoxide

SK-Tolbutamide. *See* Tolbutamide
Sleep-Eye 3. *See*
     Diphenhydramine
     hydrochloride
Sodium bicarbonate, 9, 60, 160,
     215-216
  in pediatric advanced life
     support, 253
  pediatric dosage of, 250,
     251, 252
Sodium nitrate, 216
Sodium thiosulfate, 216-217, 246
Sofarin. *See* Warfarin
Solfoton. *See* Phenobarbital
Solganal, 10f
Solu-Cortef. *See* Hydrocortisone
Solu-Medrol. *See*
     Methylprednisolone
Solurex. *See* Dexamethasone
Sominex Formula 2;. *See*
     Diphenhydramine
     hydrochloride
Somophyllin. *See* Aminophyllin;
     Aminophylline
Sonayine. *See* Chlorpromazine
Soy, 265
Sparine. *See* Promazine
Spectrobid. *See* Bacampicillin
Spironolactone (Aldactone),
     237, 246
Spirulina, 266
St. John's Wort, 265
St. Joseph Adult Chewable
     Aspirin. *See* Acetylsalicylic
     acid
St. Joseph for Children. *See*
     Dextromethorphan
Stadol. *See* Butorphanol tartrate
Stadol NS. *See* Butorphanol
     tartrate
Stanozolol (Winstrol), 271
Stelazine. *See* Trifluoperazine
Streptase. *See* Streptokinase
Streptokinase (Kabikinase;
     Streptase), 160-161, 246
Sublimaze. *See* Fentanyl citrate
Succinylcholine chloride
     (Anectine), 119-120, 237
  rapid-sequence intubation
     and, 123

Sucrets Cough Control. *See*
     Dextromethorphan
Super Totacillian. *See* Ampicillin
SuperChar. *See* Activated charcoal
Suprazine. *See* Trifluoperazine
Sus-Phrine. *See* Epinephrine
     bitartrate
Syntocinon. *See* Oxytocin

T

Talwin. *See* Pentazocine
Tambocor. *See* Flecainide
Taractan. *See* Chlorprothixene
Tavist. *See* Clemastine
Tavist-1. *See* Clemastine
Tea Tree, 266
Tegretol. *See* Carbamazepine
Temazepam (Razepam; Restoril;
     Tempay), 245, 247
Tempay. *See* Temazepam
Tempra. *See* Acetaminophen
Tenormin. *See* Atenolol
Tensilon. *See* Edrophonium
Terbutaline sulfate (Brethaire;
     Brethine; Bricanyl), 120,
     203, 238, 247
Testosterone cypionate
     (Depo-Testosterone), 271
Theo-24. *See* Theophylline
Theobid. *See* Theophylline
Theoclear. *See* Theophylline
Theo-Dur. *See* Theophylline
Theophyl. *See* Theophylline
Theophylline (Theophylline
     (Aerolate; Bronkodyl;
     Constant-T; Elixophyllin;
     Slo-bid; Somophyllin-T;
     Sustaire; Theo-24;
     Theo-Dur; Theobid;
     Theoclear; Theophyl;
     Theospan-SR;
     TheoventUniphyl), 237,
     238, 240, 246, 247. *See*
     Theophylline
Theospan-SR. *See* Theophylline
Theovent. *See* Theophylline
Thiamine. *See* Vitamin B-1
Thioridazine (Mellaril-S),
     242, 247
Thiothixene (Navane), 243, 247

Thorazine. *See* Chlorpromazine
Thor-Prom. *See* Chlorpromazine
Timolol (Blocadren; Timoptic),
     238, 247
Timoptic. *See* Timolol
Tindal. *See* Acetophenazine
Tissue plasminogen activator
     [t-PA] (Activase),
     133-134, 181
Tocainide (Tonocard), 247
Tolazamide (Ronase; Tolinase),
     246, 247
Tolbutamide (Oramide; SK-
     Tolbutamide), 244, 246, 247
Tolinase. *See* Tolazamide
Tonocard. *See* Tocainide
Toradd. *See* Ketorolac
Toradol. *See* Ketorolac
Tornalate Aerosol. *See* Bitolterol
     mesylate
Tracrium. *See* Atracurium
     besylate
Trandate. *See* Labetalol
Tranmep. *See* Meprobamate
Transderm Nitro. *See*
     Nitroglycerine
Tranxene-SD. *See* Clorazepate
Tranylcypromine (Parnate),
     244, 247
Triamcinolone (Azmacort), 120,
     238, 247
Triazolam (Halcion), 241, 247
  as street drug, 268
Tridil. *See* Nitroglycerine
Tridione. *See* Trimethadione
Trifluoperazine (Suprazine;
     Stelazine), 246, 247
Trilafon. *See* Perphenazine
Trimethadione (Tridione), 247
Trimox. *See* Amoxicillin
Triptil. *See* Protriptyline
Truphylline. *See* Aminophyllin;
     Aminophylline
Ttimolol (Blocadren), 238
Tubocurarine chloride,
     120-121, 247
  rapid-sequence intubation
     and, 123
Tusstat. *See* Diphenhydramine
     hydrochloride